T0177677

Life-Course Smoking Behavior

Life-Course Smoking Behavior

Patterns and National Context in Ten Countries

EDITED BY DEAN R. LILLARD

AND

REBEKKA CHRISTOPOULOU

OXFORD
UNIVERSITY PRESS

Oxford University Press is a department of the University of
Oxford. It furthers the University's objective of excellence in research,
scholarship, and education by publishing worldwide.

Oxford   New York
Auckland   Cape Town   Dar es Salaam   Hong Kong   Karachi
Kuala Lumpur   Madrid   Melbourne   Mexico City   Nairobi
New Delhi   Shanghai   Taipei   Toronto

With offices in
Argentina   Austria   Brazil   Chile   Czech Republic   France   Greece
Guatemala   Hungary   Italy   Japan   Poland   Portugal   Singapore
South Korea   Switzerland   Thailand   Turkey   Ukraine   Vietnam

Oxford is a registered trademark of Oxford University Press
in the UK and certain other countries.

Published in the United States of America by
Oxford University Press
198 Madison Avenue, New York, NY 10016

© Oxford University Press 2015

All rights reserved. No part of this publication may be reproduced, stored in
a retrieval system, or transmitted, in any form or by any means, without the prior
permission in writing of Oxford University Press, or as expressly permitted by law,
by license, or under terms agreed with the appropriate reproduction rights organization.
Inquiries concerning reproduction outside the scope of the above should be sent to the
Rights Department, Oxford University Press, at the address above.

You must not circulate this work in any other form
and you must impose this same condition on any acquirer.

Library of Congress Cataloging-in-Publication Data
Life-course smoking behavior : patterns and national context in ten countries / edited by Dean R. Lillard,
Rebekka Christopoulou.
   p. ; cm.
Includes bibliographical references.
ISBN 978-0-19-938910-0
I. Lillard, Dean R. (Dean Reginald), 1959-, editor.   II. Christopoulou, Rebekka, editor.
[DNLM: 1. Smoking—epidemiology.   2. Behavior, Addictive—epidemiology.   3. Cohort Studies.
4. Cross-Cultural Comparison. WM 290]
RA645.T62
362.29′6—dc23
2014046436

9 8 7 6 5 4 3 2 1
Printed in the United States of America
on acid-free paper

Dean Lillard dedicates this book to Gary Becker, mentor, advisor, and intellectual role model. His devotion to scholarship was exemplary.

Rebekka Christopoulou dedicates this book to her husband, Manolis Papadakis.

CONTENTS

PREFACE

As a topic, tobacco consumption remains vitally important to ongoing public health initiatives worldwide. Despite great interest, researchers still do not fully understand how smoking behavior evolves. Our point of departure for this work was the observation that the bulk of the existing literature relies on cross-sectional descriptions (snapshots) of smoking behavior, which we believe mask important dynamics in smoking initiation and cessation. Our work builds on the premise that a life-course perspective is critical in the study of smoking. By following individuals and tracking their smoking status in every year over the course of their lives, one obtains a richer picture of what drives their smoking behavior.

In this book, we use retrospectively reported individual-level data from 10 countries to describe how men and women smoked from birth until the date they were interviewed. For each country, our data cover up to seven generations of individuals who took their smoking decisions as early as the 1920s and as late as 2011. The set of countries draws from both the developed and the developing world and includes four formerly or currently socialist economies.

To give context to the economic environment in which individuals decided whether or not to smoke, we present long time-series data on per capita gross domestic product, the average cigarette price, and/or cigarette taxes. In some of the countries—notably Turkey and two countries that were part of the former Soviet Union, Russia and Ukraine—we present price data that, to the best of our knowledge, few researchers have ever seen. For each of the 10 countries, we also list a timeline of key historical, informational, regulatory, political, and socioeconomic events that might have affected smoking behavior.

By presenting the two types of data (i.e., on smoking behavior and national context) simultaneously, we develop hypotheses about possible determinants of the smoking patterns. At the same time, the patterns are rich and varied enough that many puzzles remain for readers to understand and solve. Thus, our book serves a dual purpose. It is a reference book that describes and compares novel data, and it is also a research book that proposes and provokes new interesting hypotheses.

The book is directed mostly at academic economists and public health scientists. However, it will also interest other academicians in the many disciplines that study smoking behavior, such as epidemiology, sociology, anthropology, psychology, demography, women's and gender studies, and cultural studies. Students in all these fields will find this book a useful introduction to smoking issues and a rich source of research ideas. Furthermore, this book will appeal to companies seeking to profit from the growing awareness of the risk of smoking, such as firms that sell pharmaceutical and other products to help people quit smoking. Understanding the patterns of smoking behavior over the life course, over time, across generations, and across countries will help these firms target their products more efficiently. Finally, our book will inform technical staff within governments and international agencies that are engaged in tobacco control policy.

With such a diverse readership in mind, we put a lot of thought into how to best present our data, how to structure each chapter, and how analytical we should be in our discussion of the data. One challenge was to offer a methodical documentation of smoking patterns without being repetitive and tiresome. A second challenge was to offer convincing discussions of explanatory scenarios without being overly technical. We hope we have struck the right balance by keeping the analysis largely descriptive, standardizing the graphical depictions of the data throughout the book, and emphasizing national specificities in the text. Although we assigned a team of country specialists the task of writing chapters for some of the countries, our working group has collaborated closely and we, as editors (and authors), have worked to ensure uniformity.

Our training as economists unavoidably influences the way we approach the data. However, it is clear to us that people decide to smoke for a host of economic and noneconomic reasons. Therefore, although we naturally recognize economic factors that might explain the patterns we describe, we also discuss other possible determinants of smoking behavior that lie outside of most economic models. In fact, many of our proposed hypotheses are related to social, political, or cultural forces, such as feminism and democratic freedom. Although we have tried to cover a broad range of factors that we think are important, we invite the readers to delve deeper and interpret patterns through the prism of their own training. Given the richness of the data, we believe we have only scratched the surface of narratives that might explain similarities and differences in life-course smoking behavior between men and women, across cohorts, and within and across countries.

Dean R. Lillard
Rebekka Christopoulou

ACKNOWLEDGMENTS

Over the course of this project, several undergraduate and graduate students assisted us in our research. We especially thank Ahmed Jaber, Karen Calabrese, Duk Gyoo Kim, Dalida Akhmedova, Olga Pavlenko, and Elizaveta Blagodeteleva. The contribution of two students stands out. Jeffrey Han offered invaluable research assistance at the early and middle stages of the project, and the work of Jacob W. Fahringer was instrumental and timely in ensuring that we completed the book. We sincerely thank them for their work and devotion to careful research.

We are also grateful to those who helped us access necessary data. Former vice president of the American Cancer Society, Michael J. Thun, generously provided us with the CPS-II 1982–1988 cause-specific mortality data. We used those data to correct cohort and gender-specific smoking prevalence trajectories for bias due to differential mortality of smokers and nonsmokers. Klara Sabirianova Peter of the University of North Carolina generously provided us with data on mean wages in Russia and the USSR in many years and pointed us to sources for other data we were missing. Mustafa Seyidogullari generously provided historical cigarette price data for Turkey.

We also thank the staff, whose work is often appreciated but unacknowledged. We recognize our debt to Janet Heslop at the Cornell Institute for Social and Economic Research for helping us with state-of-the art computer processing capacity and support. We also thank the librarians at Cornell University and The Ohio State University who helped us with the countless interlibrary loans that allowed us to compile our data.

Finally, we gratefully acknowledge research funding from National Institute on Aging grant 5R01AG030379 (years 1–5) that funded the project titled "Cross-National Patterns and Predictors of Life-Course Smoking Behavior."

ABOUT THE EDITORS

Dean R. Lillard is Associate Professor at the Department of Human Sciences at The Ohio State University and Director and Project Manager of the Cross-National Equivalent File, a study that produces cross-national longitudinal data. He is also a research fellow of the Health Economics group of the National Bureau of Economic Research and a research professor at the German Institute for Economic Research in Berlin, Germany. He was trained as an economist at the University of Chicago (PhD) and the University of Washington (BA), and he has worked as a senior researcher for more than a decade at Cornell University. His research focuses on health economics, the economics of schooling, and international comparisons of economic behavior. His work has been published in leading scholarly journals, including the *Journal of Political Economy*, the *Journal of Health Economics*, the *Journal of Labor Economics, Health Economics, Statistics in Medicine, Preventive Medicine*, and *Social Science and Medicine*. Funding for his projects has been provided by grants from the National Institute of Aging, the National Institute on Alcohol Abuse and Alcoholism, the National Cancer Institute, the National Institute of Child Health and Human Development, the Robert Wood Johnson Foundation, and the Spencer Foundation.

Rebekka Christopoulou has been recently appointed as a lecturer at the Economics Department of the University of Macedonia, Greece. She holds a PhD in Economics from the University of Cambridge and has worked as a researcher at The Ohio State University, Cornell University, the London School of Economics, and the European Central Bank. Although she was trained and started her career as a labor economist, she soon moved into the areas of health economics and economic demography, and she currently has more than 5 years of research experience in international smoking patterns. She has presented her work extensively at academic conferences and has published her research in edited books and scholarly journals, including *Preventive Medicine*, the *International Journal of Public Health,* and the *Journal of Economic Behavior and Organization*.

ABOUT THE CONTRIBUTING AUTHORS

Philip DeCicca is Associate Professor and Canada Research Chair in Public Economics at the Department of Economics of McMaster University. He is also a research associate of the Program in Health Economics of the National Bureau of Economic Research.

Logan McLeod is Assistant Professor in the Department of Economics at Wilfrid Laurier University, Canada. He is also a faculty associate at the Canadian Centre for Health Economics.

Ana I. Gil Lacruz is Associate Professor in the Department of Business Organization and Management at Zaragoza University, Spain.

Feng Liu is Associate Professor in the School of Economics at Shanghai University of Finance and Economics, China.

Zlata Dorofeeva is a researcher in the Higher School of Economics at the National Research University. She is also a researcher in the Russian Academy of Sciences at the Institute of Sociology, Russia.

Zeynep Önder is Associate Professor in the Faculty of Business Administration at Bilkent University, Turkey.

NOTE TO THE READER

This work is part of a larger project, funded by the U.S. National Institute of Aging, whose purpose is to describe and model life-course smoking behavior in and across countries. Here, we describe patterns. In the second phase of the project, we will exploit the cross-country and temporal variation in the available data to estimate models of smoking behavior and compare results across countries. Our project has an associated page on the website of The Ohio State University (http://smoking-research.ehe.osu.edu), on which we make freely available codes that we developed to process our data. At a later stage, we will also post all policy and smoking data, supplementary material (e.g., alternative depictions of the smoking patterns), and new research papers as they become available.

1

Introduction

DEAN R. LILLARD AND REBEKKA CHRISTOPOULOU

BACKGROUND

Starting in the 1920s, scientists began to accumulate evidence that smoking and the consumption of tobacco dramatically damages health (Proctor, 1997, 1999). As the amount and statistical strength of that evidence grew steadily over time, groups with vested interests in promoting and selling tobacco fought its dissemination and governmental actions on the evidence (Fields and Chapman, 2003). By 1962, the proponents of tobacco could no longer prevent scientific organizations and governments from officially recognizing the evidence. Led by the United Kingdom Royal College of Physicians of London (RCPL) in 1962 and followed by the US Surgeon General in 1964, the UK and US governments officially acknowledged that the evidence strongly supported the hypothesis that smoking causes not only cancer but also a host of other illnesses and conditions (RCPL, 1962; US Department of Health, Education, and Welfare, 1964). As we show later in the timeline of selected smoking-related events for each country, the explicit recognition of a causal link between smoking and disease led governments to start to regulate when, where, to whom, and how companies could market tobacco and, much later, where in public people were allowed to smoke.

Although these reports motivated the UK, US, and other governments to regulate tobacco within their own countries relatively soon after their publication, governments worldwide did not act collectively for another three decades. Eventually, the disease and mortality burden associated with tobacco consumption prompted action. In 1998, the World Health Organization (WHO) announced that tobacco consumption caused more than 3.5 million premature deaths in that year and projected that, absent some change in consumption patterns, by 2020 smoking would annually kill more than 10 million people worldwide (WHO, 1999). In 2003, the United Nations drafted the Framework Convention for Tobacco Control—a global treaty that aimed to reduce the demand for and supply of tobacco. A majority of the world's governments, 172 to date, have ratified this treaty. Although the treaty has spurred governments in many countries to pass and implement new tobacco control policies, in all but the most developed countries there is as yet little indication that the policies have been effective in reducing either the consumption or disease and mortality burden of tobacco. The latest estimates of smoking-attributable mortality by the WHO remain dismal. In 2011, tobacco use caused more than 5 million premature deaths, and this death toll was projected to exceed 8 million annually by 2030, mostly in developing countries (WHO, 2012). A pessimist might conclude that even in the economically developed world, governments have made little progress in combating the health costs of tobacco consumption. For example, in its Healthy People 2010 initiative (updated in the Healthy People 2020 initiative), the United States has set and failed to meet a number of public health targets related to tobacco.

OUR PLACE IN THE LITERATURE

Given these developments, it comes as no surprise that scientists from a range of academic disciplines study how and why people smoke and the continuing spread of the habit. To describe the degree of smoking diffusion in a particular country in any given year, the public health community typically relies on the "cigarette epidemic" model by Lopez et al. (1994). Using time-series data on smoking in the United States, these authors identified a stylized hump-shaped pattern in how the overall smoking prevalence rate evolved as the US economy grew. Informed by this pattern, they hypothesized that, starting from low levels, aggregate cigarette demand and supply grow as a country's economy develops, but this relationship eventually reverses after the population smoking prevalence rate reaches some peak level. To explain the switch in the sign of the relationship, they note that on average as a country gets richer, its residents see more information about the health risks of smoking and the government is more likely to enact and implement tobacco control policies to limit cigarette consumption. Lopez et al. also observe that in early stages of this smoking diffusion process, people with higher socioeconomic status smoke more than people of lower socioeconomic status. Over time, this pattern gradually reverses. Eventually, more people with less education and/or income smoke relative to people of higher status. Although the authors observed that this pattern typically emerges in later cohorts for women than for men, in their recent update of the model, they note that smoking patterns of men and women need to be independently analyzed, especially in developing countries (Thun et al., 2012). Although stylized, these patterns figure importantly in policy considerations when, as these authors do, one recognizes that smoking-attributable mortality exhibits strikingly similar patterns a few decades later. That connection strongly suggests that policymakers can more effectively prevent smoking-related mortality through tobacco control policies if they act to limit the diffusion of the smoking habit in the early stages of its adoption in a given society or even in a given cohort.

Of course, the degree to which this model accurately represents what happens in real life is an empirical question specific to every country. The answers to that question are becoming easier to provide because of impressive efforts to collect the necessary data. In many countries, researchers and public health officials are compiling historical data on cigarette sales, cigarette consumption, and smoking prevalence rates, which they use to monitor smoking diffusion (c.f. Pierce, 1989; Nicolaides-Bouman, 1993; Forey et al., 2002, 2009). A growing number of health surveys throughout the world provide micro-level data with which scientists produce evidence on whether and how individuals adjust their smoking behavior to tobacco control policies such as cigarette taxes (Chaloupka et al., 2011; Lillard et al., 2013), smoking bans (Shetty et al., 2010), and advertising (Nelson, 2010). Qualitative research documents smoking determinants that are difficult to measure, such as culture (Nichter, 2003).

The large literature that sprang up as these resources became available has been reviewed in a number of works that relate to our book. Goodman (1994) surveys the history of tobacco and smoking from its discovery to the development of the modern tobacco industry and tobacco prevention policies. Jha and Chaloupka (2000) review extant tobacco control policies, discuss how they affect the economy, and provide new evidence on their effectiveness. They also point researchers to sources of data on tobacco consumption, prices, trade, and employment. Feldman and Bayer (2004) compare, across eight advanced economies, the legal, political, and social landscape in conflicts over tobacco control. Boyle et al. (2004, 2010) review evidence from developed and developing economies about the diffusion of smoking, its health consequences, and tobacco control policies. Finally, Cairney et al. (2012) document the extent to which governments have regulated tobacco over time, identify a major policy change from the post-war period, and use theories of public policy to help explain the change.

Our book complements this body of evidence and simultaneously adds a unique perspective because it uses data that follow individuals over their whole lives. All other books report or rely on cross-sectional smoking data. Although useful, cross-sectional data do not reveal much about dynamics of life-course smoking. For example, in any given population, the rate of smoking prevalence at a point in time reflects a complicated mixture of smoking initiation and cessation. Thus, it is difficult to separate new smokers from continuing smokers. In this book, we document temporal patterns of smoking over the life cycle of particular cohorts, and we can compare life-course smoking trajectories for men and women across different birth cohorts. This life-course perspective is also very useful for cross-country comparisons because it allows us to more richly describe the context—economic and social—that different groups of smokers experienced over the whole period that they were taking smoking decisions and during critical life-cycle years. Certainly, we are not the first to use this approach. Scholars have been long engaged in research on life-course smoking behavior through the publication of articles,[1] but no available book systematically documents this behavior and discusses its determinants in a cross-national context.

OUR APPROACH

In our book, we examine and contrast patterns of life-course smoking behavior of seven generations of men and women in 10 countries, spanning more than 80 years of history. We also discuss how governments interacted with the tobacco industry and public health advocates to establish or alter barriers to trade and to regulate the consumption and marketing of tobacco. Because tobacco excise taxes and tariffs generate government revenue—especially during economic downturns—various public agencies often face conflicting incentives about tobacco consumption of citizens. One agency may seek to eliminate smoking to improve public health while another agency simultaneously supports the cultivation, processing, and sale of tobacco to generate tax revenue. We shed light on such processes by (1) presenting time-series data on cigarette taxes or prices and economic development and (2) describing key events, some common across countries and others specific to a particular country, that plausibly affected smoking habits.

To document smoking patterns, we take advantage of data on lifetime smoking behavior, collected from retrospective questions in cross-sectional and longitudinal surveys. These national surveys collect information on respondents' current and past smoking habits. Specifically, they ask respondents to report whether they ever smoked regularly and whether they currently smoke. They also collect information about the timing of smoking initiation and, if relevant, cessation. We use these data to construct an indicator of smoking status for all surveyed individuals in each year of their lives. With the retrospective data on start and quit ages, we code a person as a smoker in every year between those two ages. If a person is currently a smoker, we code him or her to have smoked in every year since he or she started up to the year of the survey. We then compute smoking prevalence rates over the life course as the mean smoking status indicator in each year by gender and 10-year birth cohort (using sampling weights). Finally, we correct our smoking rates for bias due to differential mortality of smokers and nonsmokers. Our sample sizes typically comprise thousands of individuals and hundreds of thousands of person-year observations. Not only does our use of these data demonstrate their many advantages but also it is timely. Until now, relatively few researchers used these data. However, many existing surveys ask these retrospective questions, and a growing number of countries are mounting and maintaining longitudinal panel surveys that can or do ask them.

To put the life-course smoking patterns into their historical and economic context, we describe selected events in five major categories—informational, regulatory, social, political, and economic. They include the discovery and dissemination of important information about the health risks of smoking, important regulations that affected how cigarettes could be marketed or consumed, and important historical events that shifted the economic fortunes of a country's residents. Informational events, such as the 1950 *British Medical Journal* publication of scientific evidence that linked smoking and cancer, plausibly affected decisions of people in all countries because they revealed new evidence that could be communicated in different languages at very low cost (Doll and Hill, 1950). Other events were country-specific, such as the 1987 Turkish government ruling making it legal for domestic firms to import and sell cigarettes produced abroad. Together, these events and forces shaped when and how much men and women smoked over the course of their lives and how life-course patterns of smoking evolved over successive generations. We present these events not to establish a causal link between them and the smoking patterns. Rather we use them as a way to frame the patterns and to stimulate ideas.

The country sample of this book consists of 10 developing and developed economies, including 4 formerly or currently socialist economies. We describe smoking patterns in Australia, Canada, China, Germany, Spain, Turkey, the Russian Federation, Ukraine, the United Kingdom, and the United States. Australia, Canada, Germany, Spain, the United Kingdom, and the United States are economically mature economies that allow us to compare and contrast patterns of smoking in and across countries that currently occupy similar stages of economic development. The economies of the remaining countries are developing and have been changing, sometimes very dramatically, over the period of study. Often these changes occurred because their political systems changed. In the early years of the period we analyze, governments in China, East Germany, Russia, Turkey, and Ukraine more directly controlled economic production. In later years, governments in all of these countries allowed resources and production, including the production of cigarettes and tobacco, to be directed more by market forces. Finally, governments in each of the 10 countries have regulated the sale, taxation, marketing, and consumption of cigarettes and tobacco in different ways at different times.

BOOK OUTLINE AND ORGANIZATION OF CHAPTERS

We have organized the book around 12 main chapters and an appendix. Each of the first 9 chapters corresponds to a different country. We collect those chapters into three geographically defined groups. We group together the Anglo-Saxon countries, countries of Western Europe, and countries of Eastern Europe and Asia. Although there are alternative ways to group the countries, we believe that our selected grouping relies on the most important dimensions along which the countries resemble and differ from each other. As mentioned previously, the first two country groups are economically more advanced compared to the last group. Also, countries that are in the same group have historical connections and share language or culture. In fact, as we discuss in the respective chapters, the Anglo-Saxon countries also share a common tobacco industry. In the remaining 3 chapters of the book, we compare across countries smoking patterns of different population groups. Three appendix chapters provide technical details.

To facilitate comparisons of patterns over time and across countries, we report findings for each country in comparably defined figures and tables. Specifically, each country-specific chapter includes four standardized figures and one standardized table.

In the first figure, we plot over time the smoking prevalence rate of each 10-year birth cohort defined by age at the most recent national survey. These trajectories generally follow a bell-shaped pattern, reflecting a common pattern of smoking initiation that occurs in a fairly narrow chronological age window—during puberty and early adolescence—and a longer period that stretches over the decades of adulthood during which smokers quit (at a much lower annual rate). Figure 1 always includes two subfigures that appear together; the one on the top shows results for men (Figure 1a), and the one on the bottom shows results for women (Figure 1b). In each subfigure, we also mark years during which informational, regulatory, economic, or historical events occurred that might have affected or be related to smoking behavior. Because the figures are "busy," we show only a few events. From the large set of potentially important events, we select and display events we judge to provide the most relevant context for the life-course smoking trajectories of each cohort. We mark events that might have affected smoking behavior generally or events that might have affected smoking behavior of a particular sex. Even when we list different events for men and women, the two subfigures are plotted on the same scale so one can trace events up or down from either figure to the other.

In the second figure, we plot, as data are available, annual time-series data on cigarette taxes and/or prices and per capita gross domestic product (GDP). Again, these data are but a few of the economic factors that potentially affect smoking decisions.

We show them to provide information about each country's level of economic development and prosperity, the affordability of cigarettes in each country, and, as importantly, to provoke our readers to think and speculate about other economic factors that might matter for smoking decisions.

In the third figure, we plot the same smoking trajectories shown in Figure 1 but this time on an age scale. We present the data on this scale to allow readers to more easily compare across cohorts how smoking trajectories of different cohorts of men and women differed or resembled each other when all members of each cohort were the same chronological age. Here, one can directly and more easily observe how rates of smoking initiation and smoking cessation compared over the life course across sex cohort groups.

In Table 1, we report data on six summary measures of smoking behavior. For each gender and cohort, we list the average of the peak smoking prevalence rate, the number of cigarettes smoked on the average day (during the time a person smoked), the number of years smoked, the age the cohort reached its peak smoking prevalence, the age current and former smokers started, and the age ex-smokers quit. Except for the data on average cigarette consumption, one can observe or infer the average of each measure from the trajectories presented in Figures 1 and 3. But for most measures, it is not easy to do so. We highlight these summary measures to call attention to particular aspects of life-course smoking. The peak prevalence rate reflects how popular smoking was among members of a given cohort. The average daily cigarette consumption reflects how intensively the cohort smoked. The number of years a cohort smoked reflects the duration of the smoking habit for that cohort. The mean age at which a cohort reached its peak smoking prevalence rate reflects when the smoking habit was most popular in that cohort and corresponds to the age at which the rate of quitting first exceeded the rate of smoking initiation in that cohort. Four of these measures are essentially fixed for every cohort. The fixed measures are the peak prevalence rate, average cigarette consumption, age at peak smoking prevalence, and the average start age. One can directly compare these measures across genders and across birth cohorts. Because we observe each cohort from birth until the time of interview and not from birth until death, one cannot directly compare smoking duration and quit age across all cohorts. However, one can compare the level of these variables of men and women from a given cohort.

In the fourth and final figure of each chapter, we use the data in Table 1 to plot, for each birth cohort, the ratio of the value of each indicator of men to the value of each indicator for women. We do so because in the plots of the male/female ratio of the indicators, it is much easier to identify differences and similarities in the smoking behavior of men and women.

In the three final chapters, we respectively compare across countries patterns of smoking behavior of men, women, and men relative to women. To ensure that smoking outcomes by cohort are comparable across countries, we define birth cohorts using their age in 2002, which is the earliest year of all available country surveys. In doing so, we summarize the smoking history of individuals born between 1913 and 1982. Because in the country-specific chapters cohorts are defined by the age at the most recent national survey, the smoking indicators in the figures presented in those chapters may differ from the ones we present in the comparative chapters.

Each of the three comparative chapters starts with a brief summary of the existing related literature. The authors then describe cross-country similarities and differences in four measures of smoking behavior: the peak smoking prevalence rate, the mean number of cigarettes consumed each day, the average age smokers started, and the average age ex-smokers quit. The authors conclude each chapter by discussing potential explanations of the observed patterns. To inform their discussion, they present correlations between the data on life-course smoking prevalence rates and a set of factors that are plausible determinants of smoking decisions.[2]

The technical appendix concludes the book. In its three chapters, we describe the data and document data sources; explain how we construct our measure of smoking prevalence; and present a brief history of each country's regulation of tobacco, country-specific events, and references that can guide readers to more extensive documentation.

CORE FINDINGS

Our analysis reveals both expected and unexpected patterns in life-course smoking. Some of the patterns replicate previous work that relies on cross-sectional snapshots of smoking behavior. The unexpected patterns arise because we have longitudinal data, which offer special insights to individual smoking behavior over each person's life course.

We find the following general patterns:

- The popularity of smoking (as reflected in the peak smoking prevalence rate of each cohort) follows the hump-shaped pattern predicted by the smoking epidemic model; it rises and falls earlier in more advanced economies and, for women, lags behind that of men by a few generations.
- In contrast, and contrary to expectations, the intensity of smoking (as reflected in the mean number of cigarettes consumed by smokers in each cohort) follows a hump-shaped pattern across generations that is consistently timed both across countries and across genders.
- Differences in the timing and duration of the smoking pattern (as reflected in the mean age at smoking initiation and cessation by cohort) do not follow a clear pattern across more and less developed countries. However, cross-country differences in the age smokers quit largely persist across generations, whereas mean initiation age declines across generations in most countries, converging to a common low value between 16 and 19 years.
- Across practically every country (in most cohorts), smoking is less prevalent among women than it is among men. In fact, when women smoke, they typically start later in life and smoke fewer cigarettes on average. Somewhat surprisingly, female smokers quit at roughly the same age as men.
- Whereas the popularity and timing of the smoking habit is generally converging across successive cohorts of men and women in almost every country, we observe no such convergence in the number of cigarettes smoked.

Although not unique, there are two particularly striking exceptions to the aforementioned patterns. China and the United Kingdom are the only countries in which the popularity of smoking among women does not seem to follow a hump-shaped pattern. Instead, in China peak smoking rates consistently decline across successive cohorts of women, thus causing the smoking rates of Chinese men and women to diverge in younger cohorts. In the United Kingdom, women's smoking rates increase and then decline sporadically across successive generations.

Studying these patterns in light of the national and international contexts has allowed us to speculate about factors that might explain them. As previously mentioned, we interpret the hump-shaped pattern in the peak smoking rates across generations to be consistent with changing economic development—the idea at the core of the cigarette epidemic model. That is, we believe that smoking rates increase with factors that co-evolve as a country's economy grows (e.g., disposable income, education, formal employment, political stability, and democratic freedom) when the health consequences of smoking are unknown, and people are exposed to cigarette advertising. The relationship switches from positive to negative when the information on the health risks of smoking becomes widely available and, by consequence, governments understand the need to protect public health and adopt tobacco control policies.

The fact that the data in cigarette consumption do not fit this scenario presents a puzzle. Because we find that cigarette consumption reaches its peak in those generations that were first exposed to the information shock on the health consequences of smoking (i.e., individuals born between 1932 and 1962), we hypothesize that individuals may respond to information shocks more by adjusting their level of cigarette consumption and less so by changing their smoking participation status.

Finally, for all other patterns in smoking behavior that are not consistent with the "usual suspect" forces, we identify one important factor that many scientists—especially economists—had been overlooking for a long time. Repeatedly, the smoking patterns we observe have suggested an important role for cultural norms in general and on gender roles in particular.[3] As we argue in the respective chapters, societal norms about gender roles may have driven the striking patterns in female smoking behavior in China and the United Kingdom.

We hope these patterns inspire our readers to develop other hypotheses and conjectures about the factors that cause men and women to smoke or quit. We also hope that the studies we inspire will lead to a new and better understanding of smoking behavior so that policymakers can both anticipate and better respond to evolving patterns of smoking across the life course of their citizens.

NOTES

1.   A non-exhaustive list of articles follows here: Harris (1983), La Vecchia et al. (1986), Warner (1989), Brenner (1993), Ronneberg et al. (1994), Escobedo and Peddicord (1996), Birkett (1997), Burns et al. (1998), Laaksonen et al. (1999), Anderson and Burns (2000), Kemm (2001), Fernández et al. (2003), Marugame et al. (2006), Federico et al. (2007), Perlman et al. (2007), Ahacic et al. (2008), Park et al. (2009), Kenkel et al. (2009), Christopoulou et al. (2013), and Holford et al. (2014).

2. Note that it does not make sense to regress cigarette consumption, age quit, and age start on the predictors because these indicators vary very little over time.
3. In other work, we formally test the hypothesis that culture affects smoking behavior and offer evidence that it does (Christopoulou and Lillard, 2015).

REFERENCES

Ahacic, K., R. Kennison, and M. Thorslung. 2008. "Trends in smoking in Sweden from 1968 to 2002: Age, period and cohort patterns." *Preventive Medicine* 46:558–564.

Anderson, C., and D. M. Burns. 2000. "Patterns of adolescent smoking initiation rates by ethnicity and sex." *Tobacco Control* 9:ii4–ii8.

Birkett, N. J. 1997. "Trends in smoking by birth cohort for births between 1940 and 1975: A reconstructed cohort analysis of the 1990 Ontario Health Survey." *Preventive Medicine* 26:534–541.

Brenner, H. 1993. "A birth cohort analysis of the smoking epidemic in West Germany." *Journal of Epidemiology Community Health* 47:54–58.

Boyle, P., N. Grey, J. Henningfield, J. Seffrin, and W. Zatonski, eds. 2004 (1st ed.), 2010 (2nd ed.). *Tobacco: Science, Policy and Public Health*. New York: Oxford University Press.

Burns, D. M., L. Lee, and L. Z. Shen. 1998. "Cigarette smoking behavior in the United States." In *Changes in Cigarette-Related Disease Risk and Their Implications for Prevention and Control*, edited by D. Burns, L. Garfinel, J. Samet, pp 13–112. Bethesda, MD: National Institutes of Health.

Cairney, P., D. T. Studlar, and H. M. Mamuda, eds. 2012. *Global Tobacco Control: Power, Policy, Governance and Transfer*. New York: Palgrave Macmillan.

Chaloupka, F. J., K. Straif, and M. E. Leon. 2011. "Effectiveness of tax and price policies in tobacco control." *Tobacco Control* 20:235–238.

Christopoulou, R., and D. R. Lillard. 2015. "Is smoking behavior culturally determined? Evidence from British Immigrants." *Journal of Economic Behavior and Organization* (forthcoming).

Christopoulou, R., D. R. Lillard, and J. R. Balmori de la Miyar. 2013. "Smoking behavior of Mexicans: Patterns by birth-cohort, gender, and education." *International Journal of Public Health* 58:335–343.

Doll, R., and A. B. Hill. 1950. "Smoking and carcinoma of the lung." *British Medical Journal* 2:739–748.

Escobedo, L. G., and J. P. Peddicord. 1996. "Smoking prevalence in US birth cohorts: The influence of gender and education." *American Journal of Public Health* 86:231–236.

Federico, B., G. Costa, and A. E. Kunst. 2007. "Educational inequalities in initiation, cessation, and prevalence of smoking among 3 Italian birth cohorts." *American Journal of Public Health* 97:838–845.

Feldman, E. A., and R. Bayer, eds. 2004. *Unfiltered: Conflicts Over Tobacco Policy and Public Health*. Cambridge, MA: Harvard University Press.

Fernández, E., A. Schiaffino, J. M. Borras, O. Shafey, J. R. Villalbi, and C. La Vecchia. 2003. "Prevalence of cigarette smoking by birth cohort among males and females in Spain, 1910–1990." *European Journal of Cancer Prevention* 12:57–62.

Fields, N., and S. Chapman. 2003. "Chasing Ernst L. Wynder: 40 years of Philip Morris' efforts to influence a leading scientist." *Journal of Epidemiology and Community Health* 578:571–578.

Forey, B., J. Hamling, P. Lee, and N. Ward, eds. 2002 (2nd ed.), 2009 (online ed.). *International Smoking Statistics*. New York: Oxford University Press.

Goodman, J. 1994. *Tobacco in History*. New York: Routledge.

Harris, J. E. 1983. "Cigarette smoking among successive birth cohorts of men and women in the United States during 1900–80." *Journal of the National Cancer Institute* 71:473–479.

Holford, T. R., D. T. Levy, L. A. McKay, L. Clarke, B. Racine, R. Meza, et al. 2014. "Patterns of birth cohort-specific smoking histories, 1965–2009." *American Journal of Preventive Medicine* 46:e31–e37.

Jha, P., and F. Chaloupka, eds. 2000. *Tobacco Control in Developing Countries*. New York: Oxford University Press.

Kemm, J. R. 2001. "A birth cohort analysis of smoking by adults in Great Britain 1974–1998." *Journal of Public Health Medicine* 23:306–311.

Kenkel, D., D. R. Lillard, and F. Liu. 2009. "An analysis of life-course smoking behavior in China." *Health Economics* 18:S147–S156.

Laaksonen, M., A. Uutela, E. Vartiainen, P. Jousilahti, S. Helakorpi, and P. Puska. 1999. "Development of smoking by birth cohort in the adult population of eastern Finland 1972–97." *Tobacco Control* 8:161–168.

La Vecchia, C., A. Decarli, and R. Pagano. 1986. "Prevalence of cigarette smoking among subsequent cohorts of Italian males and females." *Preventative Medicine* 15:606–613.

Lillard, D. R., E. Molloy, and A. Sfekas. 2013. "Smoking initiation and the iron law of demand." *Journal of Health Economics* 32:114–127.

Lopez, A. D., N. E. Collishaw, and T. Piha. 1994. "A descriptive model of the cigarette epidemic in developed countries." *Tobacco Control* 3:242–247.

Marugame, T., K. Kamo, T. Sobue, S. Akiba, S. Mizuno, H. Satoh, et al. 2006. "Trends in smoking by birth cohorts born between 1900 and 1977 in Japan." *Preventive Medicine* 42:120–127.

Nelson, J. P. 2010. "What is learned from longitudinal studies of advertising and youth drinking and smoking? A critical assessment." *International Journal of Environmental Research and Public Health* 7:870–926.

Nichter, M. 2003. "Smoking: What does culture have to do with it?" *Addiction* 98:139–145.

Nicolaides-Bouman, A. 1993. *International Smoking Statistics: A Collection of Historical Data From 22 Economically Developed Countries*. New York: Oxford University Press.

Park, E. J., H. K. Koh, J. W. Kwon, M. K. Suh, H. Kim, and S. I. Cho. 2009. "Secular trends in adult male smoking form 1992 to 2006 in South Korea: Age-specific changes with evolving tobacco-control policies." *Public Health* 123:657–664.

Perlman, F., M. Bobak, A. Gilmore, and M. McKee. 2007. "Trends in the prevalence of smoking in Russia during the transition to a market economy." *Tobacco Control* 16:299–305.

Pierce, J. P. 1989. "International comparisons of trends in cigarette smoking prevalence." *American Journal of Public Health* 79:152–157.

Proctor, R. N. 1997. "The Nazi war on tobacco: Ideology, evidence, and possible cancer consequences." *Bulletin of the History of Medicine* 71:435–488.

Proctor, R. N. 1999. *The Nazi war on Tobacco: Ideology, evidence, and possible cancer consequences*. Princeton, NJ: Princeton University Press.

Ronneberg, A., K. E. Lund, and A. Hafstad. 1994. "Lifetime smoking habits among Norwegian men and women born between 1890 and 1974." *International Journal of Epidemiology* 23:267–276.

Royal College of Physicians of London (RCPL). 1962. *Smoking and Health: Summary and Report of the Royal College of Physicians of London on Smoking in Relation to Cancer of the Lung and Other Diseases*. London: Pitman.

Shetty, K. D., T. DeLeire, C. White, and J. Bhattacharya. 2010. "Changes in US hospitalization and mortality rates following smoking bans." *Journal of Policy Analysis and Management* 30:6–28.

Thun, M., R. Peto, J. Boreham, and A. D. Lopez. 2012. "Stages of the cigarette epidemic on entering its second century." *Tobacco Control* 21:96–101.

US Department of Health, Education, and Welfare (USDHEW). 1964. *Smoking and Health: Report of the Advisory Committee to the Surgeon General of the Public Health Service*. Public Health Service Publication No. 1103. Rockville, MD: USDHEW.

Warner, K. E. 1989. "Effects of the antismoking campaign: An update." *American Journal of Public Health* 79(2):144–151.

World Health Organization (WHO). 1999. *The World Health Report 1999: Making a Difference*. Geneva: WHO.

World Health Organization (WHO). 2012. *WHO Global Report: Mortality Attributable to Tobacco*. Geneva: WHO.

PART I

The Anglo-Saxon World

Australia, Canada, the United Kingdom, and the United States

Smoking in Australia

DEAN R. LILLARD

INTRODUCTION

Australia's tobacco history differs from that of other countries because so much of Australia's population arrived as colonists (forced and willing). Tobacco arrived in 1788 when England established its penal colony (Walker, 1984). The sailors and free settlers brought not only tobacco, tobacco seeds, and knowledge of how to grow tobacco but also a ready-made culture of tobacco use. As a result, the cultivation and culture of tobacco rapidly took root among both residents and governments of the Australian colonies.

From its beginning, and through the latter half of the 20th century, Australian governments supported the tobacco industry. For example, in 1936, the Commonwealth Government introduced the Statutory Leaf Percentage system that reduced tariffs on imported tobacco when domestic factories used a minimum fraction of Australian-grown tobacco to produce cigarettes.[1] The percentage increased from 2.5 percent in 1936 to a maximum of 50 percent on January 1, 1966 (Commonwealth Parliamentary Debates, 1936; Australia Tariff Board, various years). The Commonwealth Government also established and maintained a tradition of regulating industries through quasi-governmental organizations that included representatives of each industry. In 1941, they formed the *Australian Tobacco Board* to buy and market Australian-grown tobacco (Australia Commonwealth, 1947).[2] This close collaboration benefitted both the industry and Commonwealth and state governments.

Australia imported much of its tobacco industry and culture from the United States and Great Britain, but not completely. For example, in the 1970s, the Australian industry created its own version of the "Marlboro Man," choosing an up-and-coming actor named Paul Hogan to serve as the embodiment of a quintessential Aussie character (*Jobson's Yearbook*, 1977). His commercials for the Winfield brand, created to compete head-to-head with Marlboro, were wildly successful, and within 2 years of being launched, Winfields were Australia's top-selling cigarettes.[3] Many Australians who grew up seeing television cigarette commercials can still recite the slogan Hogan delivered to close every spot: ". . . anyhow, have a Winfield." At the same time, tobacco consumption in Australia differed from the patterns among American and British smokers. For example, unlike their US and British counterparts, Australian feminists did not adopt the cigarette as a symbol of their emancipation, and, in the first half of the 20th century, Australians smoked far fewer factory-made cigarettes than smokers did in most other countries (in part because of high taxes on factory-made cigarettes) (Australian Retail Tobacconist, 1959, 1972).

Australians' life-course smoking patterns may also differ from the UK and US patterns because the Australian medical community and government were slower to respond as information about the health risks of smoking unfolded. It was not until 1956, 6 years after the 1950 publication of Doll and Hill (1950), that the *Medical Journal of Australia* noted a link between smoking, cancer, and heart disease (Walker, 1984). To be fair, the journal had published an article as early as 1936 suggesting that smoking might play a role in chest pains associated with poor circulation.[4] However, the medical profession did not widely acknowledge or act on the warnings. In 1962, a collection of groups began to lobby the Commonwealth Government to implement policies that the UK Royal College of Physicians (RCP) suggested in their report *Smoking and Health* (RCP, 1962).[5] However, the government did not pass legislation to mandate a health warning on cigarettes until 1968, and the label did not appear until 1973 (Walker, 1984).

Public information campaigns started in 1972 when the federal government launched its first campaign to educate consumers about the health risks of smoking. In 1982, the industry voluntarily agreed to list tar and nicotine content on cigarette packs. Following developments in the United States, in 1985, the Commonwealth Government and the tobacco industry agreed on a set of four warning labels that would appear on a rotating schedule on cigarette packs and packages for cut tobacco.

During the period we study, state and commonwealth governments regulated how companies could market tobacco, who could legally buy cigarettes, and where people could smoke. Paul Hogan's reign as the television face of Australian smokers ended by 1976, when the Commonwealth Government banned advertising of cigarettes on radio and television. During the next 30 years, state and commonwealth governments limited advertising in cinemas, on billboards and vehicle displays, in print media, and also the sponsoring of "domestic" sports events (Winstanley et al., 1995). During the same period, governments regulated who could buy and where Australians could consume tobacco. By 1917, every state had made it illegal to sell tobacco to juveniles—typically defined to be those younger than the age of 16 years (*The Free Library*, 1998). Later, this age was increased to 18 years (Walker, 1984). Since 1986, the commonwealth and state governments have increasingly restricted the public places where people can smoke. They first banned smoking in workplaces, public venues, restaurants, licensed clubs, and pubs. Recently, Australian governments have begun to regulate smoking in what had formerly been considered private spaces. Between 2008 and 2010, several states (Tasmania, New South Wales, Queensland, Northern Territories, and Victoria) made it illegal for a person to smoke in a private car when any passenger younger than 16 years is present.[6]

Although cigarette prices had been more or less uniform in Australia, from 1974 to 1997, prices of cigarettes began to differ across state boundaries because state governments levied specific fees on tobacco (Australia Taxation Office, 2002). In 1974, the Government of Victoria became the first Australian state to levy a separate, state-level tobacco license fee on firms selling tobacco. Other state governments quickly followed suit. The differences persisted until 1997, when the High Court ruled that state tobacco license fees were illegal (*Ha and Anor vs. the State of New*

South Wales; Walter Hammond and Associates vs. the State of New South Wales).
Since then, cigarette taxes have not differed across states.

During this period, the industry was not idle. In late 1978, tobacco firms operating in Australia formed the Tobacco Institute of Australia Limited to "promote understanding of the tobacco industry" (Winstanley et al., 1995). In response to increasing taxes, firms experimented with and ultimately adopted different pack sizes to better target consumers with different price sensitivities. Balkan, Sobranie, and Sullivans introduced packs containing 25 cigarettes in 1975 and a pack size of 50 in 1976. Rothmans followed suit in 1976. Philip Morris effectively discounted the price of cigarettes in 1983 when it introduced a pack size of 30 with a list price similar to the price charged for the 25-cigarette packs. In 1985, Philip Morris introduced packs of 15 cigarettes at a price of approximately $1 per pack.

Unsurprisingly, as the regulatory burden on tobacco increased, smokers also changed their behavior. In the face of increased taxes and tobacco license fees, groups formed to legally evade them. In 1993, Western Australian smokers formed the "Tobacco Smokers Freedom Movement Inc." to buy cigarettes overseas. Its members paid a lower price for cigarettes because the group did not have to pay the state tobacco license fees (Winstanley et al., 1995). This type of behavior is likely to become more common because the Commonwealth, state, and territory governments plan to increase taxes. The joint federal–state National Tobacco Strategy (NTS 2012-2018), endorsed in November 2012, aims to increase the price of cigarettes as its number 3 priority, behind the battle with big tobacco and stronger mass media campaigns. Accompanying that goal is the recognition that tax avoidance and evasion will increase. Indeed, the Customs Amendment (Smuggled Tobacco) Act 2012 (Intergovernmental Committee on Drugs, 2012)

> creates new offences of smuggling tobacco or tobacco products and conveying or possessing smuggled tobacco products, and will allow a penalty of up to 10 years imprisonment to be imposed, in addition to the existing monetary penalty of up to five times the amount of duty evaded. (p. 20)

These and other historical events shaped and continue to shape whether, when, and how intensively Australian men and women smoke. We document this association in what follows. Specifically, in this chapter, we describe patterns in life-course smoking rates of seven different cohorts of men and women and put them in the national context.

SMOKING PREVALENCE RATES IN HISTORICAL PERSPECTIVE

In Figure 2.1, we mark a selection of smoking-related economic and regulatory events, on which we overlay the life-course smoking trajectories of men and women born in different 10-year birth cohorts. We mark the years during which Australia actively committed troops to the Allied forces during World War II (WWII) because, like governments in almost every country, the Australian government issued tobacco to soldiers. In addition, the war generally disrupted the domestic supply of tobacco. We also mark the years when the third and fourth major tobacco firms began to do business in Australia. Philip Morris (Australia) entered the Australian market in 1954.[7] A year later, Rothmans arrived (*Jobson's Yearbook,*

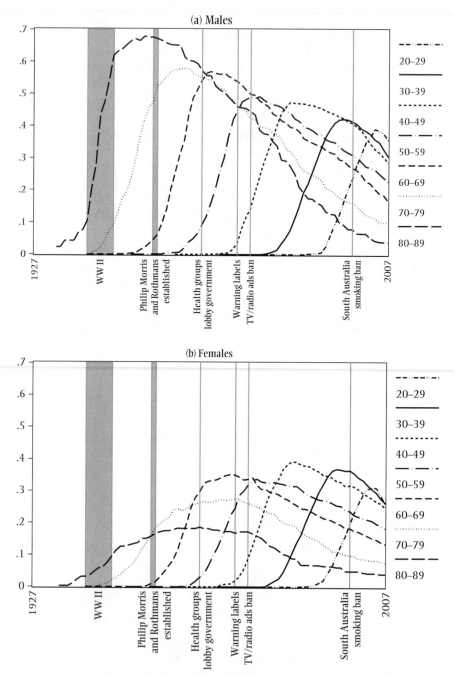

Figure 2.1 Smoking prevalence rates over the life course by gender and birth cohort.
SOURCE: Household, Income, and Labour Dynamics in Australia (HILDA) Survey. 2007.
Melbourne Institute of Applied Economic and Social Research, University of Melbourne.

1977; Rothmans, 1980). Their arrival introduced more competition, new marketing strategies (Rothmans aired the first television advertisement for cigarettes in 1956), and likely led to price discounting observed in the newly developed supermarkets starting in 1958 (Walker, 1984). During the 1950s, UK and US scientists were accumulating evidence about the health risks of smoking. As noted previously, the publication of the 1962 Royal College of Physician's report caused health groups in Australia to petition the government to more actively inform Australians about the health risks of smoking. We list that event here. We also list the regulatory events that subsequently unfolded, including the requirement in 1973 that warning labels appear on cigarette packs and the full implementation in 1976 of the ban on advertising of cigarettes on radio and television (passed in 1972 and applied in 1973) (National Archives of Australia, 2013). Finally, we mark 1995 because it is the first year after the Australian Capital Territory implemented Australia's first ban on smoking in public places. Although it took another 10 years for other states to follow suit, observers consider the passage of that legislation to be a landmark event (Goodin, 1995).[8]

The most striking pattern is that peak smoking prevalence rates declined almost monotonically from the high peak prevalence rate of 68 percent among the oldest cohort of men (age 80–89 years in 2007) to 39 percent among the cohort of men who were 20–29 years old in 2007. What might be less obvious is the difference in the initiation behavior between the oldest and later cohorts of men. By coincidence, it is the case that the average man in the oldest cohort turned 17 years old in 1939, the year Australia entered World War II. Figure 2.1 also shows that there was a break in the trend of life-course smoking in that year for the oldest cohort of men—a break that one does not observe in any other cohort. Although association does not equal causation, the timing of this break with World War II suggests that policies and market conditions associated with the war may explain differences between the smoking behaviors of men in the oldest cohort relative to the behavior of those born in later cohorts.[9]

Figure 2.1b reveals further insights about this and other patterns because it allows the reader to examine whether there was a similar break in the trend in the smoking behavior of the oldest cohort of women in the years of World War II. There is no obvious break in the trend. If anything, it appears that the increase in smoking prevalence of the oldest cohort of women decelerated during the years of World War II.

At the same time, Figure 2.1 shows that, across successive cohorts, the smoking prevalence rate of Australian women fluctuated more than the rate for Australian men. In the 1950s and early 1960s, the cigarette industry grew more competitive, firms were marketing more aggressively, and supermarkets were capturing an increasing share of cigarette sales (at substantially discounted prices). The two cohorts of women who matured in this period—women who were 50–59 and 60–69 years old in 2007—smoked more than women in the cohorts that preceded them. During the time that women in these two cohorts came of age, the 1962 RCP was published and Australian public health groups were actively lobbying the government to warn smokers about health risks of smoking, and yet a greater fraction of the next cohort smoked. This increase seems somewhat at odds with the assertions and hopes of the public health advocates who successfully lobbied to get the government to ban radio and television advertising of cigarettes. That ban was fully implemented by 1976, but relative to the immediately preceding cohort, the rate of smoking prevalence was higher, not lower, among the cohort that came of age after the ban was fully in place.

One possible explanation for this is that, during this time period, rates of labor participation by women steadily increased, especially for younger cohorts. For example, in 1966, approximately 58 percent of Australian women between 20 and 24 years old were working, whereas in 1984, 73 percent of women of the same age were working. By 1988, the female labor force participation rate of women in this age group had reached what appears to be its long run steady-state rate. Between 1988 and 2010, on average, approximately 77 percent of women aged 20–24 years worked.[10] Furthermore, between 1969 and 1975, subsequent to the 1969 Equal Pay case, Australia eliminated pay discrimination by sex that allowed employers to legally pay women 25 percent less than the wage they paid men (Eastough and Miller, 2004). Gregory and Duncan (1981) document that the share of wages paid to women increased from 18 percent in 1964 to 28 percent in 1976. In 1976, the average woman earned approximately 85 percent of the wage of the average man. Since then, it has risen slowly and now fluctuates, more or less with the business cycle, around that figure (Cassells et al., 2009).

The rising wages and labor force participation rate of women were occurring at a time when the government was more actively informing the public about the health risks of smoking, requiring warning labels, and banning advertising. Thus, during the period from 1973 to 1988, it is possible that countervailing forces were influencing smoking decisions of women. On the one hand, they were earning more, working in offices rather than staying at home, and had control over more of the household budget. On the other hand, they stopped being exposed to television and radio advertising of cigarettes, and they began to see warning labels. At the same time, surveys conducted between 1983 and 1989 found that Australian men and women shared similar attitudes about smoking (Clarke et al., 1993). It is plausible that the rise in incomes of women and gender-neutral attitudes about smoking explain the increase in the level of smoking in successive cohorts of women; an increase that ended with the cohort of women who turned 23 years old in 1984. Peak smoking prevalence fell in the two cohorts that followed.

Of course, the smoking behaviors of both men and women were also subject to changes in cigarette prices and overall economic growth. In Figure 2.2, we plot time-series data on the average price of cigarettes and per capita gross domestic product (GDP) in Australia from 1945 to 2009. It is striking, and again suggestive, that real cigarette prices were either constant or generally falling from the end of World War II until the beginning of the 1980s. During the same period, real per capita GDP grew much faster than the price of a pack of cigarettes. This period coincides with the increasing smoking rates among Australian women and with their increased labor force participation rate. From 1982 until 2000, cigarette prices increased much faster than per capita GDP, in part because tobacco taxes dramatically increased. One could plausibly relate this increase to the simultaneous fall in smoking rates of both men and women. From 2001 to 2007, cigarette prices increased at about the same rate as per capita GDP, but after 2007 they increased explosively.

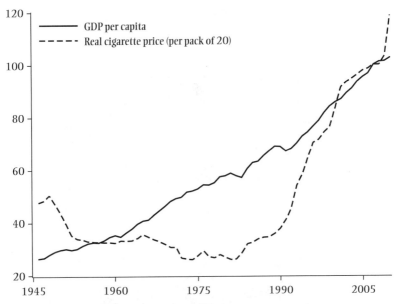

Figure 2.2 Economic development and cigarette prices (2007 = 100).
SOURCES: Barro, R. J., and J. F. Ursua. 2008. "Macroeconomic crises since 1870." NBER
Working Paper No. 13940. Cambridge, MA: National Bureau of Economic Research;
Australian Ministry of Labour Gazette (various issues).

COHORT AND GENDER DIFFERENCES

Next, we present data that more clearly show the convergence in the smoking patterns of men and women across successive cohorts. We start by lining up each cohort's smoking prevalence rate by chronological age in Figure 2.3, which reveals two patterns already mentioned and two patterns that were not so obvious.

Over the course of their lives, Australian men of different cohorts smoked in broadly similar ways at similar ages, but, as noted previously, the oldest cohort of men smoked more at almost every age. Figure 2.3 shows the less obvious result that this statement is only true from age 17 years onward. Up until age 17, the oldest cohort of men smoked less at every age than the men in cohorts that followed them. Figure 2.1 indicated that the average man in the oldest cohort turned 17 years old in 1939—the year Australia entered World War II. Together these patterns suggest that supply and demand conditions during World War II differentially affected the smoking behavior of Australian men.

In addition, Figure 2.3 makes more clear the more or less monotonic reduction in smoking at every age for men and the up-and-down pattern of smoking participation for women. Women in the oldest cohort smoked less at every age than did women of successive cohorts. As observed previously, smoking among Australian women peaked in the middle cohorts. Importantly, Figure 2.3 clearly shows that the higher rate of smoking participation of these cohorts is limited to higher rates of participation in the early part of the life course. Women in middle-aged cohorts started smoking earlier than women in cohorts before or after them. Among women in the cohorts that were 30–39 and 40–49 years old in 2007, approximately 37 and

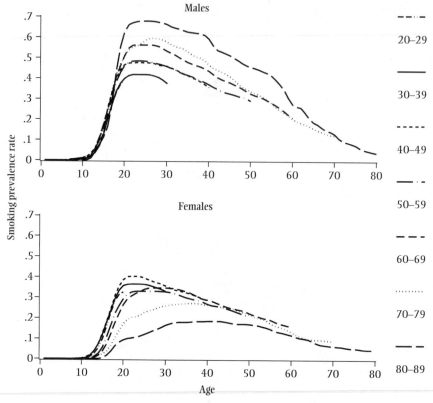

Figure 2.3 Change in smoking prevalence rate with age by birth cohort.
SOURCE: Household, Income, and Labour Dynamics in Australia (HILDA) Survey. 2007.
Melbourne Institute of Applied Economic and Social Research, University of Melbourne.

40 percent, respectively, were smoking at age 20. But, in cohorts aged 40 years and
older, by age 30 and after, the smoking prevalence rates did not substantially differ
in any year. This perhaps surprising conclusion suggests that these middle cohorts
of Australian women faced conditions that affected their initiation behavior but not
their quitting behavior.

   In Table 2.1, we present the six summary measures of smoking behavior described
in Chapter 1 that expose differences in smoking behavior of different cohorts that
are less easy to notice both in Figure 2.1 and in Figure 2.3. The comparisons reveal
interesting patterns. As observed for other countries, although more men in the oldest cohort smoked than in all other cohorts, they smoked fewer cigarettes on average.
Smoking intensity was highest among men aged 60–69 years in 2007. On the average
day, smokers in that cohort consumed more than a pack a day. In every cohort of
men that followed, fewer men smoked, and, when they did, they smoked fewer cigarettes on the average day. The pattern differs for women. As noted previously, smoking prevalence was highest among the cohort of women who turned 40–49 years
old in 2007, and the smokers in this cohort smoked more on average than women
smokers in every other cohort.

Table 2.1. SUMMARY INDICATORS OF SMOKING BY GENDER AND BIRTH COHORT

Gender/ cohort	Sample size	Peak prevalence rate	Cigarettes per day	Years smoking	Average age at		
					peak	start	quit
MALES							
80–89	126	0.68	12	36	28	19	52
70–79	371	0.58	12	32	28	19	46
60–69	580	0.57	23	32	24	18	43
50–59	789	0.49	20	26	26	18	38
40–49	1003	0.47	19	22	23	18	33
30–39	863	0.42	17	16	25	18	29
20–29	825	0.39	15	9	21	17	23
FEMALES							
80–89	212	0.19	11	36	41	24	54
70–79	417	0.27	13	33	40	23	50
60–69	657	0.35	15	30	29	21	44
50–59	900	0.34	15	26	25	20	37
40–49	1119	0.39	17	21	23	18	31
30–39	1004	0.37	13	15	23	18	28
20–29	892	0.31	13	9	21	17	23

SOURCE: Household, Income, and Labour Dynamics in Australia (HILDA) Survey. 2007. Melbourne Institute of Applied Economic and Social Research, University of Melbourne.

One can also characterize a cohort's smoking behavior by the age at which smoking prevalence reached its peak. For men, the oldest two cohorts were approximately 28 years of age when the cohorts' smoking prevalence rate reached its peak. There was no obvious pattern in the age of highest smoking prevalence for men in the following three cohorts. The age at peak smoking prevalence of the next four cohorts of men bounced between 23 and 26 years. We do not discuss the youngest cohort because not all members of that cohort were old enough by 2007 to have reached their peak smoking prevalence. Among women, each successive cohort reached its peak smoking prevalence rate at increasingly younger ages.

Finally, one can describe trends across cohorts in the average age at which smokers started to smoke and the average age at which ex-smokers quit. The average age of smoking initiation has fallen for each successive cohort of both men and women. Again, it becomes clear that women in older cohorts started at much older ages than did their male counterparts. However, as in the United States, the United Kingdom, and other countries, relative to the older cohorts, men and women in younger birth cohorts are starting to smoke at younger and more similar ages. Furthermore, women achieved "equality" with men in their age of initiation because the average age of smoking initiation of women fell faster across successive cohorts than it did across the corresponding cohorts of men. This "equality" was

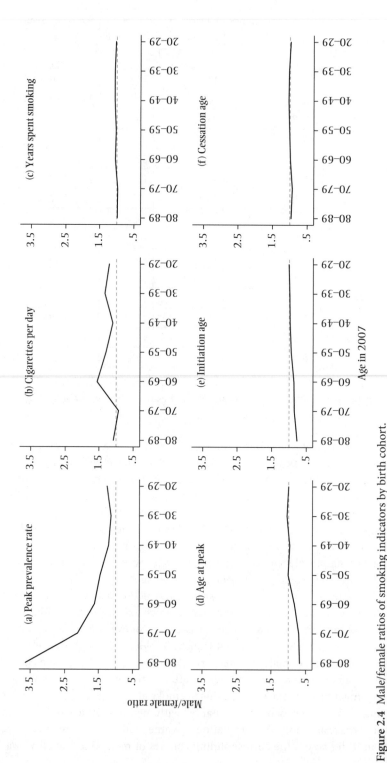

Figure 2.4 Male/female ratios of smoking indicators by birth cohort.
SOURCE: Household, Income, and Labour Dynamics in Australia (HILDA) Survey. 2007. Melbourne Institute of Applied Economic and Social Research, University of Melbourne.

reached in the cohort of men and women who were 40–49 years old in 2007. All subsequent cohorts of men and women smokers started at the same average age. Interestingly, the average age of quitting, conditional on being a smoker, was more broadly similar for men and women. The difference is troubling because it implies that, relative to men (and relative to older cohorts of women), younger cohorts of women will likely face an increasing risk of smoking-related health problems and mortality as they age.

Figure 2.4 more starkly highlights similarities and differences in the smoking behavior of Australian men and women. In each panel, we use the data reported in Table 2.1. Figure 2.4 more clearly shows that men and women in each birth cohort smoked approximately for the same number of years and quit at approximately the same ages. Women in older cohorts started later than their male counterparts, and these older cohorts reached their peak smoking prevalence rate when they were older. More men than women smoked in almost every cohort and smoked more cigarettes on the average day.

These gender differences were not tied to any changes in social and cultural norms associated with feminism. In the previous section, we mentioned that Australian feminists lobbied hard for equal rights to work and be paid commensurate with their work, which may have increased their smoking participation by increasing their financial independence. They also lobbied for the abolition of arcane rules that constrained social behaviors—other than smoking—to be different than men's. For example, until the mid-1970s, social norms dictated that hotel pubs not serve women alcohol in the same room as men (Lake, 1999; Wright, 2003). However, they did not promote smoking as an act of female liberalization, as groups did in other countries (e.g., the United Kingdom). Perhaps the Australian feminist movement chose gender-specific social norms attached to drinking rather than smoking because Australian culture does not center so strongly on tobacco. In any event, gender differences in smoking patterns do not seem to flow from the cultural consequences of the Australian feminist movement but, rather, from its economic consequences.

CONCLUSION

Smoking behavior of Australians has evolved in ways similar to those in the United States and United Kingdom. This similarity is unsurprising when one realizes there were firms that operated in all three countries to produce and sell manufactured tobacco. Those firms shared technology, marketing practices, and responses to the threat posed by health information and by the efforts of public health advocates to limit when, where, and how tobacco was sold and consumed. As in the other countries, smoking patterns of Australian men and women have converged so that, in the youngest cohorts, they are practically indistinguishable. However, the regulatory environment in Australia is in many ways more active than in the other countries we study. In the past 10 years, Australian governments have more strictly and more stringently regulated when and where people can smoke than have any other governments. These patterns suggest that there are systematic influences on smoking behavior that remain to be modeled to explain what caused the behavioral changes discussed in this chapter and when and how these changes occurred.

NOTES

1. Similar concessionary duties applied to imported tobacco that was to be mixed and sold as cut tobacco.
2. In 1965, the government established this board by statute and renamed it the Australian Tobacco Marketing Advisory Committee (Australian Government, 1965).
3. In later years, people throughout the world would recognize Hogan's face after the commercially successful movie "Crocodile Dundee" appeared.
4. See University of Sydney online resource http://www.tobaccoinaustralia.org.au/appendix-1/a1-6-history-of-tobacco-in-australia-timeline- (accessed in 2010).
5. The groups include the Australian Medical Association, the Royal Australian College of Physicians, the Royal Australian College of Surgeons, the Royal Australian College of General Practitioners, and the Anti-Cancer Council of Victoria (Walker, 1984).
6. c.f. New South Wales Public Health (Tobacco) Act 2008 No. 94.
7. See http://www.pmi.com/marketpages/pages/market_en_au.aspx.
8. Although 6 months after the government implemented the ban only 22 percent of businesses had complied with its provisions (Goodin and McAllister, 1997), a 2007 study found that the rate of observed compliance in Queensland, Tasmania, and Western Australia was more than 90 percent (Cooper et al., 2010).
9. The smoking prevalence rates of the older cohorts match well with contemporaneous smoking prevalence rates from various surveys reported in Gray and Hill (1975), Hill and Gray (1977, 1982), Hill (1988), Hill et al. (1988, 1991), and Gartner et al. (2009). We matched prevalence rates from men from these sources to men in our data that were 50–59, 60–69, and 70 years old and older in 2007. We then regressed the year-specific rates from the previously mentioned cross-sectional surveys to the rates in the same calendar years that we generated retrospectively. Although the age groupings did not exactly correspond across the data sources, the ordinary least squares coefficients from these regressions were 0.92, 0.92, and 1.08 for these three groups, respectively. The difference of 8 percent for the younger two age groupings corresponds closely with a result reported by Kenkel et al. (2003). They compared prevalence rates from retrospectively reported data to contemporaneously measured prevalence 20 years earlier and found a difference of 5–7 percent.
10. Organization for Economic Cooperation and Development labor force statistics by sex and age are available at http://stats.oecd.org/Index.aspx?DataSetCode=LFS_D.aspx?DataSetCode=LFS_SEXAGE_I_R. Accessed September 12, 2013.

REFERENCES

Australia Commonwealth Bureau of Census and Statistics. 1947. *Official Year Book of the Commonwealth of Australia: No. 37 1946 and 1947.* Australian Capital Territory: Australia Commonwealth Bureau of Census and Statistics.

Australia Tariff Board. various years. *Annual Report.* Canberra: Commonwealth Government Printer.

Australian Auditor General. 2001. *The Auditor-General Audit Report No. 55 2001-02.* Barton, Australian Capital Territory: Australian National Audit Office.

Australian Government. 1965. "Tobacco Marketing Act 1965. Act No. 85 of 1965 as amended, taking into account amendments up to Act No. 48 of 1982." Prepared January 6, 1994. Available at http://www.comlaw.gov.au/Details/C2004C07616.

Australian Retail Tobacconist. 1959. *New South Wales Retail Tobacco Traders' Association* April:11.

Australian Retail Tobacconist. 1972. *New South Wales Retail Tobacco Traders' Association* January:42.

Australian Taxation Office. 2002. *Administration of Tobacco Excise; Australian National Audit Office, The Auditor-General, Audit Report No.55 2001–02, Performance Audit.* Commonwealth of Australia: Australian Taxation Office.

Barro, R. J., and J. F. Ursua. 2008. "Macroeconomic crises since 1870." NBER Working Paper No. 13940. Cambridge, MA: National Bureau of Economic Research.

Cassells, R., Y. Vidyattama, R. Miranti, and J. McNamara. 2009. *The impact of a sustained gender wage gap on the economy: Report to the Office for Women, Department of Families, Community Services, Housing and Indigenous Affairs.* Canberra, Australia: National Centre for Social and Economic Modelling, University of Canberra.

Clarke, V., V. White, J. Beckwith, R. Borland, and D. Hill. 1993. "Are attitudes towards smoking different for males and females?" *Tobacco Control* 2:201–208.

Commonwealth Parliamentary Debates. 1936. *Commonwealth Government of Australia* 152:2764.

Cooper, J., R. Borland, H. Yong, and A. Hyland. 2010. "Compliance and support for bans on smoking in licensed venues in Australia: Findings from the International Tobacco Control Four-Country Survey." *Australian and New Zealand Journal of Public Health* 34:379–385.

Doll, R., and A. B. Hill. 1950. "Smoking and carcinoma of the lung." *British Medical Journal* 2:739–748.

Eastough, K., and P. W. Miller. 2004. "The gender wage gap in paid- and self-employment in Australia." *Australian Economic Papers* 43:257–276.

Gartner, C. E., J. J. Barendregt, and W. D. Hall. 2009. "Predicting the future prevalence of cigarette smoking in Australia: How low can we go and by when?" *Tobacco Control* 18:183–189.

Goodin, M. 1995. "Clean indoor air legislation in Australia." *Tobacco Control* 4:294.

Goodin, M., and I. McAllister. 1997. "Evaluating compliance with Australia's first smoke-free public places legislation." *Tobacco Control* 6:326–331.

Gray, N. J., and D. J. Hill. 1975. "Patterns of tobacco smoking in Australia." *Medical Journal of Australia* 2:819–822.

Gregory, R. G., and R. C. Duncan. 1981. "Segmented labor market theories and the Australian experience of equal pay for women." *Journal of Post Keynesian Economics* 3:403–428.

Hill, D. J. 1988. "Australian patterns of tobacco smoking in 1986." *Medical Journal of Australia* 149:6–10.

Hill, D. J., and N. J. Gray. 1977. "Patterns of tobacco smoking in Australia." *Medical Journal of Australia* 2:327–328.

Hill, D. J., and N. J. Gray. 1982. "Patterns of tobacco smoking in Australia." *Medical Journal of Australia* 1:23–25.

Hill, D. J., V. M. White, and N. J. Gray. 1988. "Measures of tobacco smoking in Australia 1974–1986 by means of a standard method." *Medical Journal of Australia* 149:10–12.

Hill, D. J., V. M. White, and N. J. Gray. 1991. "Australian patterns of tobacco smoking in 1989." *Medical Journal of Australia* 154:797–801.

Household, Income, and Labour Dynamics in Australia (HILDA) Survey. 2007. Melbourne Institute of Applied Economic and Social Research, University of Melbourne. Available at http://www.melbourneinstitute.com/hilda.

Intergovernmental Committee on Drugs. 2012. *National Tobacco Strategy 2012–2018.* Canberra, Australia: Intergovernmental Committee on Drugs.

Jobson's Yearbook of Public Companies of Australia and New Zealand. 1977. Melbourne: Jobson's Financial Services.

Kenkel, D., D. R. Lillard, and A. Mathios. 2003. "Smoke or fire? Are retrospective smoking data valid?" *Addiction* 98:1307–1313.

Lake, M. 1999. *Getting Equal: The History of Australian Feminism Address.* St. Leonards, New South Wales, Australia: Allen & Unwin.

National Archives of Australia. 2013. "Tobacco advertising ban in Australia: Fact sheet 252." Available at http://www.naa.gov.au/collection/fact-sheets/fs252.aspx. Accessed September 17, 2013.

Rothmans. 1980. *Rothmans of Pall Mall (Australia) Limited, 1955–1980.* Australia: Rothmans.

Royal College of Physicians of London (RCP). 1962. *Smoking and Health: Summary and Report of the Royal College of Physicians of London on Smoking in Relation to Cancer of the Lung and Other Diseases.* London: Pitman.

The Free Library. S.v. The anti-tobacco reform and the temperance movement in Australia: connections and differences. Retrieved December 24, 2014 from http://www.thefreelibrary.com/The+anti-tobacco+reform+and+the+temperance+movement+in+Australia%3a...-a021231027

Walker, R. 1984. *Under Fire: A History of Tobacco Smoking in Australia.* Melbourne: Melbourne University Press.

Winstanley, M., S. Woodward, and N. Walker. 1995. *Tobacco in Australia: Facts and Issues* (2nd ed.). Carlton South, Victoria, Australia: Victorian Smoking and Health Program.

Wright, C. 2003. "Doing the beans: Women, drinking and community in the ladies' lounge." *Journal of Australian Studies* 27:5–16.

3

Smoking in Canada

PHILIP DECICCA AND LOGAN MCLEOD

INTRODUCTION

The unique history of tobacco in the lands Canada now occupies is deeply inter-twined with the history of Canada's First Nations (i.e., aboriginal or indigenous) peoples who predate the modern Canadian state. Although nobody knows exactly when the indigenous peoples of Canada first began to consume tobacco, seeds from an archaeological site in southern Ontario date the earliest tobacco use to the 8th century (Facteau, 1983). Researchers believe that the seed's plant, *Nicotania rustica*, originated in South America and that traders brought it to North America (Brandt, 2007). But most historians also believe that it was not until the 16th century, when Europeans brought large quantities of tobacco to trade in the southernmost por-tions of Canada, that First Nations peoples consumed tobacco more widely (Winter, 2000). Most First Nations peoples smoked tobacco in corncob or clay pipes, and they smoked *N. rustica*, not *Nicotiana tabacum*, the latter of which accounts for nearly all of today's commercially produced cigarettes (Physicians for a Smoke-Free Canada, 2007). When smoked, *N. rustica* produces mild hallucinogenic effects (Rudgley, 1998). Such pharmacological properties served well in native belief systems that focused on interactions between the spirit and natural worlds, a focus that was com-mon to many First Nations tribes (von Gernet, 1989). In both North and South American tribes, tobacco served as an important tool that tribes needed to practice these beliefs, principally as a gift that people in the natural world could offer deni-zens of the spirit world, and as a medium humans could use to communicate with ancestral spirits (Winter, 2000).

However, Canadian natives used tobacco differently than South American natives, primarily because, in South America, it was more difficult to get. In South America, because people perceived tobacco as the gateway to the spirit world, its use was often limited to holy persons termed shamans (Wilbert, 1987). In Canada, however, this restricted access to tobacco—an early form of "tobacco control"—did not apply. Despite popular misconceptions, tobacco use among Canadian natives was not reserved exclusively for religious and/or ceremonial occasions but, rather, was an ever-present feature of everyday life (Physicians for a Smoke-Free Canada, 2007). Indeed, historians believe that much of the male aboriginal population was addicted to tobacco. Although tobacco's pharmacological effects are now known, early native tobacco users interpreted those effects to be spiritual in nature (Winter, 2000).

For most Canadian aboriginals, tobacco was generally available to men but not women. Women were not allowed to grow, harvest, or smoke tobacco (von Gernet, 2000). Although the reasons for this early bit of tobacco control are unclear, this female-specific prohibition had the perhaps unintended effect of protecting women from tobacco addiction and the other hazards that are often associated with smoking (von Gernet, 2000; Winter, 2000). Such prohibitions, although in this case limited to aboriginal Canadians, may inform gender-specific patterns in smoking in the cohorts we examine later in this chapter. Indeed, as discussed later, in Canada's broader society, the consumption of tobacco developed as a predominately male activity.

Near the turn of the 20th century, Montreal was, and still remains, the center of Canada's tobacco industry. At this time, most people smoked tobacco in pipes and cigars, although it was also popular for men to chew tobacco and take "snuff." Although cigarettes were available, they were not generally popular (Collishaw, 2009). As in the early First Nations societies, smoking was largely an activity restricted to men in part because social norms strongly discouraged smoking by women (von Gernet, 1989). These social norms about smoking may have also caused the social behavior of women and men to differ in other ways. For example, women were discouraged from entering fields of endeavor such as politics or journalism with a stated goal of keeping them away from tobacco smoke (Cook, 2012). Women were also not allowed in smoking rooms, cigar stores, or the back rows of city tramcars (Rudy, 2005). At the same time, social norms sanctioned men who smoked in front of women. The general support for this particular social norm set the stage for some of Canada's first tobacco control policies. After an intense lobbying campaign, the Women's Christian Temperance Union (WCTU), a group who viewed themselves as "moral crusaders," helped persuade Montreal's government to completely ban smoking on Montreal's tramcars (Brandt, 2007; Cook, 2012).

One of the dominant lobbying groups of the time, the WTCU, sought to eradicate the consumption of alcohol, tobacco (particularly cheaper cigarettes), drugs, and other commodities it perceived to be vices, immoral, and unhealthy (Cook 2003, 2012; Eliott, 2007). Although by 1922, the WCTU helped persuade 16 state governments in the United States to ban cigarettes, it was less successful in Canada. It did help bring a bill (Bill 128) to the Canadian parliament in 1904 that would have banned cigarettes in all of Canada. However, despite passing initial committee votes, parliament failed to adopt the bill (Rudy, 2005). Interestingly, the WCTU and other interest groups focused most of their efforts on cigarettes rather than cigars and pipes because they feared that the low cost of widely available cigarettes would tempt young boys to use tobacco. Such concerns echo in today's modern public health campaigns that aim to reduce youth smoking (Brandt, 2007). In 1908, the Canadian government passed the Tobacco Restraint Act of 1908 and, in so doing, prohibited the sale of cigarettes to individuals younger than 16 years of age and prohibited youth from possessing cigarettes. Relative to the earlier Bill 128, which would have banned cigarettes outright, the Act was weaker and the government failed to enforce it, causing it to quickly fall into disuse (Rudy, 2005). By the mid-1910s, public attention shifted away from moral crusades as the public focused its attention on World War I.

After 1908, the Canadian parliament would not seriously consider tobacco control for another 60 years (Rudy, 2005; Cook, 2012).

Although Canadians did smoke cigarettes prior to World War I, the tobacco companies used the war—and the public sentiment surrounding it—to develop and implement strategies to increase the demand for cigarettes (Collishaw, 2009). For example, Canadian tobacco companies sent free cigarettes to the troops stationed in Europe. To capitalize on national sentiment, they injected patriotic themes into their cigarette advertising. These efforts appeared to pay off handsomely. Between 1896 and the early 1920s, cigarette sales increased nearly 30-fold, from approximately 87 million cigarettes in 1896 to approximately 2.4 billion cigarettes in the early 1920s (Cunningham, 1996). As in the United States, World War I also changed women's roles in Canadian society. In 1916, women gained the right to vote. During and after World War I, many women worked in office and factory jobs that had previously been difficult for them to get. For some women, smoking represented freedom from social strictures. Perhaps unsurprisingly, the advertising of the time attests to the fact that tobacco companies were quick to encourage demand among women (Cook, 2012). For example, in 1920, Imperial Tobacco advertised its Pall Mall cigarette brand in women's magazines as "the best cigarette after a cup of tea," which was interpreted as a direct salvo at the female audience (Rudy, 2005).

During World War II, in the early to mid-1940s, the tobacco companies ramped up their strategy of supporting the war effort, both monetarily and by sending cigarettes to troops overseas (Rudy, 2005). Unlike earlier periods, there were no large social advocacy organizations, such as the WCTU, and no government activity/ regulation to check the growth of smoking in the Canadian population (Collishaw, 2009). Indeed, cigarette consumption increased roughly 10-fold between the early 1920s and late 1940s, when it hit roughly 28 billion cigarettes sold in 1949 (Cunningham, 1996).

Canadians continued to smoke at very high rates into the 1950s, despite a "cancer scare" in the early 1950s that was linked to research of Canadian medical student William DeLarue (Collishaw, 2009). In the same period, the government and tobacco industry fought over a proposed cigarette tax of three cents per pack. The government imposed the tax in 1951 but rolled it back by 1953 after strong industry lobbying (Cunningham, 1996). Meanwhile, medical science was beginning to link smoking to an increased likelihood of lung cancer. Public awareness was limited until 1952 when *Reader's Digest* published an article titled "Cancer by the Carton" that described the research in layman's terms. To assuage the resulting fears of the public, tobacco companies produced filtered cigarettes—hoping that consumers would feel reassured. The strategy worked. Sales continued to increase after the filters were added (Cunningham, 1996). However, the accumulating evidence of the harmful health effects of cigarettes was also increasing the probability that the government would regulate the tobacco industry (Collishaw, 2009).

To protect itself, the tobacco industry developed a research and development program, the results of which it strongly guarded as secrets. The industry also cultivated discreet relationships with government officials to more effectively lobby them as it tried to thwart regulation. The industry's overall strategy worked, as annual per capita consumption increased from approximately 3000 cigarettes in 1950 to 4000 cigarettes in 1963 (Cunningham, 1996). Although information on the health effects of cigarettes slowly accumulated throughout the 1950s, it was not until 1962 and 1964 when the United Kingdom's Royal College of Physicians and the US Surgeon General respectively issued official government reports linking smoking and cancer. These reports reviewed the best available evidence. That evidence included findings from the Canadian Veterans' Study, which followed the smoking behavior and subsequent mortality and morbidity of Canadian veterans from the Korean War. The Canadian government's initial response to these reports was relatively timid. In November 1963, tobacco industry officials and anti-smoking activists were called to Parliament to meet with government representatives. Following a meeting in 1964, the government earmarked $600,000, to be spent over 5 years, for a "smoking and health" public education program. The goal of the program was to inform the Canadian public of the dangers associated with cigarette smoking (Cunningham, 1996).

In the late 1960s, a large number of private member's bills circulated in Parliament that the industry vigorously and largely successfully fought (Collishaw, 2009). In 1968, to deal with the large number of such bills, the government created the "Standing Committee on Health, Welfare, and Social Affairs." The committee, chaired by Dr. Gaston Isabelle of Hull, Quebec, soon came to be known as the "Isabelle Commission." After a year of work, the committee issued its "Isabelle Report" in December 1969. Among the more notable items, the Isabelle Commission recommended that the government completely ban cigarette advertising and promotion, increase its efforts to educate the public about ways to reduce smoking, and require firms to print health warnings on all cigarette packages and to track and publish the maximum levels of tar and nicotine in cigarettes. Although the industry did agree, in 1972, to a voluntary ban on cigarette advertising in broadcast media, none of the other major recommendations of the "Isabelle Report" were implemented until almost 20 years later (Cunningham, 1996).

Although there was a paucity of activity on the tobacco control front in Canada in the 1970s, the early 1980s represented a re-emergence of sorts for anti-tobacco forces, sparked largely by research that showed that passive or "secondhand" smoke might also have detrimental health effects (Collishaw, 2009). Faced with this evidence, the public demanded more restrictions on smoking. As a result, not only did some Canadian municipalities enact their own smoking bans but also two bills were proposed in Parliament—the Non-Smokers Health Act (Bill C-204) and the Tobacco Products Control Act (Bill C-51). The Non-Smokers Health Act, proposed in the fall of 1986, aimed to ban tobacco advertising and smoking in workplaces that were under federal government jurisdiction. In the spring of 1987, legislators submitted the Tobacco Products Control Act. The Act also sought to ban advertising and, in addition, required that firms print labels on cigarette containers that warned smokers about the hazards of smoking. Both pieces of legislation were passed on May 31, 1988—World No-Tobacco Day. Unlike earlier legislation and private agreements that were largely watered down in nature, these Acts imposed significant restrictions. Although a significant victory for anti-smoking forces, the tobacco industry fought back in the courts. The gains were put in jeopardy in 1995 when the Supreme Court of Canada ruled in a 5–4 decision that much of the 1988 legislation violated the Canadian Charter of Rights and Freedoms. During this same period, the government dramatically reduced tobacco taxes to combat the persistent smuggling from the United States caused by the high taxes (Gruber et al., 2003). Taken together, the Supreme Court ruling and the reduction in taxes dealt a substantial blow to anti-smoking forces (Cunningham, 1996).

After the 1995 Supreme Court ruling, the Government of Canada crafted the Tobacco Act of 1997. They wrote the Act to again ban advertising and workplace smoking but to do so with wording and a form that would pass judicial review (Collishaw, 2009). Once again, the tobacco industry fought the legislation in court, but this time the government prevailed in a 2001 decision (Rudy, 2005). Although many people considered many provisions of the 1997 Tobacco Act to be watered down relative to the earlier legislation, some were stronger. For example, the Act required not only that firms print warning labels on cigarette packaging but also that they print graphic images of physical damage ostensibly caused by smoking, such as photos of diseased mouths. These images first appeared in 2001 (Rudy, 2005). The Tobacco Act of 1997 also seems to have laid the groundwork for further legislation at the provincial level. Indeed, from 2004 to 2008, with very limited exceptions, all Canadian provinces and territories banned smoking in public places and in workplaces.

This history and these events are but a small subset of changes in Canadian history that have likely affected patterns of life-course smoking behavior, even though many occurred prior to the birth of any of the cohorts we examine. Given their nature, it is also very likely that these events differentially impacted the smoking decisions of men and women, especially when the gender and social contexts of smoking are taken into consideration (Dedobbeleer et al., 2004). In the next section, we present patterns of life-course smoking of seven generations of Canadian men and women, noting the timing of several of the events mentioned previously in order to give better context to the patterns we display.

SMOKING PREVALENCE RATES IN HISTORICAL PERSPECTIVE

Figure 3.1 presents, for successive birth cohorts, life-course smoking prevalence rates of men and women from 1929 to 2009. In the figure, we mark the year or range of years that potentially important events occurred. In particular, we denote World War II (WWII), the UK smoking report (1962), the US Surgeon General report (1964), the Smoking and Health Program implementation (1966), the voluntary ban on advertising in broadcast media (1972), the two pieces of legislation (Bill C-204 and Bill C-51, 1988), the Canadian Supreme Court overturning these bills (1995), the Tobacco Act (1997), the introduction of graphic image package warnings (2001), and the plethora of provincial-level bans on smoking in public places and workplaces (2004–2008).

Figure 3.1a shows that patterns of life-course smoking of men in the first four cohorts strongly resemble each other (i.e., men aged 50–89 years in 2009). Among these cohorts, smoking prevalence tends to peak at approximately 65–75 percent. Life-course smoking patterns of the three youngest cohorts, those aged 20–49 years, also resemble each other but, relative to the older cohorts, peak at successively lower rates of smoking prevalence that decline from 55 percent to approximately 45 percent among the youngest cohort.

Clearly, smoking patterns did not always change when events occurred. For example, male smoking prevalence in Canada did not change much before or after the

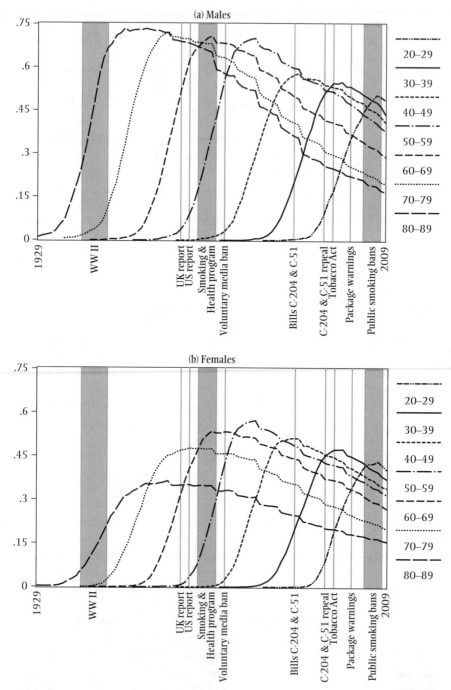

Figure 3.1 Smoking prevalence rates over the life course by gender and birth cohort.
SOURCE: Canadian Community Health Survey (CCHS). 2009. Ottawa, Ontario, Canada: Statistics Canada.

information shocks of the US and UK reports in the early 1960s. This apparent lack of response is interesting because, historically, Canada has had strong cultural ties to both the United Kingdom and the United States, so one presumes that Canadians would respond to information from the UK and US health authorities. By contrast, male smoking prevalence did appear to change in the years surrounding legislative bills C-204 and C-51 and the events preceding and following their passage. The 50- to 59-year-old cohort reached its peak smoking prevalence rate in the latter part of the 1970s—before these events. The next adjacent cohort of 40- to 49-year-old males reached their peak in the late 1980s—after tobacco control legislation had been passed and after the firestorm of public debate that led this legislation. Between the cohort of 50- to 59-year-old males and the cohort of 40- to 49-year-old males, the peak smoking prevalence rate decreased from greater than 70 percent to less than 60 percent. Of course, events other than legislation occurred during this time, including a rapid increase in real cigarette prices (see Figure 3.2).

Figure 3.1b presents life-course smoking prevalence rates for corresponding cohorts of women. In contrast to the cross-cohort smoking patterns of men, smoking prevalence increases sharply across the oldest four cohorts of women, from a peak of approximately one-third in the oldest cohort to a lifetime peak of nearly 60 percent for women in the 50- to 59-year-old cohort. Starting with the 40- to 49-year-old cohort, women's peak smoking prevalence rate begins to decline and does so in ways that mirror the decline in smoking rates in the corresponding cohorts of men. This decline continues across the three youngest cohorts. Smoking prevalence in the youngest cohort (those who were 20–29 years old in 2009) peaked at just over 40 percent. Thus, relative to men who experience a decline in peak smoking prevalence that is at first gradual in the oldest four cohorts and accelerates in the youngest three, women's peak smoking prevalence first rises and then falls over successive birth cohorts. This pattern is consistent with the notion that smoking cigarettes was predominantly the province of men rather than women in older cohorts.

As with men, female smoking prevalence in Canada seems to have been unaffected by the reports of UK and US health authorities in the early 1960s. Furthermore, although female smoking prevalence began declining after the 40- to 49-year-old cohort, the decline seems rather secular in nature. That is, it is very gradual over time, consistent with a gradual decline in the demand for cigarettes rather than a change that was caused by particular events. It is also possible, as discussed later, that women's smoking decisions were less affected by information or changes in government policies partly because females smoked to signal that they were liberated from social strictures imposed on women (Cook, 2012).

In Figure 3.2, we plot trends in the average price of Canadian cigarettes and per capita gross domestic product (GDP) between 1921 and 2013 to highlight periods during which real per capita GDP rose faster, with, or slower than the real cigarette price. During most of the period from 1921 to 1981, GDP grew faster than cigarette prices. Starting in 1981, cigarette prices began to grow somewhat faster than the economy. This difference accelerated until the early 1990s when governments dramatically reduced cigarette taxes in an attempt to capture tax revenue they were losing when the high taxes had caused smokers to buy cheaper smuggled cigarettes. Those tax decreases translated into a sudden and quite substantial real price decrease. Within a very short time, starting again in the mid-1990s, prices began to again increase much faster than per capita GDP. Growth rates in the two series diverged in the early 1980s mostly because provincial and federal governments increased excise taxes (except for the tax reduction of the early 1990s noted previously).

Although Figures 3.1 and 3.2 do not establish that these trends drove patterns in smoking prevalence, together they highlight contemporary trends. Peak smoking prevalence was much lower among men age 40–49 years in 2009 than it was among men who were 50–59 years old in 2009. The former cohort was entering its phase of smoking initiation precisely during the years that real cigarette prices were rising fastest. Also, they were the first cohort to face those higher prices. The peak smoking prevalence rate continued to drop in successive cohorts of males—those ages 30–39 and 20–29 years in 2009—but they dropped by a smaller amount. Patterns among cohorts of women were similar in the younger cohorts. The peak smoking prevalence rate was highest among women aged 50–59 years in 2009. In each successive cohort of women, the peak smoking prevalence rate dropped. This steady decline coincided with the (mostly) steady increase in the real price of cigarettes—a pattern consistent with the notion that cigarette price inflation led to a decrease in smoking participation. However, the decrease moving from the 50- to 59-year-old cohort to the 20- to 29-year-old cohort is much more gradual than the decline in smoking prevalence of Canadian males. Of course, one cannot determine if price causally affected the observed trends from only a simple comparison of these trends. However, the comparison is nonetheless useful because it suggests that price and other factors likely played a role in the cohort-to-cohort decline in smoking prevalence. Also, it inspires a search for the other factors.

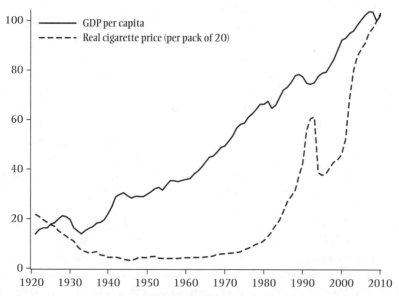

Figure 3.2 Economic development and cigarette prices (2009 = 100).
NOTES: GDP, Bolt, J., and J. L. van Zanden. 2013. "The first update of the Maddison Project; Re-estimating growth before 1820." Maddison Project Working Paper 4; cigarettes prices: 1921–1948, imputed with Dominion Bureau of Statistics data (see Appendix); 1949–2010, Statistics Canada.

COHORT AND GENDER DIFFERENCES

In Figure 3.3, we plot cohort-smoking trajectories on an age scale to highlight the similarities and differences in each cohort's smoking behavior when they were all the same age. The top panel plots the smoking trajectories of men, and the bottom panel plots corresponding trajectories for women. The top panel of Figure 3.3 reveals a pattern not easy to observe when the trajectories are plotted on the calendar scale of Figure 3.1. It shows that the four oldest cohorts of Canadian men have strikingly similar patterns of initiation. In those cohorts, the earliest initiators are approximately 10 years old, and nearly three-fourths of those who smoke start to do so by age 20. Figure 3.3 also reveals cohort trends in smoking cessation that are not easily noticed in Figure 3.1. Smokers in older cohorts waited longer to quit. Men in the three youngest cohorts, those aged 20–49 years in 2009, start at slightly older ages than did men in the oldest cohorts. Even in these cohorts, however, men who are going to smoke will have done so by the time they are 20–22 years old—similar to older cohorts. In summary, although smokers in younger cohorts were starting at slightly older ages, the overall smoking behavior of all cohorts of men follows a similar age pattern across cohorts.

The bottom panel of Figure 3.3 plots cohort-smoking trajectories of women on an age scale. Here, one observes tremendous variation, especially between the oldest (80–89 years old in 2009) and second oldest (70–79 years old in 2009) cohorts. In successive cohorts of women, the peak smoking prevalence rate not only increases dramatically, as seen in Figure 3.1, but also occurs at increasingly younger ages in successive cohorts (not so easily seen in Figure 3.1).

This last pattern and others are highlighted in Table 3.1. There, we summarize the six measures of smoking behavior described in Chapter 1 to more clearly show how smoking patterns of men and women both resemble and differ from each other. Again, the upper portion of Table 3.1 refers to the behavior of men, and the lower portion refers to the smoking behavior of women.

Table 3.1 demonstrates yet again that the oldest four cohorts of Canadian men smoked in remarkably similar ways. Their peak rate of smoking prevalence ranges from 0.70 to 0.74. In addition, these cohorts smoked a similar amount each day—about a pack or between 19 and 21 cigarettes during the average day. There are some interesting, and perhaps counterintuitive, differences in the age of initiation among these first four cohorts. In particular, the average age of initiation decreases from 17 years for the oldest cohort to approximately 15 years among men ages 50–69 years in 2009. Despite these differences in the age of initiation, the rate of smoking prevalence in the four oldest cohorts reached its peak when the average man in each cohort was roughly the same age—23 or 24 years old. Whereas Figure 3.3 shows that fewer men smoked in the youngest three cohorts (their peak smoking prevalence rates range from 0.50 to 0.58), Table 3.1 more clearly shows that smokers in these cohorts smoked less on average. The average number of cigarettes smoked per day decreases from 17 to 13, a major decrease from the 40- to 49-year-old cohort to the 20- to 29-year-old cohort. In terms of initiation, these three youngest Canadian male cohorts closely resemble men in older cohorts. The average male smoker in Canada starts and, except for the oldest cohort, has always started when he is 15 or 16 years old.

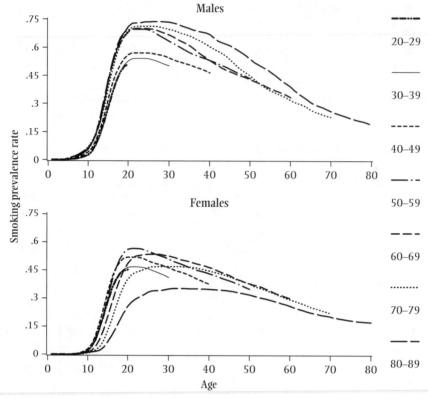

Figure 3.3 Change in smoking prevalence rate with age by birth cohort.
SOURCE: Canadian Community Health Survey (CCHS). 2009. Ottawa, Ontario,
Canada: Statistics Canada.

Table 3.1 also shows how much the peak smoking prevalence rate increases across female cohorts, from a low of approximately 36 percent for the oldest cohort to the highest rate of 57 percent in the cohort of women ages 50–59 years in 2009 and then decreasing across the remaining three youngest cohorts to a low of 43 percent among Canadian females aged 20–29 years. Interestingly, the pattern in smoking intensity mirrors the pattern in peak smoking prevalence, first rising then falling. Perhaps most interesting of all, the data are consistent with the hypothesis that changing expectations of women's social behavior has made tobacco smoking more socially acceptable for women over time. Among women who smoked in each cohort, the average age of smoking initiation has decreased steadily from age 22 in the oldest cohort (i.e., ages 80–89 years in 2009) to age 15 in the youngest cohort (i.e., ages 20–29 years in 2009).

Finally, Figure 3.4 illustrates these trends graphically by plotting, for each cohort, the ratio of each statistic for men relative to the corresponding statistic for women. A ratio of 1 indicates that men and women in that cohort smoke in the same way. It appears that, on all but two aspects of smoking represented here, younger cohorts of Canadian women have neared "equality" with younger cohorts of Canadian men. The two notable exceptions for which Canadian men still smoke more than

Table 3.1. Summary Indicators of Smoking by Gender and Birth Cohort

Gender/ cohort	Sample size	Peak prevalence rate	Cigarettes per day	Years smoking	Average age at		
					peak	start	quit
MALES							
80–89	1152	0.74	19	42	23	17	51
70–79	2500	0.72	21	38	24	16	47
60–69	4089	0.71	21	36	24	15	42
50–59	4439	0.70	20	31	24	15	37
40–49	3601	0.58	17	25	25	16	33
30–39	3464	0.55	14	18	25	16	29
20–29	2840	0.50	13	10	22	15	23
FEMALES							
80–89	2041	0.36	12	45	33	22	53
70–79	3322	0.48	15	41	29	19	50
60–69	4896	0.54	17	36	24	18	44
50–59	5348	0.57	16	30	24	16	36
40–49	3921	0.51	14	24	24	16	31
30–39	4046	0.47	12	18	25	16	28
20–29	3291	0.43	10	10	23	15	23

SOURCE: Canadian Community Health Survey (CCHS). 2009. Ottawa, Ontario, Canada: Statistics Canada.

Canadian women are the peak rate of smoking prevalence and the number of cigarettes smoked per day. Younger cohorts have closed the gap in what used to be large differences between men and women in both of these aspects of smoking, but complete convergence does not appear to be imminent. The convergence in peak rate of smoking prevalence appears to be happening mostly because the peak smoking prevalence rate fell faster across successive cohorts of men than it fell across successive cohorts of women. Although it is difficult to explain these divergent rates of decline, recent research on female smoking in Canada suggests that, in the past, women smoked as a way to flout earlier social conventions that held smoking as something of a taboo for women (Cook, 2012). To the extent this was true, it suggests that women smoked not only because they enjoyed doing so but also to signal their "liberation" from patriarchal norms (Cook, 2012). If true, the slower reduction in smoking participation, relative to males, is understandable because female smoking would be more resilient to changes in public policy and information on the possible deleterious effects of cigarette smoking. Interestingly, this logic suggests that, as women's social roles become less restrictive, younger cohorts may no longer need to send such signals. If so, then younger cohorts of Canadian women will have one less reason to smoke. Although it is not possible to know if this hypothesis operates in a causal sense, these patterns are very interesting and worthy of rigorous future study.

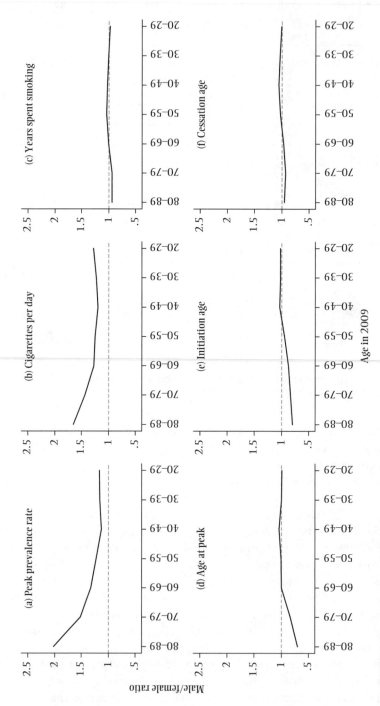

Figure 3.4 Male/female ratios of smoking indicators by birth cohort.

SOURCE: Canadian Community Health Survey (CCHS). 2009. Ottawa, Ontario, Canada: Statistics Canada.

CONCLUSION

Canada's long history with tobacco stretches from the First Nations' peoples who predated the current Canadian state to recent provincial-level bans on smoking in nearly all public and workplaces enacted in the past 10 years. We examined the smoking histories of seven ten-year cohorts of Canadian men and women born from 1920 until 1989. Many interesting patterns have emerged. The oldest four cohorts smoked in similar ways. There is suggestive evidence that public policy may have altered smoking behavior of men, starting with the cohort aged 40–49 years in 2009 who came of age during a time when knowledge of tobacco's potentially deleterious health effects and general anti-smoking sentiment began to grow. The experience of Canadian women was substantially different and followed a pattern of increasing smoking, consistent with a rise in the social acceptability of female smoking, proceeded by a decline that mirrors a more general and increasing societal disapproval of smoking. In essence, younger cohorts of women behaved similarly to younger cohorts of men in that they reduced their peak smoking prevalence rates over time, albeit at a slower rate than men, even though older cohorts of men and women behaved very differently, with male smoking remaining constant at a high level and female smoking increasing.

In summary, the descriptions of life-course smoking that we have provided, along with their framing in the context of the events and forces that shaped them, reveal patterns that point toward future research. That research should investigate what gender-specific factors and what factors shared in common caused men and women to start or not start smoking and what factors induced smokers to quit. Although the descriptive research informs our broad understanding of patterns, it is the latter research that will inform legislators as they design policies to better serve the public interest.

REFERENCES

Bolt, J., and J. L. van Zanden. 2013. "The first update of the Maddison Project; Re-estimating growth before 1820." Maddison Project Working Paper 4. Available at http://www.ggdc.net/maddison/maddison-project/home.htm.

Brandt, A. M. 2007. *The Cigarette Century: The Rise, Fall and Deadly Persistence of the Product That Defined America.* Atlanta: Basic Books.

Canadian Community Health Survey (CCHS). 2009. Ottawa, Ontario, Canada: Statistics Canada. Available at http://www23.statcan.gc.ca/imdb/p2SV.pl?Function=getSurvey&SDDS=3226.

Collishaw, N. 2009. *History of Tobacco Control in Canada.* Ottawa, Ontario, Canada: Physicians for a Smoke-Free Canada.

Cook, S. A. 2003. "Smoking in the boys' room." In *Out of the Ivory Tower: Feminist Research for Social Change,* edited by A. Martinez and M. Stuart, pp. 25–48. Toronto: Sumach Press.

Cook, S. A. 2012. *Sex, lies and cigarettes: Canadian women, smoking and visual culture, 1880–2000.* Montreal, Quebec: McGill-Queen's University Press.

Cunningham, R. 1996. *Smoke and mirrors: The Canadian tobacco wars.* Ottawa, Ontario, Canada: International Development Research Centre.

Dedobbeleer, N., F. Beland, A. P. Contandriopoulos, and M. Adrian. 2004. "Gender and the social context of smoking behavior." *Social Science and Medicine* 58:1–12.

Eliott, R. 2007. *Women and Smoking Since 1890*. New York: Routledge.

Facteau, R. 1983. "A preliminary report on plant remains from three early Iroquoian sites in Southwestern Ontario." Report submitted to Archaeology Unit, Heritage Branch, Ontario Ministry of Citizenship and Culture, London, Ontario, Canada.

Gruber J., A. Sen, and M. Stabile. 2003. "Estimating price elasticities when there is smuggling: The sensitivity of smoking to price in Canada." *Journal of Health Economics* 22:821–842.

Physicians for a Smoke-Free Canada. 2007. *Towards Effective Tobacco Control in First Nations and Inuit Communities*. Ottawa, Ontario, Canada: Physicians for a Smoke-Free Canada.

Rudgley, R. 1998. *The Encyclopedia of Psychoactive Substances*. New York: St. Martin's Press.

Rudy, J. 2005. *The Freedom to Smoke: Tobacco Consumption and Identity*. Montreal, Quebec, Canada: McGill–Queen's University Press.

Von Gernet, A. 1989. "Hallucinogens and the origins of the Iroquoian pipe/tobacco/smoking complex." In *Proceedings of the 1989 Smoking Pipe Conference*, edited by C. F. Hayes III, pp. 171–185. Rochester, NY: Rochester Museum & Science Center.

Von Gernet, A. 2000. "Origins of nicotine use and global tobacco diffusion." In *Nicotine and Public Health*, edited by R. Farrance, J. Slade, R. Room, and M. Pope, pp. 3–16. Washington, DC: American Public Health Association.

Wilbert, J. 1987. *Tobacco and Shamanism*. New Haven, CT: Yale University Press.

Winter, J. C. 2000. *Tobacco Use by Native North Americans: Sacred Smoke and Silent Killer*. Norman, OK: University of Oklahoma Press.

4

Smoking in the United Kingdom

REBEKKA CHRISTOPOULOU

INTRODUCTION

Tobacco was introduced to the United Kingdom as early as the 15th century, when British colonists sent it from the Americas (Goodman, 1993). Shops that produced and traded tobacco products quickly multiplied. Some, like W.D. & H.O. Wills, not only survived but also grew large enough over the following centuries that they shaped the evolution of the domestic industry (Alford, 1973). As in other countries, the industry evolved in response to technological innovations, particularly to the invention of the cigarette-rolling machine, which dramatically reduced cigarette production costs. What followed was a dramatic decline in cigarette prices and an equally dramatic increase of supply, which caused the number of smokers to rapidly increase. At the dawn of the 20th century, the profit potential of the British market was so high that it attracted the attention of James Duke, the founder and genius behind the American Tobacco Company. After his success dominating the US market, Duke laid the groundwork to repeat his strategy in the British market. To fend off this US invasion, in 1901, directors of 13 British companies, led by W.D. & H.O. Wills, agreed to merge, forming the Imperial Tobacco Company of Great Britain and Ireland. Their strategy succeeded in rendering Duke uncompetitive. In 1902, the Imperial and American Tobacco Companies agreed to operate solely in their respective domestic markets and to share trade elsewhere by entering a joint venture—the British–American Tobacco Company (Corina, 1975).

In the ensuing decades, the British industry prospered not only because it was protected from competition from abroad but also because the British government collaborated with the tobacco industry to support the domestic market. The government did so because it derived a large share of its revenue from tobacco taxes, tariffs, and duties. This reliance was especially strong during the two World Wars when the government needed extra revenue to fund war operations. Therefore, the British government collaborated closely with the tobacco industry, often enacting specific government policies that expanded the demand for cigarettes. For example, although the government rationed trade of many goods during World War II, it neither rationed tobacco nor restricted the price at which firms could sell it (Corina, 1975). On the contrary, like other Allied and Axis governments, the British government distributed cigarettes to troops during both World Wars—ostensibly as a means to boost troop morale. It was a tactic that helped to establish a culture of smoking in the country. Arguably, this string of policies and events helped expand the domestic market for cigarettes so that, by the late 1940s, UK tobacco industry sales reached a historical high (Nicolaides-Bouman et al., 1993).

At the same time, the British government was ignoring the accumulating scientific evidence about the detrimental health effects smoking causes. In 1950, British researchers published an epidemiological study that identified a strong correlation between smoking and cancer (Doll and Hill, 1950).[1] Although that study received widespread attention in the English language press, the UK government ignored the evidence. In fact, during the 1950s, the National Government left responsibility for the content and intensity of public health education campaigns in the hands of local authorities (Berridge and Loughlin, 2005). Still relying heavily on the millions of pounds of revenue generated by the tobacco industry, the Central Government not only failed to discourage smoking but also sometimes subsidized it. For example, after World War II it distributed tokens to pensioners through a Tobacco Duty Relief scheme that could be used to pay for tobacco products (Tinkler, 2006).

It was not until the 1960s that the UK government began to actively campaign against tobacco consumption. The foundation of that change was laid by the publication of the Royal College of Physicians 1962 report on smoking and health (RCPL, 1962). It is perhaps telling that the RCPL report was aimed more at the (voting) public than the medical community. Its success in sparking an official anti-smoking campaign may have been due to the fact that the report was widely circulated and it received much media attention. The publication of the RCPL report even prompted the US Department of Health, Education, and Welfare to compile its own body of scientific papers and to publish a similar official report 2 years later (US Department of Health, Education, and Welfare, 1964).

As information spread about the health risks of smoking, the tobacco industry was not idle. It launched a coordinated counteroffensive that included (dis)information campaigns, lobbying, and new marketing strategies. The industry published articles to discredit or question the validity of the medical evidence, arguing that the government needed to undertake more research before any official policies could be enacted. In 1956, the industry formed the Tobacco Manufacturers' Standing Committee, which cooperated on such research. To launch that effort, the industry donated £250,000 to the Medical Research Council. However, the publication of the 1962 RCPL report clearly signaled that the tide of favorable treatment by the government had shifted against the industry. Although the Standing Committee insisted that the scientific evidence remained contradictory and inconclusive, UK manufacturers began to shift production to filtered "healthier" cigarettes that were becoming increasingly popular, and they intensified their diversification of investments in other industries (Corina, 1975).

In the decades following the RCPL report, the UK government began to regulate the consumption and sale of tobacco in several ways. It gradually restricted when, where, and how firms could advertise or market tobacco; made it illegal for firms to sell tobacco products to children and teenagers; required firms to print health warnings on cigarette packs; used mass media to educate the public about the health consequences of smoking; and banned smoking in public places.

Today, the UK Department of Health continues to spend considerable resources to reduce smoking prevalence in the United Kingdom, investing—among others—in hard-hitting public awareness campaigns. These campaigns emphasize themes common in tobacco control campaigns throughout the world: that smoking is addictive, causes early mortality, and is physically punishing for smokers and those around them. For example, the 2007 "Get unhooked" campaign shows smokers getting snatched by fishhooks in their mouths. The 2008 "Scared" campaign illustrates the fear parents engender in their children when they smoke. In it, a schoolgirl admits that her only fear is that her mother will die because she smokes. In the 2009 "Fight back" campaign, a smoker lights a cigarette and is brutally beaten by an invisible attacker. The latest campaign is equally graphic and more extensive, encompassing several different advertisements. For example, one shows a cancerous tumor growing on a cigarette as it is smoked, and a second shows that smoking by a window or a back door still allows a large amount of smoke to remain indoors, exposing children to health risks. This latter campaign, launched in December 2012, cost £2.7 million and aims to convince smokers to avail themselves of National Health Service assistance that will help them quit, including specialized "quit kits" from pharmacies.

As elsewhere, in Britain, the development of clinically effective pharmaceutical treatments that help smokers quit and the regulatory changes that made it easier for smokers to buy those products has spawned a dynamic sector in the over-the-counter pharmaceutical product market. The first products to be introduced were "nicotine-replacement" therapies (NRT), which required a doctor's prescription. In the early 1990s, the UK Medicines and Healthcare Products Regulator Agency (MHPRA) reclassified the NRT gum products so that smokers could buy them from pharmacies; in the late 1990s, the regulatory authority concluded that smokers did not need the advice of a pharmacist and allowed nonpharmacy retail outlets to sell them. Currently, gums, patches, and lozenges can be sold over-the-counter (officially designated as "general sales list" status). To get other forms of smoking cessation products, smokers must still buy the products in a venue in which they can get advice from a healthcare professional (MHPRA, 2005).

With spreading anti-smoking information, policies, and smoking cessation products, people were increasingly less likely to start smoking and existing smokers were quitting. As a result, smoking prevalence consistently fell over time. By the early 2000s, the overall UK smoking prevalence rate had declined to half of the 1950 rate (Robinson and Bugler, 2008; Cancer Research UK, 2009). It is notable that the rate of smoking prevalence declined primarily because younger generations of men were smoking less. Rates of smoking among women have been stubbornly persistent. Despite the significant decline of smoking rates over time, more than one-fifth of British adults still smoke regularly. In this chapter, we document in detail and from a life-course perspective how smoking behavior has evolved in Britain since the early 1920s in light of the aforementioned contextual forces.

SMOKING PREVALENCE RATES IN HISTORICAL PERSPECTIVE

As in every chapter, Figure 4.1 plots smoking prevalence rates by gender and birth cohort over time. In Figure 4.1, we also mark selected historical events to put these smoking patterns in context. We flag the years of World War II (WWII) because

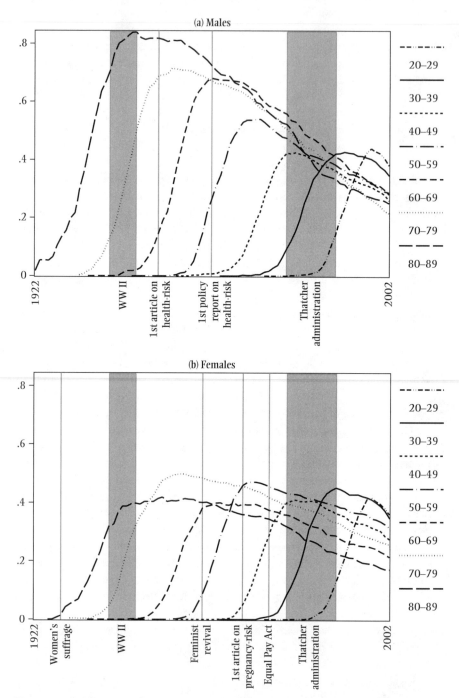

Figure 4.1 Smoking prevalence rates over the life course by gender and birth cohort.
SOURCE: British Household Panel Survey (BHPS). 1999, 2002. Institute for Social and Economic Research, University of Essex.

the UK government distributed cigarettes to (mostly male) members of the armed forces. We also identify the years of the Thatcher administration (1979–1990) because that administration drastically cut income taxes. Furthermore, Margaret Thatcher was the first and, to date, only woman to have been Prime Minister of the United Kingdom. Researchers argue that her visible leadership role altered how British women perceived their roles in society and in the household (Loach, 1987; Wilkinson, 1999).

In Figure 4.1a, we highlight 1950 and 1962 because those years saw the publication of new information about the health risks of smoking (Doll and Hill, 1950; RCPL, 1962). In Figure 4.1b, we mark years associated with the three phases of feminism (up to the 1930s, 1960–1980, and from the 1980s onward). Specifically, we mark 1928 as the year women were given voting rights equal with men; 1960 as the year the feminism movement began its revival after an extensive period of decline (1945–1959); and 1975 as the year compliance with the Equal Pay Act became compulsory and was also extended, through the Sex Discrimination Act, to enforce equal treatment in spheres other than the workplace (e.g., in education and training). In Figure 4.1b, we also identify the year of publication of the first scientific article that specifically identified the health risks of smoking during pregnancy (Butler and Alberman, 1969).

Figure 4.1 reveals interesting patterns. Specifically, it shows substantial variation in the smoking prevalence rate by gender and cohort. It confirms the commonly held wisdom that older cohorts of men smoked more than women and that this difference has disappeared among younger cohorts. Smoking was most prevalent in the oldest cohort of men—the one that entered adulthood during World War II. Every successive cohort of men smoked less. By contrast, smoking among women was most prevalent in the cohort that followed the cohort of men who smoked the most—a pattern that has been documented before with UK data by Kemm (2001). In addition, peak smoking prevalence rates among successive cohorts of women did not follow the same downward trend that we observe for men. The cohort of women who came of age just after World War II smoked more than the cohorts that immediately preceded and followed them. Furthermore, smoking rates were almost as high among the women who came of age two cohorts later—during the so-called second wave of feminism. Whereas rates of smoking fell in the next successive cohort, they increased again in the cohort that came of age during the Thatcher administration. One observes a similar, but smaller, relative rise in smoking prevalence of the cohort of men who came of age during this period.

To provide some economic context for the smoking patterns, we plot, in Figure 4.2, the evolution of per capita gross domestic product (GDP), cigarette taxes, and the price of Capstan cigarettes from 1922 to 2006. Capstan is a brand of unfiltered cigarettes made by Imperial Tobacco (and originally launched by W.D. & H.O. Wills in 1894), which was very popular before the 1970s. Although Capstan is not a representative cigarette brand during the most recent decades, we have verified that its price over 1997–2007 is highly correlated with that of Benson & Hedges Gold, a more mainstream brand (correlation coefficient is greater than 0.9).[2]

While per capita GDP rose more or less monotonically over the whole period, the real cigarette taxes and prices rose and fell dramatically in different periods. Tax and prices generally moved in the same direction (with a correlation coefficient of 0.94),

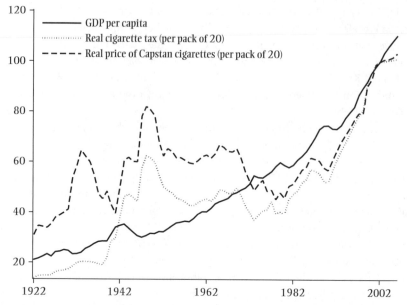

Figure 4.2 Economic development, cigarette taxes, and cigarette prices (2002 = 100). SOURCES: GDP, Bolt, J., and J. L. van Zanden. 2013. "The first update of the Maddison Project; Re-estimating growth before 1820." Maddison Project Working Paper 4; cigarette tax, *Ministry of Labor Gazette, U.K. Index of Retail Prices* (various issues); price of Capstan cigarettes, Tobacco Manufacturers' Association.

apart from the period around the Great Depression, when the inflation-adjusted price rose while taxes remained roughly constant. Between 1941 and 1947, the government dramatically raised the cigarette tax, most likely to finance debt accumulated during the war. Researchers have shown that the need for more revenue during and after the war led to an impressive increase in overall taxation (Clark and Dilnot, 2002). After the war, the government did not raise the cigarette tax again until 1960. Consequently, in real terms, the tax per pack of cigarettes declined. Starting in 1960, the government again increased the cigarette tax so that it rose each year at approximately the same rate that real per capita GDP increased. From 1977 to 1979, the cigarette tax fell dramatically because the government reduced the nominal cigarette tax. Finally, the cigarette tax increased at a rate higher than the rate of increase of real per capita GDP during the Thatcher administration and thereafter. In all these years, the trend of the cigarette tax mirrors the trend in price.

Interestingly, the substantial variation in cigarette taxes and prices is not reflected in the observed changes in smoking prevalence of different cohorts as one might expect. Smoking prevalence seems to rise for some cohorts just as real taxes are increasing. This association suggests that other determinants of smoking behavior also played a significant role, at times counteracting the effect of taxation. For example, the general downward trend in peak smoking prevalence of men is consistent with the growth and spread of information about the health impact of smoking. The uptick in smoking rates of both men and women during the Thatcher administration is consistent with the decline in income taxes during those years. It is also possible that changing social norms, perhaps resulting from the feminist movement, might help explain the pattern of peak prevalence rates that rise and fall in different cohorts of women. Finally, the changing structure of the retail markets may also explain smoking rates of women, particularly those who reached adulthood in the 1960s. It was at that time when women gained access to cheap cigarettes because the newly established supermarket sector offered impressive discounts on bulks of cigarettes, especially following the collapse of resale price maintenance in 1965 (Corina, 1975). It is plausible that women were more exposed to such offers than men (given that they were typically the ones who did the grocery shopping for the family) and/ or that women were more responsive to such offers than men (consistent with earlier evidence that cigarette demand by British women is more price elastic than cigarette demand by British men (Townsend et al., 1994)).

Clearly, there is a plethora of other factors that are potential determinants of smoking rates. In the Appendix, we list a timeline of major events and dates when major anti-smoking policies were adopted. Interested readers can consult it to identify years in which particular events occurred.

To continue to tease out interesting patterns, we plot cohort-smoking trajectories on an age scale. Figure 4.3 shows that, over their life course, men and women of every birth cohort smoke in broadly similar ways at similar ages. All men and women start smoking in a fairly narrow chronological window from approximately

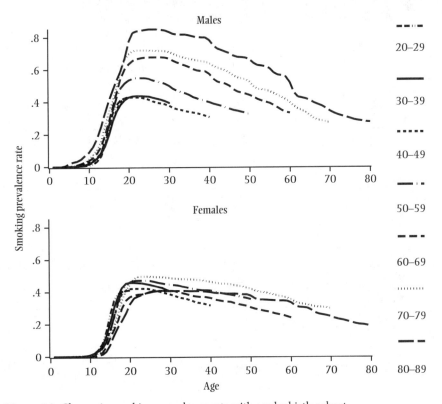

Figure 4.3 Change in smoking prevalence rate with age by birth cohort.
SOURCE: British Household Panel Survey (BHPS). 1999, 2002. Institute for Social and Economic Research, University of Essex.

age 14 until approximately age 20. After age 20, both men and women (to a lesser degree) quit at mostly similar rates. Although the peak smoking prevalence rates differ (especially for men), the slope of the trajectories after those peaks is (mostly) constant; that is, the differences in the smoking prevalence rates of different cohorts stay relatively constant to the right of the peak smoking prevalence age. A striking exception to this pattern concerns the very oldest cohort of women. Smokers in that cohort appear to persist in their smoking habit over their life course; that is, once they start smoking, they rarely quit. As a result, the smoking trajectory of that cohort only starts to slope downward when the average smoker is approximately 60 years old.

COHORT AND GENDER DIFFERENCES

Despite the apparent similarity of life-course smoking behavior in Figure 4.3, the plots mask some important differences. We expose those differences in Table 4.1 by comparing the six summary measures of smoking behavior described in Chapter 1. The comparisons reveal interesting patterns. Among men, smoking was most popular for the oldest cohort, but smoking intensity was highest for the cohorts in the middle of the age range. That is, more 80- to 89-year-old men smoked regularly than men in later cohorts, but among the men who smoked, the oldest cohort and

Table 4.1. SUMMARY INDICATORS OF SMOKING BY GENDER AND BIRTH COHORT

Gender/ cohort	Sample size	Peak prevalence rate	Cigarettes per day	Years smoking	Average age at		
					Peak	Start	Quit
MALES							
80–89	161	0.84	19	44	27	18	48
70–79	353	0.71	21	41	25	17	49
60–69	441	0.68	22	36	24	17	44
50–59	645	0.54	22	29	25	16	36
40–49	740	0.43	20	22	23	16	31
30–39	749	0.43	15	17	25	16	27
20–29	637	0.44	10	10	21	16	21
FEMALES							
80–89	266	0.42	13	45	33	22	53
70–79	431	0.50	14	43	28	19	49
60–69	473	0.40	15	33	29	20	42
50–59	747	0.47	15	31	24	17	37
40–49	772	0.41	15	22	23	17	31
30–39	859	0.45	14	17	23	16	27
20–29	695	0.42	11	10	21	15	22

SOURCE: British Household Panel Survey (BHPS). 1999, 2002. Institute for Social and Economic Research, University of Essex.

the next four birth cohorts smoked approximately the same number of cigarettes on average. Among women, smokers in the middle three cohorts smoked the same amount on average, and unlike men, the prevalence of smoking varied more and exhibited no monotonic trend across older cohorts. In general, the popularity and intensity of smoking by both men and women do not move in the same direction across different generations. This observation is consistent with econometric findings from UK data that smoking participation and demand of cigarettes per smoker respond differently to determinants of smoking behavior, such as price, income, and health scares (Jones, 1989; Yen and Jones, 1996).

Another striking pattern, which is not immediately obvious from Figure 4.3, is that, relative to the older cohorts, men and women in younger birth cohorts have been starting to smoke at younger ages. At the same time, women have been catching up with men in their age of initiation, as the average age of initiation has been falling faster across successive female cohorts than it has across the corresponding cohorts of men. For example, in the oldest cohort of smokers, the average male started to smoke at age 18, whereas the average female started at age 22. Five cohorts later, among smokers who were 30–39 years old in 2002, both the average male and the female smoker started to smoke at age 16. More troubling is that the average smoker in the youngest cohort of women started at an even younger age than her male counterparts. Furthermore, whereas smoking prevalence for men has decreased substantially across cohorts, there is no clear negative trend for women. Consistently, men and women in the youngest three cohorts are quitting at similar rates. In each of the youngest three cohorts, women have smoked, on average, exactly as long as men in their same age group. Together, these facts point to a troubling implication: Relative to older cohorts, younger cohorts of women will likely face an increasing risk of smoking-related health problems and mortality as they age.

To more easily compare gender similarities and differences, in Figure 4.4, we plot the value of each indicator in Table 4.1 for men in each birth cohort relative to the value of the indicator for women in the same birth cohort. Figure 4.4 more clearly shows that men and women in each birth cohort smoked approximately the same number of years and started and quit at approximately the same ages. The only notable differences are that the oldest three cohorts of women started to smoke later and they reached their peak smoking prevalence rate at an older age than men. However, because they also quit smoking later than men, they smoked a similar number of years in total. Figure 4.4 also reveals more sharply that men and women of different birth cohorts differed dramatically in how popular smoking was and how much each gender smoked on average. In older cohorts, men smoked more often and more heavily than women, whereas women in younger cohorts achieved "equality" with their male counterparts on all these dimensions. The data in Table 4.1 show that this convergence happened because male smoking participation almost halved from the oldest to the youngest cohort, whereas female smoking participation rates persisted and even increased.

Although we cannot settle the issue of what drives the persistence in the smoking behavior of women, we can speculate about possible reasons. In the previous section, we identified three factors specific to women that might influence their smoking behavior independently of men. Namely, we suggested that women might have

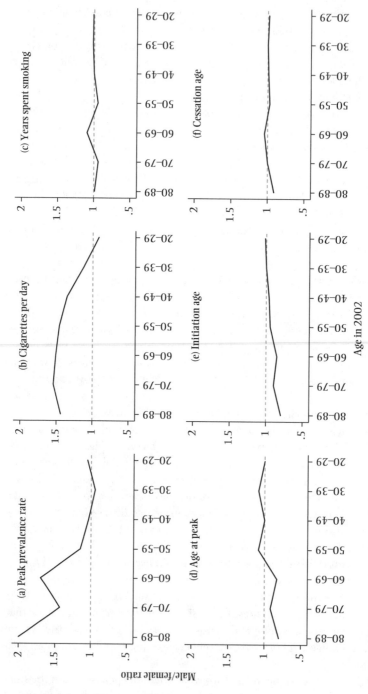

Figure 4.4 Male/female ratios of smoking indicators by birth cohort.
SOURCE: British Household Panel Survey (BHPS). 1999, 2002. Institute for Social and Economic Research, University of Essex.

changed their smoking behavior in response to new attitudes brought by feminism, in response to new information about how smoking during pregnancy affects an unborn fetus, and because supermarket stores made cigarettes accessible to them at low prices. It is unlikely that the health information drives the observed trends because it should have caused fewer women to start smoking and more women to quit (at earlier ages) consistently over the relevant period. Similarly, the supermarket effect, although plausible, is likely weak or short-lived. Thus, of these three possible factors, we are inclined to give more weight to the possible role of changes in social norms and attitudes that the feminist movement caused.

Historical evidence supports such a role. In 1910, the Women's Press shop sold "Votes for Women" cigarettes and encouraged women to smoke as a way to signal society and to general authority that they were independent (Tinkler, 2006). Despite this evidence, the up and down pattern of female smoking prevalence across different birth cohorts does not coincide very well with the timing of the three waves of feminism. The end of the suffragette movement in the United Kingdom was officially marked in 1928, when women finally achieved the same voting rights as men. At that time, people in the oldest cohort in our data—the only cohort that could have been directly affected by that movement—were just entering puberty. However, we observe that it is the next cohort that smokes most. Furthermore, that cohort of women reached its peak smoking prevalence rate in the mid-1950s—when British feminism was at its nadir (Pugh, 2000). Indeed, some observers claim that authorities tried, from 1930 to 1960 and especially after World War II, to shift social attitudes in favor of the nuclear family and to re-establish the norm that a woman's primary occupation should be the management of domestic affairs (Pugh, 1990; Ward, 2004). However, that period also marked the redefinition of the stigma that women bore if they smoked. The attitude that considered women who smoked as unladylike and in possession of "loose morals" shifted in favor of the attitude that women who smoked had liberated themselves from the traditional social norms (Tinkler, 2006). Tobacco companies and feminists actively promoted this cultural shift by using mass media to visually represent women who smoked as classy, sophisticated, and modern. In particular, tobacco companies used advertisements and new cigarette brands that specifically targeted women. Wills, the largest UK tobacco company, started this marketing strategy in the late 1930s, approximately the same time that Philip Morris was doing the same in the United States. Concomitant with those campaigns, feminists adopted the image of a smoking woman as the prototypical liberated woman. Up through the 1970s, feminist activism aligned with the interest of the tobacco companies. However, as information spread about how nicotine affects unborn children, smoking became a stigmatized social practice. By the end of the century, the common perception was that women who smoke are predominantly "low-class" women, who use smoking for self-medication (Graham, 1994; Elliot, 2008).

CONCLUSION

Historical trends in smoking behavior in the United Kingdom have been subject to influences that pushed smoking prevalence in opposite directions. These influences seem to have differentially affected the smoking patterns of men and women across different birth cohorts. On the one hand, increasing information about the health risks associated with smoking and recent tobacco control policies have reduced smoking participation. On the other hand, relatively low levels of cigarette taxes from the 1950s to the 1990s and changing social and political norms about women and smoking—sometimes promoted by early feminist movements—pushed smoking participation rates to increase.

Since the 1920s, the rate of smoking among men in successive birth cohorts decreased significantly. However, smoking prevalence rates of women increased, declined somewhat, and then persisted. From a public health perspective, it is notable that smoking prevalence of the most recent cohort of adults in our data (ages 20–29 years in 2002) peaked at greater than 40 percent for both men and women. It is also notable that men and women in younger cohorts appear to be taking up smoking at increasingly younger ages. These results suggest that tobacco control should continue to be a policy priority in Britain and that special efforts should be made to target women and minors.

NOTES

1. Although German scientists had established that relationship for more than 50 years (Proctor, 1997, 1999), the Doll and Hill publication was the first time it appeared in an English language journal.
2. In fact, due to missing data, the prices of Capstan reported during 1980–1996 are imputed based on their correlation with Benson & Hedges.

REFERENCES

Alford, B. W. E. 1973. *W.D. & H.O. Wills and the Development of the UK Tobacco Industry, 1786–1965*. London: Methuen.

Berridge, V., and K. Loughlin. 2005. "Smoking and the new health education in Britain 1950s–1970s." *American Journal of Public Health* 95:956–964.

Bolt, J., and J. L. van Zanden. 2013. "The first update of the Maddison Project; Re-estimating growth before 1820." Maddison Project Working Paper 4. Available at http://www.ggdc.net/maddison/maddison-project/home.htm.

British Household Panel Survey. 1999, 2002. Institute for Social and Economic Research, University of Essex. Available at https://www.iser.essex.ac.uk/bhps.

Butler, N. R., and E. D. Alberman. 1969. *Perinatal Problems*. Edinburgh, UK: Livingstone.

Cancer Research UK. 2009. *Lung Cancer Incidence Projections to 2024: Future Rates and Numbers of New Cases in Great Britain and the UK*, by the Statistical Information Team. London: Cancer Research UK.

Clark, T., and A. Dilnot. 2002. "Long-term trends in British taxation and spending." Note No. 25. London: Institute for Fiscal Studies.

Corina, M. 1975. *Trust in Tobacco: The Anglo-American Struggle for Power*. London: Michael Joseph.

Doll, R., and A. B. Hill. 1950. "Smoking and carcinoma of the lung." *British Medical Journal* 2:739–748.

Elliot, R. 2008. *Women and Smoking Since 1890*. London: Routledge.

Goodman, J. 1993. *Tobacco in History: The Cultures of Dependence*. London: Routledge.

Graham, H. 1994. "Surviving by smoking." In *Women and Health: Feminist Perspectives*, edited by S. Wilkinson and C. Kitzinger, pp 102–123. London: Taylor & Francis.

Jones, A. 1989. "The UK demand for cigarettes 1954–1986, a double-hurdle approach." *Journal of Health Economics* 8:133–141.

Kemm, J. R. 2001. "A birth cohort analysis of smoking by adults in Great Britain 1974–1998." *Journal of Public Health Medicine* 23:306–311.

Loach, L. 1987. "Can feminism survive a third term?" *Feminist Review* 27:23–35.

Medicines and Healthcare Products Regulatory Agency (MHPRA). 2005. *Report of the Committee on Safety of Medicines Working Group on Nicotine Replacement Therapy*. London: MHPRA, Committee on Safety of Medicines.

Nicolaides-Bouman, A., N. Wald, B. Forey, and P. Lee. 1993. *International Smoking Statistics*. Oxford: Oxford University Press.

Proctor, R. N. 1997. "The Nazi war on tobacco: Ideology, evidence, and possible cancer consequences." *Bulletin of the History of Medicine* 71:435–488.

Proctor, R. N. 1999. *The Nazi war on tobacco: Ideology, evidence, and possible cancer consequences*. Princeton, NJ: Princeton University Press.

Pugh, M. 1990. "Domesticity and the decline of feminism 1930–1950." In *British Feminism in the Twentieth Century*, edited by H. L. Smit, pp 144–162. Amherst, MA: University of Massachusetts Press.

Pugh, M. 2000. *Women and the Women's Movement in Britain*, 2nd ed. New York: Palgrave Macmillan.

Robinson, S., and C. Bugler. 2008. "Smoking and drinking among adults, 2008." General Lifestyle Survey. Newport, South Wales, UK: Office for National Statistics.

Royal College of Physicians of London. 1962. *Smoking and Health: Summary and Report of the Royal College of Physicians of London on Smoking in Relation to Cancer of the Lung and Other Diseases*. London: Pitman Medical.

Tinkler, P. 2006. *Smoke Signals: Women, Smoking and Visual Culture in Britain*. Oxford: Berg.

Townsend, J., P. Roderick, and J. Cooper. 1994. "Cigarette smoking by socioeconomic group, sex, and age: Effects of price, income, and health publicity." *British Medical Journal* 309:923–927.

US Department of Health, Education, and Welfare (USDHEW). 1964. *Smoking and Health: Report of the Advisory Committee to the Surgeon General of the Public Health Service*. Public Health Service Publication No. 1103. Rockville, MD: USDHEW.

Ward, P. 2004. *Britishness Since 1870*. London: Taylor & Francis.

Wilkinson, H. 1999. "The Thatcher legacy: Power feminism and the birth of girl power." In *On the Move: Feminism for a New Generation*, edited by N. Walter, pp 27–47. London: Virago.

Yen, T., and A. M. Jones. 1996. "Individual cigarette consumption and addiction: A flexible limited dependent variable approach." *Health Economics* 5:105–117.

5

Smoking in the United States

DEAN R. LILLARD

INTRODUCTION

As an indigenous plant of the Americas, it is unsurprising that tobacco figures prominently in the history of the United States and American culture. Soon after Columbus introduced tobacco to Europeans, merchants and settlers in the Americas—mostly in the Spanish colonies in the West Indies, Cuba, and Mexico—cultivated and transported tobacco to meet a growing European demand. But it was not until the early 17th century, when demand for tobacco in England grew rapidly, that the cultivation and exportation of tobacco took root in the mid-Atlantic British colonies (Kluger, 1996). The development and growing popularity of the cigarette led 18th- and 19th-century entrepreneurs to create a new industry—factories in which workers rolled cigarettes by hand. But the real spread of cigarettes began in 1881 when James Bonsack invented a machine that could roll cigarettes faster and cheaper than humans. Major tobacco firms in the United States and Britain quickly recognized the machine's potential, bought it, and ramped up production. Between 1890 and 1900, US firms increased the number of cigarettes they exported by 366 percent—from 319 million to 1.16 billion sticks (Cox, 2000). Because the new machines not only sped up rates of production but also lowered costs, revenues increased much faster—by approximately 1200 percent. For example, sales revenue of the American Tobacco Company increased from $25 million in 1890 to $316 million in 1903 (Burns, 2007). Historians often credit James B. Duke, founder of the American Tobacco Company, as the force that organized, controlled, and significantly expanded the market for cigarettes and tobacco in the United States. It took the concentrated effort of Republican President Theodore Roosevelt to dissolve the American Tobacco Company. The antitrust lawsuit that his Justice Department filed in 1907 resulted in a Supreme Court ruling, handed down in 1911, that dissolved the company soon thereafter (Kluger, 1996).

Narrowly defined, the dissolution of the tobacco cartel was a success. The resulting industry, without a controlling dominant firm, quickly competed to attract existing smokers and to entice others to start. To compete for customers, firms lowered prices, increased advertising, developed new products, and exploited new technologies to create and sustain a place for smoking in American culture. Firms also launched advertising campaigns to induce more women and minority populations to smoke (Cox, 1933).

For its part, the US government used its fiat power to both indirectly and directly expand the consumption of tobacco. For example, Crowell (1919) describes the US Army's decision to introduce tobacco into troop rations. During World War I, the US government first issued tobacco and cigarette papers to overseas troops as part of their "reserve ration."[1] In May 1918, the government began to issue a daily ration of tobacco to all troops and allowed them to buy cigars, cigarettes, and tobacco at Army and military canteens at prices "lower than the price paid by the biggest wholesalers in the United States." During this period, the Subsistence Division shipped to France an average of 20 million cigars and 425 million cigarettes each month. Firms in the industry willingly sold at cost to the government not only because they were investing in a new crop of smokers but also because the government divided the contracts among the most popular brands according to their share of sales in the US market. For the industry, it was an eye-opening innovation: 95 percent of troops stationed abroad (1 million at its peak in 1918) consumed tobacco—a per capita average of 22 packs and 21 cigars per month. The industry also benefitted because the troops traded and shared cigarettes with natives. That trade helped firms to increase their brand name recognition abroad.

This arrangement continued when the United States entered World War II. The US government issued cigarettes as part of the combat rations troops carried (the so-called K rations and C rations), and the military continued to sell cigarettes and tobacco free of tax in its commissaries worldwide. Despite the growing information about the health risks of smoking, both practices continued through the Korean and Vietnam Wars. It was not until 1975 that the government stopped issuing cigarettes to troops. Starting in 1978, the Department of Defense (DoD) began to regulate where troops could smoke. In 1992, the DoD banned military commissaries and exchanges from using promotions that the tobacco companies targeted at military personnel. It was only in December 2002 that the DoD fully implemented a 1997 Executive Order that banned smoking in government-owned, rented, or leased interior spaces (Joseph et al., 2005).

As in the United Kingdom, even before 1950, information about the health risks of smoking was starting to spread. For example, in 1938, 1939, and 1940, the magazine *Science News Letter* published articles titled, "Smoking causes cancer of the lung" (October 29, 1938), "Cigaret smoking causes rise in blood pressure" (July 17, 1939), and "Heart disease more frequent among tobacco smokers" (November 2, 1940). Although these articles were sharing with their readers evidence that scientists were accumulating, the information likely had little effect because in the average month in 1940, only 32,466 people (0.02 percent of the US population) read *Science News Letter*. The public, politicians, and the industry paid more attention as articles began to appear in more widely circulated consumer magazines. The report by Doll and Hill (1950) sparked articles in *Reader's Digest* and *Newsweek*, respectively titled "How harmful are cigarettes?" (*Reader's Digest*, January 1950) and "Smoker's lungs" (*Newsweek*, May 8, 1950). In 1950, 6.8 and 1.1 percent of the US population read *Reader's Digest* and *Newsweek*, respectively.[2] As scientists accumulated and presented more evidence, articles such as these became increasingly common during the 1950s. For the United States, a watershed event occurred in 1964 when the

US Surgeon General issued the first official US government report on "health and smoking," in which the government linked smoking, cancer, and many other detrimental health consequences (US Department of Health, Education, and Welfare, 1964). Other federal reports published in the 1960s linked cigarette smoking with lung cancer, underweight newborns, and heart disease.

As information accumulated, the US authorities began to more strictly regulate the tobacco industry. In passing the federal Cigarette Labeling and Advertising Act of 1965, Congress required firms to print labels on cigarette packages that warned smokers, "Caution: Cigarette Smoking May be Hazardous to Your Health." The act also mandated that the Department of Health, Education, and Welfare and the Federal Trade Commission (FTC) report annually about smoking and health (Action on Smoking and Health (ASH), 2011; Centers for Disease Control and Prevention (CDC), 2011). Subsequently, both federal and state governments more actively regulated the sale and consumption of tobacco products. By 1969, every state levied a tax on cigarettes in addition to the federal cigarette tax. Between 1964 and 1971, state governments changed their cigarette tax 95 times (Lillard et al., 2013). In 1967, the Federal Communications Commission ruled that the so-called "fairness doctrine" required that television and radio broadcasters air anti-smoking messages in proportion to the time that cigarette advertisements appeared. The airing of such messages ended on January 1, 1971, when the federal Public Health Cigarette Smoking Act of 1969 took effect. In that federal legislation, Congress banned all advertising of cigarettes on television and radio.

Private industry also started to react to the growing information. Insurance companies began to offer nonsmokers a discount on life insurance premiums. By 1987, the US government had allowed a federal health management organization to charge smokers a higher premium (ASH, 2011; CDC, 2011). On January 13, 1984, the US Food and Drug Administration (FDA) approved SmithKline Beecham's application to market Nicorette, the first clinically effective nicotine replacement therapy (NRT) whose approved purpose is to help smokers quit. Other companies were developing similar treatments. By 1992, the FDA had approved the sale of four more pharmaceutical NRT products (Avery et al., 2007). Today, the set of products that the FDA has approved to aid in smoking cessation includes six types of NRTs and two types of nicotine agonists. In addition, for many of these products, the FDA no longer requires that consumers get a doctor's prescription. Instead, they allow firms to sell the products "over-the-counter."

Starting in 1964, the US government began to devote more resources to educate its citizens about the health risks of smoking. Between 1964 and 2014, the US Surgeon General issued 35 separate reports that specifically focused on the state-of-the-art knowledge about the health risks of smoking and tobacco consumption. As it became apparent that women's smoking prevalence rate was rising, the Surgeon General tailored reports to convey information specific to women. The 1980 and 2001 reports focus specifically on smoking and women's health issues. In 1985, the FTC required new wording on cigarette pack warning labels—including a warning for women that smoking while pregnant causes low birth weight. Starting in approximately 1988, many states began their own information campaigns.

The flow of information from states and the federal government increased rapidly in 1998 when Congress negotiated an agreement between 46 state governments and the four major tobacco companies. Four states had previously settled with the tobacco companies. That agreement, known as the "Master Settlement Agreement" (MSA), ended a lawsuit that the state governments had filed to recover public monies spent to treat smoking-related illnesses. As part of the MSA, tobacco companies paid state governments a part of the revenue from sales in each state (National Association of Attorneys General, 1998). Most of those governments devoted some of the money to public awareness/education campaigns. State and national campaigns broadcasted television and radio commercials and paid for billboards depicting how smoking affects health. Despite these efforts to discourage smokers and nonsmokers alike from tobacco use, more than 45.3 million American adults in 2010 still chose to smoke (CDC, 2012).

These and other historical events shaped and continue to shape whether, when, and how intensively Americans smoke. We next describe patterns in life-course smoking rates of different cohorts of men and women and discuss them in the aforementioned context.

SMOKING PREVALENCE RATES IN HISTORICAL PERSPECTIVE

In Figure 5.1, we plot smoking prevalence rates by gender and birth cohort over time, and we highlight selected historical events that may be relevant. We draw attention to the World War II years because the US government included cigarettes in rations to (male) soldiers and because female labor force participation rates increased then and in subsequent years. In the figure for men (Figure 5.1a), we also highlight several events that likely affected both men and women, but we show them only in the figure for men to avoid too much clutter in the figure for women (Figure 5.1b). These events are the year of the first US Surgeon General's report on smoking (1964), the start of the fairness doctrine (1967), the end of that doctrine and TV and radio advertising of cigarettes (1971), and the Master Settlement Agreement (November 1998). For men, we also list the end of the Vietnam War (1975) because that event likely affected smoking behavior of men more than it affected the smoking behavior of women. For women, we separately mark some events that are related to female labor force participation. In particular, we mark 1963—the year Congress passed the Equal Pay Act of 1963—and 1972 because it was in this year that activists concentrated most on trying to pass the Equal Rights Amendment.[3] Finally, we list the years the Surgeon General published reports on smoking that focused specifically on women (1980 and 2001).[4]

Figure 5.1 presents smoking patterns that closely correspond to patterns presented in Harris (1983), Escobedo and Peddicord (1996), and Burns et al. (1998).[5] One of the most striking patterns in this figure is the steady decrease in the peak prevalence of smoking among US men from the oldest to the youngest cohorts, whereas for women, the peak prevalence rate increases up to the cohort that is 60–69 years old in 2007. For cohorts of women younger than 60–69 years in 2007, the peak smoking prevalence rate steadily declines—albeit at a much slower rate than does the rate for men.

It is likely that the smoking patterns of men were driven in part by developments in the military documented in the introduction. One possibility is that rates of smoking among men were higher because a substantial fraction of men served in the

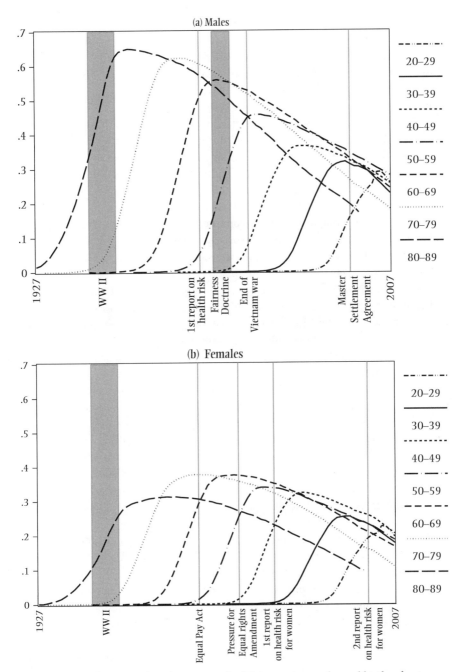

Figure 5.1 Smoking prevalence rates over the life course by gender and birth cohort.
SOURCE: Tobacco Use Supplement to the Current Population Survey (TUS-CPS). 1967, 1968, 1985, 1989, 1992, 1993, 1995, 1996, 1998–2003, 2006, 2007. Washington, DC: US Census Bureau.

military, in which they could buy cigarettes at deeply discounted prices. Military service peaked during World War II. Thereafter, with the exception of a period from 1965 to 1971 during the Vietnam War, the fraction of the US population serving worldwide in the military fell steadily from a high of 2.2 percent in 1953 during the Korean War to 0.4 percent in 2012 (US Department of Defense, n.d.). Because most of these military personnel were men, this steady decline in their military service may partly explain the gender differences in smoking prevalence rates of successive cohorts.

At the same time, several factors specific to women were operating. As noted previously, the US Surgeon General released information about health risks of smoking specific to women. The pattern in women's smoking rates does not necessarily mean that they did not respond to the health risk information that was unfolding because they may also have responded to other factors that increased their smoking participation. For example, feminists lobbied for and won legal changes to federal and state laws that expanded women's social and labor market rights. In 1920, Congress passed and the states ratified the 19th Amendment—banning sex-based restrictions on voting in state and federal elections. Women were also campaigning for basic economic rights—to work, to enter any occupation, and to be paid a wage equal to the wage paid to an equally qualified man. Their successes (e.g., the Equal Pay Act of 1963), and even their failures (e.g., the Equal Rights Amendment), increased women's educational attainment, opened occupations that had previously been closed to them, and gave them command over more economic resources. For example, the labor force participation rates of younger women rapidly increased starting in approximately 1960, in which 46.5 percent of US women age 20–24 years participated in the labor force. That figure increased to 57.7 percent in 1970, 68.9 percent in 1980, and then more or less leveled off (it was 71.3 percent in 1990 and 67.8 percent in 2011).[6]

In Figure 5.2, we plot the per-pack cigarette tax and cigarette price faced by the average US resident and per capita gross domestic product (GDP) in each year from 1927 onward.[7] To show these time series on the same figure, we plot the annual value for each time series relative to the value of that series in 2007. The cigarette tax is the sum of federal and state cigarette tax and, for years after 1998, adds in state-specific MSA escrow payments that are effectively the same as a per-pack cigarette tax (Viscusi and Hersch, 2011; Lillard and Sfekas, 2013).

Figure 5.2 highlights that different cohorts experienced quite difference economic conditions, cigarette prices, and taxes, which do not always co-vary with smoking rates in the expected direction. In the oldest cohorts that experienced the Great Depression, cigarette prices and taxes were increasing while per capita GDP fell. Starting in approximately 1937, per capita GDP rose much faster than cigarette prices and taxes—which were either constant or falling. The end of the war saw a substantial reduction in per capita GDP and the real cigarette tax. Both price and tax moved more or less together with per capita GDP until approximately 1960. For the next 20 years, per capita GDP rose much faster than the average cigarette price or cigarette tax. In fact, starting in 1971 and lasting until 1982, the real tax on cigarettes (and real price of cigarettes) fell dramatically at a time when real per capita GDP was growing rapidly. From 1998 onward, starting from the time of the Master Settlement Agreement, states began to tax cigarettes heavily. During this period, cigarette taxes and cigarette prices rose much faster than per capita GDP.

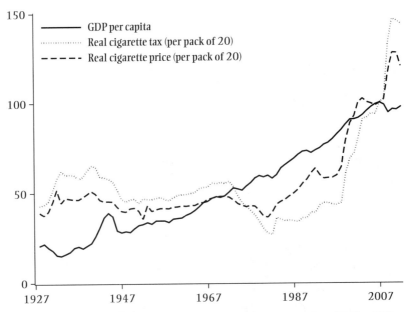

Figure 5.2 Economic development, cigarette taxes, and cigarette prices (2007 = 100).
SOURCES: GDP, Bolt, J., and J. L. van Zanden. 2013. "The first update of the Maddison Project; Re-Estimating growth before 1820." Maddison Project Working Paper 4; cigarette taxes and prices, Orzechowski and Walker (2012) and US Bureau of Labor (various years).

Whether these developments have causal effects on smoking patterns is of course an empirical question. Although the price elasticity of smoking behavior has been largely established (e.g., Lillard et al., 2013), there is suggestive, but not definitive, evidence that, before information was widespread, rates of smoking increased as incomes increased and that, after information become more widespread, this relationship reversed (Cheng and Kenkel, 2010).

In Figure 5.3, we plot smoking trajectories across an age scale so we can more directly compare how smoking patterns differed across cohorts when members of each cohort were the same age. That is, we plot the same trajectories shown in Figure 5.1 but use chronological age on the horizontal axis. The figure shows the well-recognized life-cycle pattern of smoking by age. Almost all people start to smoke in a narrow chronological window between the ages of 14 and 20. This is true for every cohort of US men and women, although older cohorts of men started at slightly younger ages and older cohorts of women started at slightly older ages. Practically every cohort reaches its peak smoking prevalence rate when the cohort is in its 20s. Rates of cessation are more or less constant across cohorts of men (lines remain more or less parallel). This statement is not true for women, especially for the older cohorts of women. Once the oldest cohort of women began to smoke, they quit at lower rates than did later cohorts (their trajectory remains high longer and crosses over the trajectories of other cohorts).

What is less easy to observe, but which we reveal in Table 5.1, is that the smoking trajectories of younger cohorts of US women so closely resemble the smoking

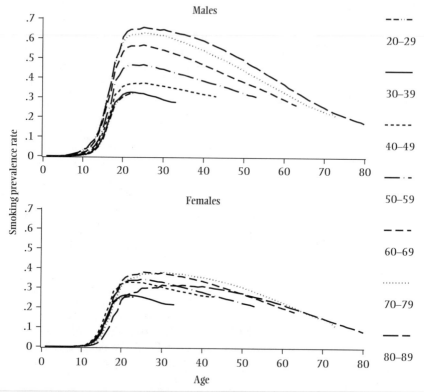

Figure 5.3 Change in smoking prevalence rate with age by birth cohort.
SOURCE: Tobacco Use Supplement to the Current Population Survey (TUS-CPS). 1967, 1968, 1985, 1989, 1992, 1993, 1995, 1996, 1998–2003, 2006, 2007. Washington, DC: US Census Bureau.

trajectories of US men so as to be indistinguishable from one another. We next present summaries that highlight this finding.

COHORT AND GENDER DIFFERENCES

In Table 5.1, we present six summary measures of smoking behavior for each cohort of men and women to highlight differences that are less easy to notice in the previously discussed plots. The comparisons reveal interesting patterns. For men, we see that not only was smoking prevalence higher in the oldest cohort but also, unlike the patterns we observe in other countries, men in the oldest cohort smoked roughly as many cigarettes per day as did men in adjacent birth cohorts. Smoking intensity was highest among men aged 60–69 years in 2007. However, the oldest four cohorts of male smokers in the United States consumed more than a pack a day. Although the peak smoking prevalence rate monotonically declines across successive cohorts of men, Table 5.1 confirms the pattern we discussed previously for women. The peak smoking prevalence rate rose to its highest level for the two birth cohorts of US women who were 60–69 and 70–79 years old in 2007 and steadily declined in all subsequent cohorts.

Table 5.1. SUMMARY INDICATORS OF SMOKING BY GENDER AND BIRTH COHORT

Gender/ cohort	Sample size	Peak prevalence rate	Cigarettes per day	Years smoking	Average age at		
					peak	start	quit
MALES							
80–89	57,741	0.65	21	39	26	18	51
70–79	59,861	0.62	22	35	27	17	46
60–69	86,870	0.56	23	33	25	17	40
50–59	117,917	0.46	21	27	24	17	35
40–49	114,785	0.37	19	20	26	17	30
30–39	84,341	0.32	16	13	25	17	25
20–29	53,324	0.29	13	7	22	16	21
FEMALES							
80–89	79,364	0.32	16	38	36	21	54
70–79	70,830	0.38	17	35	30	20	49
60–69	95,985	0.38	18	31	28	19	41
50–59	127,836	0.34	17	25	25	19	35
40–49	126,269	0.32	16	20	24	18	30
30–39	92,536	0.25	14	12	25	17	25
20–29	55,269	0.22	12	7	22	16	21

SOURCE: Tobacco Use Supplement to the Current Population Survey (TUS-CPS). 1967, 1968, 1985, 1989, 1992, 1993, 1995, 1996, 1998–2003, 2006, 2007. Washington, DC: US Census Bureau.

One can also characterize a cohort's smoking behavior by the age at which smoking prevalence reached its peak and the age at which the average smoker started to smoke regularly.[8] For men, these two measures of smoking behavior are surprisingly stable across cohorts. On average, men between the ages of 30 and 89 years in 2007 reached their peak smoking prevalence between the ages of 24 and 27 years, with no obvious pattern across different birth cohorts. Clearly, this does not hold for men in the oldest cohort, those men began to smoke regularly at approximately age 17 years. By contrast, for cohorts of US women, one observes a mostly steady downward trend in both measures of smoking age. Peak smoking prevalence fell from approximately 36 years of age for the oldest cohort of women to 25 years for the cohort that was 30–39 years old in 2007. Similarly, there is a 4-year difference between the age at which the average smoker started in the oldest cohort and the cohort that turned 30–39 years old in 2007.

These summary statistics about smoking patterns make it easy to compare patterns for men and women in the same birth cohort. To sharpen the trends, we compute the ratio of each statistic for each cohort of men relative to the statistic for the corresponding cohort of women. As Figure 5.4 shows, younger cohorts of US women have the dubious distinction of reaching "equality" with their

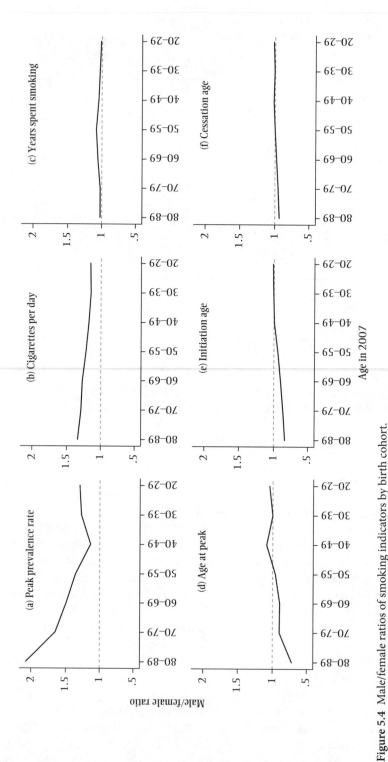

Figure 5.4 Male/female ratios of smoking indicators by birth cohort.

SOURCE: Tobacco Use Supplement to the Current Population Survey (TUS-CPS). 1967, 1968, 1985, 1989, 1992, 1993, 1995, 1996, 1998–2003, 2006, 2007. Washington, DC: US Census Bureau

male counterparts of the same age in almost every measure of smoking behavior. Furthermore, women achieved "equality" with men in their age of initiation because the average age of smoking initiation of women fell faster across successive cohorts of women than it did across the corresponding cohorts of men. This "equality" was reached in the cohort of men and women who were 40–49 years old in 2007. All subsequent cohorts of men and women smokers started at the same average age. Interestingly, the average age of quitting, conditional on being a smoker, was more broadly similar for men and women. If anything, female smokers in younger cohorts are waiting longer to quit than their male counterparts. That similarity suggests (but does not establish) that quitting behavior is partly dictated by a physiological process common to men and women (as opposed to differential targeting of advertising or social norms). The existence of such a process is supported by medical research on nicotine addiction (Benowitz, 2010). The growing similarity in the smoking behavior of younger cohorts also suggests that, when researchers specify and estimate models to identify causal determinants of smoking, sex-specific factors may play less of a role in younger than in older cohorts.

There are several potential explanations for the observed gender differences in smoking patterns. In addition to the economic rights that women secured, the feminist movement altered public and private attitudes about the proper social role of women. The cohort and gender differences we observe may be partly due to changes in those social norms.

Scholars differ on the extent to which feminism encouraged or discouraged women to smoke. In the United States, as in the United Kingdom, cigarette manufacturers tried to capitalize on the feminist movement by launching advertising campaigns (Britton, 1998; Boyd et al., 2003). Also, as in the United Kingdom, the US feminist movement adopted the cigarette as a symbol of women's emancipation. However, other authors suggest that feminism helped women fight against social norms—such as the oft portrayed thinness of women in advertising—that some argue lead women to smoke in order to control their weight (Zucker et al., 2005). Although debate continues, the evidence suggests that smoking patterns of men and women have converged over time in the United States (and elsewhere). This trend is consistent with greater equality of women in economic and social settings.

CONCLUSION

The previously discussed patterns of life-course smoking behavior, plotted for different cohorts of US men and women, reveal similarities and differences that point to various possible causes of tobacco use. Over the period for which we describe, behavior changed quite a bit. Information emerged and spread; people got richer; cigarettes got cheap and then more expensive; and governments abandoned their passive stances to more actively educate citizens and regulate the sale, consumption, and marketing of cigarettes. Over these years, social norms about the behavior of women and smokers in general also shifted. These patterns entice researchers to delve more deeply and to seek ways to estimate whether the associations suggested here are in fact causal determinants of behavior.

NOTES

1. Crowell (1919) notes that according to one (unnamed) observer, the War Department included tobacco and cigarettes in the rations because of the enterprising spirit of workers in a "large corporation." That corporation discovered that the War Office planned to pack ration containers with wood shavings so that goods would not be jostled and damaged in transit. The workers in the unnamed corporation obtained permission to fill the empty space in some of the containers with tobacco. After a trial run, the Subsistence Division mandated that the tobacco ration be placed in all reserve ration containers. Each container contained 8 oz. of tobacco and 100 cigarette papers.

2. All circulation figures are from the Audit Bureau of Circulation reports (now named Alliance for Audited Media located in Arlington Heights, IL). Circulation figures for *Reader's Digest* are from 1955, the first year that magazine accepted advertising. Population figures from the US Census of 1940 and 1950.

3. The amendment was first proposed in 1923. In 1972, Congress passed it and sent it to the states to be ratified. Twenty-two states ratified it in 1972. Eight did so in 1973. During the next 2 years, only 4 more states ratified the amendment. With only 34 of the 38 state ratifications needed to adopt the amendment, the (once-extended) deadline expired on June 30, 1982 (Lunardini, 1986; Kyvig, 1996).

4. We list other tobacco-related events in the United States in the Appendix.

5. The prevalence rates these studies report differ slightly from the prevalence rates in Figure 5.1 for technical reasons. Some studies do not correct for differences in mortality rates of smokers and nonsmokers (Escobedo and Peddicord, 1996), or they correct for those differences using a less precise method (Harris, 1983; Burns et al., 1998).

6. See Organization for Economic Cooperation and Development labor force statistics by sex and age available at http://stats.oecd.org/Index.aspx?DataSetCode=LFS_SEXAGE_I_R (accessed March 20, 2013) and the US Bureau of Labor Statistics, "Report 1040: Women in the Labor Force: A Databook," available at http://www.bls.gov/cps/wlf-databook-2012.pdf (accessed November 16, 2013).

7. See Chapter 14 for details on the source of our cigarette price data and how we construct it.

8. As noted in Chapter 1, the age at peak statistic is not meaningful among the two youngest cohorts because many individuals may still be starting to smoke.

REFERENCES

Action on Smoking and Health (ASH). 2011. "Events related to Action on Smoking and Health." Available at http://ash.org.

Avery, R., D. Kenkel, D. R. Lillard, and A. Mathios. 2007. "Regulating advertisements: The case of smoking cessation products." *Journal of Regulatory Economics* 31:185–208.

Benowitz, N. L. 2010. "Nicotine addiction." *New England Journal of Medicine* 362:2295–2303.

Bolt, J., and J. L. van Zanden. 2013. "The first update of the Maddison Project; Re-Estimating growth before 1820." Maddison Project Working Paper 4. Available at http://www.ggdc.net/maddison/maddison-project/home.htm.

Boyd, T. C., C. J. Boyd, and T. B. Greelee. 2003. "A means to an end: Slim hopes and cigarette advertising." *Health Promotion Practice* 4:266–277.

Britton, G. A. 1998. "A review of women and tobacco: Have we come such a long way?" *Journal of Obstetric, Gynecologic, and Neonatal Nursing* 27:241–249.

Burns, D. M., L. Lee, L. Z. Shen, et al. 1998. "Cigarette smoking behavior in the United States." In *Changes in Cigarette-Related Disease Risk and Their Implications for Prevention and Control*, edited by D. Burns, L. Garfinkel, and J. Samet, pp 13–112. Bethesda, MD: National Institutes of Health.

Burns, E. 2007. *The Smoke of the Gods: A Social History of Tobacco.* Philadelphia: Temple University Press.

Centers for Disease Control and Prevention (CDC). 2011. "Selected actions of the U.S. government regarding the regulation of tobacco sales, marketing, and use." Available at http://www.cdc.gov/tobacco/overview/regulate.htm.

Centers for Disease Control and Prevention (CDC). 2012. "Adult cigarette smoking in the United States." Available at http://www.cdc.gov/tobacco/data_statistics/fact_sheets/adult_data/cig_smoking/index.htm.

Cheng, K., and D. Kenkel. 2010. "U.S. cigarette demand: 1944–2004." *B. E. Journal of Economic Analysis & Policy* 10:78.

Cox, H. 2000. *The Global Cigarette: Origins and Evolution of British American Tobacco 1880–1945.* Oxford: Oxford University Press.

Cox, R. 1933. *Competition in the American Tobacco Industry, 1911–1932: A Study of the Effects of the Partition of the American Tobacco Company by the United States Supreme Court.* New York: Columbia University Press.

Crowell, B. 1919. *America's Munitions 1917–1918.* Public Health Service Publication No. 1103. Washington, DC: Government Printing Office.

Doll, R., and A. B. Hill. 1950. "Smoking and carcinoma of the lung." *British Medical Journal* 2:739–748.

Escobedo, L. G., and J. P. Peddicord. 1996. "Smoking prevalence in US birth cohorts: The influence of gender and education." *American Journal of Public Health* 86:231–236.

Harris, J. E. 1983. "Cigarette smoking among successive birth cohorts of men and women in the United States during 1900–80." *Journal of the National Cancer Institute* 71:473–479.

Joseph, A. M., M. Muggli, K. C. Pearson, and H. Lando. 2005. "The cigarette manufactures' efforts to promote tobacco to the U.S. military." *Military Medicine* 170:874–880.

Kluger, R. 1996. *Ashes to Ashes: America's Hundred Year Cigarette War, the Public Health, and the Unabashed Triumph of Philip Morris.* New York: Knopf.

Kyvig, D. E. 1996. "Historical misunderstandings and the defeat of the Equal Rights Amendment." *The Public Historian* 18:45–63.

Lillard, D. R., E. Molloy, and A. Sfekas. 2013. "Smoking initiation and the iron law of demand." *Journal of Health Economics* 32:114–127.

Lillard, D. R., and A. Sfekas. 2013. "Just passing through: The effect of the master settlement agreement on estimated cigarette tax-price pass-through." *Applied Economics Letters* 20:353–357.

Lunardini, C. A. 1986. *From Equal Suffrage to Equal Rights: Alice Paul and the National Woman's Party, 1910–1928.* New York: New York University Press.

National Association of Attorneys General. 1998. "Master settlement agreement, archived from the original on 2008-06-25." Available at http://www.naag.org/backpages/naag/tobacco/msa/msa-pdf/1109185724_1032468605_cigmsa.pdf.

Orzechowski, W., and R. Walker. 2012. *The Tax Burden on Tobacco, Historical Compilation*, Vol. 47. Arlington, VA: Authors.

Tobacco Use Supplement to the Current Population Survey (TUS-CPS). 1967, 1968, 1985, 1989, 1992, 1993, 1995, 1996, 1998–2003, 2006, 2007. Washington, DC: US Census Bureau. Available at http://catalog.data.gov/dataset/current-population-survey-tobacco-use-supplement.

United Nations Statistical Division. 2014. "National accounts estimates of main aggregates." Available at http://data.un.org/Data.aspx?d=SNAAMA&f=grID%3A101%3BcurrID%3AUSD%3BpcFlag%3A1. Accessed July 9, 2014.

US Department of Agriculture(USDA). 1938. "Annual report on tobacco statistics." Statistical Bulletin No. 67:39. Washington, DC: USDA.

US Department of Defense, Defense Manpower Data Center. n.d. "Personnel, military, military personnel statistics, annual." Internet release date September 30, 2011. Available at https://www.dmdc.osd.mil/appj/dwp/dwp_reports.jsp.

US Department of Health, Education, and Welfare (USDHEW). 1964. *Smoking and Health: Report of the Advisory Committee to the Surgeon General of the Public Health Service*. Public Health Service Publication No. 1103. Rockville, MD: USDHEW.

US Department of Labor, Bureau of Labor Statistics. 1962. *Consumer Price Index (1957–59 = 100): Price Indexes for Selected Items and Groups, Annual Averages 1935–1961, Quarterly Indexes, March 1947–December 1961*. Washington, DC: US Government Printing Office.

US Department of Labor, Bureau of Labor Statistics. 1970. *Consumer Prices in the United States 1959–1968: Trends and Indexes*. Bulletin 1647. Washington, DC: US Government Printing Office.

Viscusi, K., and J. Hersch. 2011. "Tobacco regulation through litigation: The Master Settlement Agreement." In *Regulation Versus Litigation: Perspectives From Economics and Law, National Bureau of Economic Research Conference Report*, edited by D. P. Kessler, pp 71–101. Chicago: University of Chicago Press.

Zucker, A., A. Stewart, C. Pomerleau, and C. Boyd. 2005. "Resisting gendered smoking pressures: Critical consciousness as a correlate of women's smoking status" *Sex Roles* 53:261–272.

PART II

Western Europe

Germany and Spain

6

Smoking in Germany

DEAN R. LILLARD

INTRODUCTION

Tobacco consumption and smoking in Germany evolved within and under the influence of well-known historical events—World War I, World War II, Germany's division, and its economic "miracle." Policies enacted during World War I not only affected who smoked (German troops received tobacco and cigarettes in rations) but also affected the structure of the tobacco industry. Thereafter, the National Socialist German Workers Party, commonly known as Nazis, led Germany into a second world war and also commandeered and potentially prevented the future use of a rising body of scientific evidence about the health risks of smoking that German scientists were compiling. During the war, the Allied forces destroyed much of Germany's industrial infrastructure. Paradoxically, this destruction may have set the stage for the rebuilding of that infrastructure and one of the longest periods of sustained economic growth in modern economic times. At the same time, Germany was the victim of political fighting between the US, UK, French, and Soviet governments. The Soviets disagreed with policies advocated by the other governments to reintroduce a market economy to help rebuild post-war Germany. Thus, they barricaded the eastern states of Germany that they controlled, effectively dividing the country into East and West Germany. For the next 40 years, residents in the two areas experienced different social conditions and economic policies—more or less market-based policies in the West and centrally planned economic policies in the East. The amazing economic recovery and growth of West Germany and the anemic growth in East Germany led to the eventual reunification of the country. Together, these and other events influenced who smoked and when.

Although farmers cultivated tobacco in the lands encompassed by modern Germany since approximately 1573, it is no longer one of Germany's major agricultural products (Weigel, 1993; Proctor, 1997). Initially, landowners recruited Huguenot refugees to raise tobacco as a cash crop (Weiss and Herbert, 1854). At the end of the 19th century, approximately 200,000 German farmers cultivated more than 30,000 hectares of tobacco. But the lower quality of German tobacco, relative to tobacco grown in other countries, doomed it as a domestic agricultural commodity. Despite this failure, the German tobacco manufacturing industry thrived.

Until Germany entered World War I, two companies, the Imperial Tobacco Company and the American Tobacco Company—giants in the world tobacco industry—were laying the groundwork to invade and dominate the German tobacco industry. Kurt Pritzkoleit's (1961) accounting of the evolution of the German industrial "miracle" includes a chapter that extensively documents the evolution of the German tobacco industry from the turn of the 19th century through 1960. He notes that, already in 1900, J. B. Duke, the genius behind the American Tobacco Company, had gained a toe-hold in the German industry. Using the same tactics that led to the defensive creation of the Imperial Tobacco Company in Great Britain, the American Tobacco Company was systematically buying controlling shares of German tobacco manufacturers. This practice continued through the 1910s. After the 1911 US Supreme Court-ordered breakup of the American Tobacco Company, it was the British American Tobacco Company—the firm that rose from Duke's failed effort to enter the British market—that pressed the strategy.

Two historical events derailed the company's plan. First, because the United States and Britain were officially hostile nations during World War I, the British American Tobacco Company had to suspend its acquisitions for a number of years. During that time, the German tobacco firm Reemtsma was able to establish itself as the domi-nant firm in the industry. In the period after World War I, the German government supported the industry. For example, in 1927 they founded the Federal Institute for Tobacco Research in Forchheim with the general mission of improving the quality of German tobacco (Schweiger, 2010). A second historical event was the 1932 election in which the National Socialist Party won a majority of seats in parliament. The party had advocated economic independence as part of its platform. After it took control of the government in 1933, the National Socialists adopted and pursued policies that favored German firms and industries. The protectionism and isolation of Germany up to and through the end of World War II allowed Reemtsma to completely domi-nate the German market (Pritzkoleit, 1961).

The rule of the Nazis may also have affected how legislators in post-war Germany regulated the consumption and marketing of tobacco. After World War II, the German government continued to protect its domestic tobacco industry. For exam-ple, in 1953, the West German government lowered the tax on tobacco products manufactured with a minimum percent of domestically grown tobacco.[1] This favor-ing of the tobacco industry was also reflected in other tobacco control policies (or lack thereof). Relative to other industrialized countries, the West German govern-ment waited a long time to regulate where people could smoke in public. As we describe later, the federal government did not pass a public smoking ban in post-war Germany until 2007.

It is ironic that Germany took so long to pass and implement tobacco control policies because German scientists produced some of the earliest scientific evidence about the health consequences of smoking. Robert Proctor's (1997) article, "The Nazi War on Tobacco," and book by the same title document that, from as early as the 1920s, German scientists had been accumulating evidence about the connections between tobacco use, smoking, and cancers of various types (Proctor, 1999). Some of the early publications date to the 1920s (Seyfarth, 1924; Lickint, 1929). A 1939 medi-cal dissertation by Franz Müller was one of the first studies to use a healthy "control" group and to acknowledge the role of sample selection bias (although he did not use that term; Müller, 1939). In his 1939 book, *Tabak und Organismus: Handbuch der gesamten Tabakkunde* (*Tobacco and the Organism*), Fritz Lickint surveyed 8000 articles published worldwide that investigated correlations between tobacco consumption and health. A 1943 publication by Eberhard Schairer and Erich Schöniger was a sophisticated statistical analysis whose conclusion foreshadowed later public policy pronouncements (Schairer and Schöniger, 1943). They concluded that smoking causes lung cancer.

Scholars continue to debate why the world public health community failed to cite this evidence. A plausible explanation is that all research emanating from Germany became associated with the Nazis.[2] Already in the 1930s, partly in response to the evidence about environmental causes of cancer, including smoking and tobacco use, the government led health campaigns to raise public awareness of possible causes of cancer. The Nazis continued and expanded those efforts, launching campaigns explicitly targeting smoking. In 1938 and 1939, they began to restrict places people could smoke. At approximately the same time, the German national rail service established passenger cars in which smoking was not allowed. In December 1941, the Advertising Council restricted content allowed in tobacco advertising. Among other things, the council restricted advertising content so that it could not target women, present images of men in activities "attractive to youthful males," or suggest that a low-nicotine tobacco product was less harmful to health (Proctor, 1999).

These actions are noteworthy for two reasons. First, they predated similar policies in other countries by up to 30 years. Second, and more tellingly, starting in the late 1930s, the Nazis co-opted and abused the scientific evidence in service of their racial purity agenda. The anti-smoking policies they promulgated may have become linked to the abhorrent ideology for which the Nazis are infamously known (Proctor, 1997, 1999).

The division of Germany in October 1949 further complicated the German experience with tobacco and smoking. The founding of the German Democratic Republic (GDR; Deutsche Demokratische Republik), informally known as East Germany, and its alignment with the Warsaw Pact countries meant that people living in those areas faced different conditions than people living in West Germany. For example, firms in East Germany did not advertise cigarettes, and the government set prices without apparent regard to either demand or supply conditions. These differences sharpened over time as the East German regime increasingly restricted trade between and movement of people to and from West Germany (the Berlin Wall, built in 1961, symbolized the severity of these restrictions). Immediately after separating, prices were similar in both parts of Germany and still falling from the high levels they attained during and immediately after World War II. By 1953, 5 years after separating, the price in East Germany no longer moved with market forces. Instead, the (nominal) price of cigarettes and tobacco changed only twice, in 1960 and 1969, with the "5-year" plans that were introduced at approximately the same time. Of course, inflation eroded the real price.

In West Germany, market forces did not purely determine supply and demand in the tobacco industry. Aside from the tax differential noted previously, between 1948 and 1952, as part of the Marshall Plan, the United States provided price-subsidized tobacco to Germany and other European nations (US Economic Cooperation

Administration, 1949). However, over time, and especially after the Marshall Plan ended, market forces began to operate.

In both East and West Germany, incomes and the standard of living rose after World War II. But they rose faster and more dramatically in West Germany during the years of the so-called "economic miracle" from 1950 through the 1970s. By October 1990, when Germany reunited (the Wall fell in November 1989), economic and living conditions in the two areas differed sharply. After reunification, economic conditions in the two areas began to (slowly) converge, and East and West German smokers faced increasingly similar market conditions.

Like most countries, Germany taxed tobacco and cigarettes primarily to raise revenue. Germany's modern tobacco tax began in 1906.[3] Initially, the government levied a flat tax per cigarette, setting a higher rate for higher priced cigarettes. To finance war costs of World War I, the government more than doubled the cigarette tax in some price ranges. In the 1920s, the government abandoned the specific tax in favor of ad valorem taxes whose rate varied with retail prices. During the following two decades, tax rates increased from 20 percent in 1925 to up to 90 percent in 1941—a rate that included a surcharge set to finance the war. After World War II, tobacco taxes fell for some time. The occupation administration lowered the rate to 60 percent in 1946. In 1951, the newly elected West German government reduced the rate to 58 percent of the retail price and, in 1953, reformed the structure of tobacco taxes. In 1972, the West German government reintroduced the specific tax levied on each cigarette and simultaneously lowered the ad valorem tax rate levied on the final retail price. A more significant change in tax policy occurred in 1980 when the West German government mandated that total taxes comprise a minimum amount per cigarette. With that reform, the real price of cigarettes began to steadily increase (see Figure 6.2). With reunification, the price of cigarettes in East Germany almost immediately increased to West German levels. Today, smokers pay an indirect and a consumption tax, as well as a combination of a wholesale tax and a value-added tax.

As noted previously, Germany has only recently enacted laws to limit the sale or consumption of tobacco, despite the early evidence German scientists produced that linked smoking and health degradation. Researchers conjecture that this late action may be because its association with the Nazi regime tainted the evidence and Germany's tobacco lobby is so strong (Brenner and Fleischle, 1994; Apel et al., 1997). Although the European Union (EU) banned television advertising of tobacco in its member states in 1991, its 1998 legislation to ban non-television tobacco advertising failed because Germany, under prodding from the tobacco industry, successfully sued and blocked the implementation of the ban. The ban was suspended in 1998 and the EU Court of Justice overturned it in 2001. In a similar directive passed in 2003, the EU banned print, radio, and Internet tobacco advertising and made it illegal for tobacco companies to sponsor cultural and sport events held inside the EU. Again, the German government challenged the legality of the ban (this time together with owners of a racing circuit), but the Court upheld it. The German parliament passed legislation to implement the directive in December 2006. That legislation seems to have been a watershed event for tobacco control in Germany. Starting in 2007, the federal government and various German states passed and implemented legislation that banned smoking in public places. By July 2008, every state had established smoke-free areas in public places. In Bavaria, where the smoke-free legislation was considered to be ineffective and weak, voters approved a referendum in 2010 that substantially strengthened its scope and coverage.

This special history of German science, politics, and policy shaped whether, when, and how Germans smoked. We next describe patterns in smoking behavior of different cohorts of Germans. We describe patterns for all Germans because, despite the contextual differences we discuss previously between East and West Germany, the smoking patterns only differ for the cohorts of women coming of age during the transition to a reunified Germany.[4]

SMOKING PREVALENCE RATES IN HISTORICAL PERSPECTIVE

In Figure 6.1, we plot the life-course smoking trajectories of men (Figure 6.1a) and women (Figure 6.1b) born in different 10-year birth cohorts (defined by age in 2002). To frame these trajectories, we mark selected events or ranges of years during which smoking-related events occurred.[5] We mark the years during which Germany waged World War II. In some years, and unlike other governments, the Nazi regime ostensibly banned smoking among its troops. But accounts suggest that it abandoned this diktat by 1941 (Proctor, 1999). We also list the years of World War II (WWII) because the war generally disrupted the domestic supply of tobacco. We separately mark 1948 for several reasons. In that year, the British, US, and French forces occupying Germany, with the assistance of Ludwig Erhard, reformed the German currency and lowered a broad range of taxes (Klopstock, 1949). At the same time, the German Bizonal Economic Council assisted Erhard in removing price controls and rationing. Both sets of reforms restarted the German economy (Heller, 1949; Lutz, 1949). The following year, 1949, saw free elections and the division of Germany. In addition to the sharp reduction in tobacco taxes noted previously, 1948 marks the start of the substantial economic growth in West Germany and the separation of the two parts of Germany. Furthermore, we mark 1961, the year the Berlin Wall was erected, not because it dramatically changed conditions or trends in Germany but, rather, because it flags the start of increasingly divergent conditions in the two parts of Germany. We mark 1980 because in that year the West German government began to require a minimum tax on each cigarette. Finally, we mark 1989 because the Berlin Wall fell in November of that year, starting the process that saw Germany reunified and a period during which conditions facing smokers in the two parts of Germany began to slowly converge. Unfortunately, our data end in 2002, so we cannot trace out patterns of smoking from 2002 to 2010 when German states implemented policies to establish smoke-free public areas.

Across successive cohorts, the rate of smoking prevalence of men and women moves in opposite directions. For men, it is stable or decreasing in successive cohorts of men. For women, it increases across the oldest five cohorts and falls slightly thereafter.[6] Specifically, the peak smoking prevalence more than doubles across three cohorts of women—from approximately 20 percent among those ages 60–69 years in 2002 to 49 percent among those ages 40–49 years in 2002. Among the corresponding cohorts of men, the rate of smoking prevalence remains more or less stable at approximately 60 percent. These cohorts came of smoking age during the most intense period of the West German economic miracle. We conjecture that the increase in disposable incomes partly explains the rapid rise in smoking by German women and the stability of smoking by German men—a point to which we return when we compare the rates

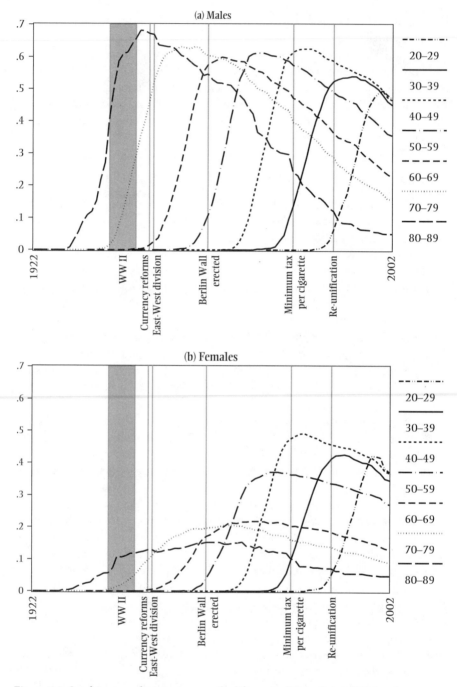

Figure 6.1 Smoking prevalence rates over the life course by gender and birth cohort.
SOURCE: German Socio-Economic Panel (SOEP). 2002. "Research data center of the SOEP." Berlin: SOEP.

of smoking for East and West Germany. This post-war peak in smoking (or plateau for men) ended with the male cohort that was 40–49 years old and the female cohort that was 30–39 years old in 2002. This latter cohort of women was 18–27 years old when Germany reunited in 1990. Subsequent cohorts smoked less (although the decrease is much less pronounced among German women than it is among German men).

To put the smoking patterns in economic context, in Figure 6.2 we plot time-series data on the average price of cigarettes and per capita gross domestic product (GDP) in Germany from 1925 to 2012. For the period 1949–1989, when Germany was divided, the price data are an average of the inflation-adjusted cigarette price in East and West Germany, weighted by the share of the total German population living in each area. We similarly average per capita GDP in East and West Germany for those years.[7] We do not plot the cigarette price for the period 1941–1948 because during these years, prices rose to many multiples of the pre-war level as the supply of cigarettes (and many other consumer goods) was severely restricted and because many Germans used cigarettes as a currency to buy other goods (Boelcke, 1986; Bignon, 2009).[8] Two events—the monetary reform of June 1948 and the passage of the US Economic Cooperation Act of 1948 (ECA; Marshall Plan)—helped to bring down the price of tobacco and cigarettes. The former event established the Deutsche Mark as a currency (Mendershausen, 1949). The latter event reduced shortages in the supply of cigarettes and tobacco. As mentioned previously, the United States not only granted aid that brought more consumer goods to residents in the US and British occupied zones but also sold tobacco to Germany at subsidized prices (Brown and Opie, 1953).[9]

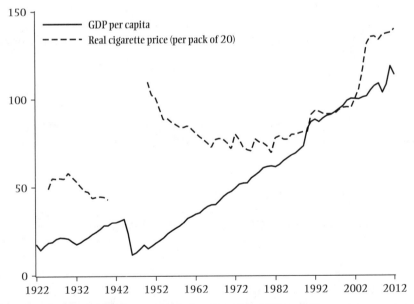

Figure 6.2 Economic development and cigarette prices (2002 = 100).
sources: GDP, Bolt, J., and J. L. van Zanden. 2013. "The first update of the Maddison Project; Re-estimating growth before 1820." Maddison Project Working Paper 4; cigarette prices, Statistisches Bundesamt Fachserie 14, Reihe 9.1.1, Absatz von Tabakwaren, and *Statistical Yearbook of the German Democratic Republic.*

Figure 6.2 shows that, as real per capita incomes were increasing during Germany's economic recovery, the real price of cigarettes fell from a high in 1949 that was more than 100 percent of the real 2002 cigarette price to a low in the early 1970s of approximately 70 percent of the 2002 price. During the same period, real per capita GDP increased from less than 20 percent of the 2012 per capita GDP in 1949 to almost 50 percent in the early 1970s. Together, the two trends are consistent with a rising smoking prevalence rate among women and the failure of smoking rates to decline among German men coming of age during these years. Starting in 1982, the price of cigarettes began to rise again in fits and starts. From 1985 until approximately 2002, the price rose at more or less the same rate as per capita GDP. Starting in approximately 2002, the real cigarette price began to rise sharply. Although our consumption data do not cover years after 2002, this figure suggests that smoking prevalence should continue to decline among recent cohorts.

In Figure 6.3, we plot the trajectories by chronological age to more clearly illustrate cross-cohort differences in smoking prevalence rates at particular ages. This figure highlights the fact that across successive cohorts of men and women, the age of initiation has fallen—dramatically so for women. In addition, it is clear that at the same chronological ages, the rate of smoking among younger cohorts of women is significantly higher than it was at the same age among older cohorts.

Although we do not plot them here, we note that these patterns are similar among men living in the former East and former West Germany but different for women in the two areas.[10] Relatively more West German women smoked than East German women. One possible explanation for this difference is that the standard of living in West Germany was rising faster than it was in East Germany. The difference in the rapid increase in smoking among women of younger cohorts is also consistent with this hypothesis. Among the women who straddled the years between World War II and the economic miracle in West Germany, one observes a much greater increase in smoking prevalence of the West Germans. In West Germany, approximately 20 percent of the 60- to 69-year-old cohort smoked, whereas almost 40 percent of women in the 50- to 59-year-old cohort smoked. By contrast, across these two cohorts of women in East Germany, smoking rates rose only slightly—from just under 20 percent to just over 20 percent. In East Germany, smoking among women jumped dramatically, to approximately 40 percent, among women of the next younger cohort—those who were 40–49 years old in 2002. This cohort of women was 28–37 years old when Germany reunified.

COHORT AND GENDER DIFFERENCES

In Table 6.1, we present six summary measures of smoking behavior, described in Chapter 1, that expose differences in smoking behavior of different cohorts that are less easy to notice in both Figure 6.1 and Figure 6.3. The comparisons reveal interesting patterns. As observed for other countries, although more men in the oldest cohort smoked than in all other cohorts, they smoked fewer cigarettes on average. Smoking intensity was highest among men aged 40–59 years in 2002. On the average day, smokers in those cohorts consumed more than a pack a day. In every cohort of men that followed, fewer men smoked, and when they did, they smoked fewer cigarettes on the average day. Similarly, smokers in the cohort of women aged 40–45 years in 2002 smoked more on average than women smokers in every other cohort.

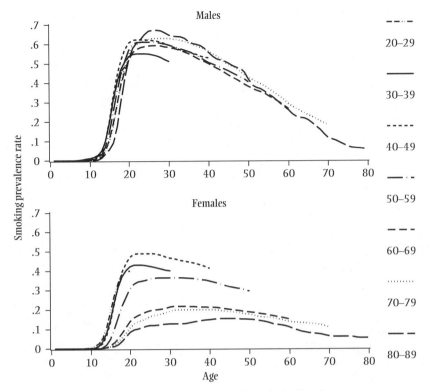

Figure 6.3 Change in smoking prevalence rate with age by birth cohort.
SOURCE: German Socio-Economic Panel (SOEP). 2002. "Research data center of the SOEP." Berlin: SOEP.

Table 6.1 also shows that men in the two oldest cohorts were approximately 27 years of age when their cohorts' smoking prevalence rate reached its peak. Men in successive cohorts reached their peak smoking prevalence at ages that were either the same or younger in successive cohorts. Among women, each successive cohort reached its peak smoking prevalence rate at younger ages over each successive birth cohorts. Finally, the average age of smoking initiation has fallen for each successive cohort of both men and women.

In addition, Table 6.1 shows that women in older cohorts started smoking at much older ages than did their male counterparts. However, as in the United States, United Kingdom, and other countries, relative to the older cohorts, men and women in younger birth cohorts are starting to smoke at younger and more similar ages. Women achieved "equality" with men in their age of initiation because the average age of smoking initiation of women fell faster across successive cohorts than it did across the corresponding cohorts of men. In fact, Germans reached this "equality" in a slightly younger cohort than in other countries (in the cohort of those who were 30–39 years old in 2002). As in countries discussed in previous chapters, smokers of both genders quit at approximately the same average age.

To highlight these patterns visually, in Figure 6.4 we plot the ratio of each indicator for men relative to the indicator for women, separately for each birth cohort.

Table 6.1. SUMMARY INDICATORS OF SMOKING BY GENDER AND BIRTH COHORT

Gender/ cohort	Sample size	Peak prevalence rate	Cigarettes per day	Years smoking	Average age at		
					peak	start	quit
MALES							
80–89	167	0.68	10	36	27	19	52
70–79	758	0.63	14	38	27	19	49
60–69	1554	0.60	19	34	26	19	45
50–59	1609	0.61	21	30	25	18	38
40–49	1976	0.63	21	25	26	17	33
30–39	1839	0.54	19	18	27	17	28
20–29	1182	0.50	16	9	22	16	22
FEMALES							
80–89	325	0.15	11	38	50	26	55
70–79	903	0.21	15	40	39	24	55
60–69	1565	0.22	14	33	34	23	46
50–59	1589	0.37	16	30	27	20	39
40–49	2111	0.49	16	24	25	18	33
30–39	1964	0.43	15	17	25	17	27
20–29	1278	0.42	14	9	20	16	22

SOURCE: German Socio-Economic Panel (SOEP). 2002. "Research data center of the SOEP." Berlin: SOEP.

Again, Figure 6.4 shows that, at the peak of smoking in every cohort, a greater fraction of men smoked than did women (Figure 6.4a). Except in the very oldest two cohorts (those age 70 years or older in 2002), men smoked more cigarettes on the average day than did women (Figure 6.4b). Interestingly, and similar to patterns in other countries, conditional on being a smoker, men and women in each birth cohort smoked approximately the same number of years (Figure 6.4c). Women in older cohorts started later than their male counterparts (Figure 6.4e), and women in these older cohorts reached their peak smoking prevalence rate when they were older than the men in their cohort (Figure 6.4d). Finally, men and women in every cohort quit at approximately the same ages (Figure 6.4f).

The gender ratios in the summary statistics are broadly similar for residents of the former East and the former West German states in all but two cases. In all but the youngest three birth cohorts, East German women reached their peak smoking prevalence rate when they were older, sometimes much older, than men in their cohort. Also, in the birth cohorts ages 60–69 and 50–59 years in 2002, East German female smokers quit at (slightly) younger ages than men, whereas in West Germany male and female smokers were quitting at approximately the same ages.[11]

A number of factors may explain these gender differentials. Some of the increase in smoking among women may be due to increasing participation of women in the

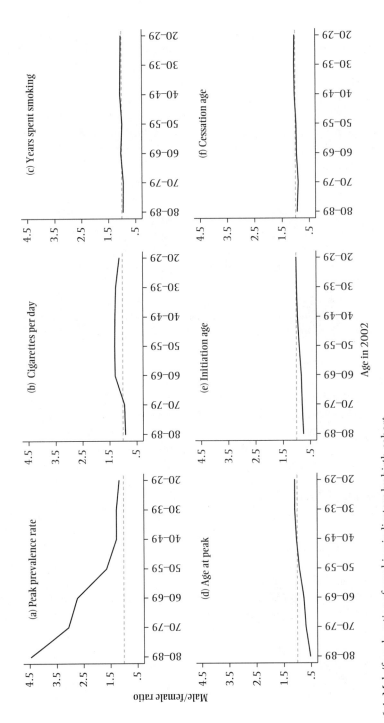

Figure 6.4 Male/female ratios of smoking indicators by birth cohort.
SOURCE: German Socio-Economic Panel (SOEP). 2002. "Research data center of the SOEP." Berlin: SOEP.

labor force and to increasing legal rights granted to women in the younger cohorts. However, at least in West Germany, women only recently gained more rights. In 1980, the Civil Code required that employers pay equal salaries to women with comparable education, training, and experience. In 1994, it made the language even more exact, requiring that employers pay women the same as men based on the work they performed, not just on their qualifications (Maier, 2007). Over time, a greater fraction of German women have been pursuing university studies. West German women's university participation rose from 31 percent of students in 1970 to 41 percent by 1989 (Solsten, 1996). At the same time, more women are working. According to the Organization for Economic Cooperation and Development, the rate of labor force participation of (West) German women increased from 50 percent in 1970 to 78 percent in 2010.[12] As in other countries, it seems that smoking patterns of women are related to the increasing economic independence of women. Despite these changes, gender wage differentials persist in Germany. Some observers suggest that the differences persist because Germany still largely follows a policy used in West Germany of the "breadwinner" model—giving economic incentives for one partner in a couple to work (usually the man) while the other partner (usually the woman) stays home to raise children. Finally, it is notable that, during the 1990s, cigarette firms targeted young German women with cigarette advertising that included images of women whose dress, demeanor, and situation suggested they were successful, westernized, and confident (Poetschke-Langer and Schunk, 2001). This likely encouraged more young women to take up smoking.

CONCLUSION

Smoking behavior of Germans was shaped by events and history linked to the Nazi regime, the social and economic turmoil during and after World War II, the division and reunification of Germany, and the economic miracle that West Germany produced. We conjecture that relatively high rates of smoking prevalence persisted in Germany in part because the anti-smoking movement—or any movement that highlighted health—got tainted by the link the Nazis established between their ideology and health campaigns. Smoking prevalence rates have begun to decline only among the most recent cohorts. Although the Nazi regime established smoke-free public areas long before they were established in other developed countries, those policies were abandoned after the end of World War II. Only recently have legislators in German states passed and begun to enforce laws that (again) establish smoke-free areas. With the passage of those laws, there appears to be a growing movement in Germany and awareness among Germans of the potential health risks associated with smoking and the protection of nonsmokers. This awareness is reflected in reforms to smoking bans that various states passed between 2010 and 2013. Although the effects of this changing economic, social, and legal environment remain to be seen, trends in other countries suggest that the higher costs and greater awareness will translate into lower smoking prevalence and better public health.

NOTES

1. The Australian government followed a similar policy for many years.
2. However, Bachinger et al. (2008) argue for a more nuanced interpretation.

3. The first documented tobacco tax dates to 1628 when the City of Köln levied an import duty on pipe tobacco (Schäfke, 1984).

4. Interested readers can find separate descriptions of the sample of residents of former East and West Germany at http://smoking-research.ehe.osu.edu/patterns-and-predictors.

5. The Appendix lists other events and websites that more exhaustively review the smoking-related German history.

6. These patterns match well with patterns reported by Westphal and Doblhammer (2012), who use the German Microcensus, and Schulze and Mons (2006), who use the German Federal Health Survey of 1998.

7. We describe the exact construction of these data in the Appendix.

8. Boelcke (1986) cites diary accounts from residents of Berlin and Hamburg who report paying a black market cigarette price in March 1945 that was 100 times the pre-war cigarette price.

9. In its first year, through December 1958, the ECA approved for purchase $106.4 million of tobacco. Of that amount, 14 percent was for the US and British occupied zones of Germany (US Economic Cooperation Administration, 1949, p. 36), with a price subsidy equal to 33.5 percent (only on sales prior to June 1948; p. 57).

10. Figures, tables, and results are available from the author on request.

11. Results are available on request.

12. See the Organization for Economic Cooperation and Development labor force statistics by sex and age available at http://stats.oecd.org/Index.aspx?DataSetCode=LFS_SEXAGE_I_R (accessed March 20, 2013). Solsten (1996) notes that 90 percent of East German women worked outside the home.

REFERENCES

Apel, M., K. Klein, R. J. McDermott, and W. W. Westhoff. 1997. "Restricting smoking at the University of Köln, Germany: A case study." *Journal of American College Health* 45:219–223.

Bachinger, E., M. McKee, and A. Gilmore. 2008. "Tobacco policies in Nazi Germany: Not as simple as it seems." *Public Health* 122:497–505.

Bignon, V. 2009. "Cigarette money and black market prices around the 1948 German Miracle." EconomiX Working Paper No. 2009-2, University of Paris West—Nanterre la Défense.

Boelcke, W. A. 1986. *Der Schwarz-Markt, 1945–1948.* Braunschweig, Germany: Westermann.

Bolt, J., and J. L. van Zanden. 2013. "The first update of the Maddison Project; Re-estimating growth before 1820." Maddison Project Working Paper 4. Available at http://www.ggdc.net/maddison/maddison-project/home.htm

Brenner, H., and B. Fleischle. 1994. "Smoking regulations at the workplace and smoking behavior: A study from southern Germany." *Preventive Medicine* 23:230–234.

Brown W. A., Jr., and R. Opie. 1953. *American Foreign Assistance.* Washington, DC: The Brookings Institution.

German Socio-Economic Panel (SOEP). 2002. "Research data center of the SOEP." Berlin: SOEP. Available at http://www.diw.de/en/diw_02.c.221180.en/research_data_center_soep.html

Heller, W. W. 1949. "Tax and monetary reform in occupied Germany." *National Tax Journal* 2:215–231.

Klopstock, F. H. 1949. "Monetary reform in western Germany." *Journal of Political Economy* 57:277–292.

Lickint, F. 1929. "Tabak und Tabakrauch als Ätiologischer Factor des Carcinoms." *Zeitschrift für Krebsforschung* 30:349–365.

Lickint, F. 1939. *Tabak und Organismus: Handbuch der gesamten Tabakkunde.* Stuttgart: Hippokrates.

Lutz, F. A. 1949. "The German currency reform and the revival of the German economy." *Economica* 16:122–142.

Maier, F. 2007, December. "The persistence of the gender wage gap in Germany." Discussion paper 01. Berlin: Harriet Taylor Mill-Institut für Ökonomie und Geschlechterforschung..

Mendershausen, H. 1949. "Prices, money and the distribution of goods in postwar Germany." *American Economic Review* 39:646–672.

Müller, F. H. 1939. "Tabakmissbrauch und Lungencarcinom." *Zeitschrift für Krebsforschung* 49:57–85.

Poetschke-Langer, M., and S. Schunk. 2001. "Germany: Tobacco industry paradise." *Tobacco Control* 10:300–303.

Pritzkoleit, K. 1961. *Auf Einer Woge von Gold.* Wien, Germany: Desch.

Proctor, R. N. 1997. "The Nazi war on tobacco: Ideology, evidence, and possible cancer consequences." *Bulletin of the History of Medicine* 71:435–488.

Proctor, R. N. 1999. *The Nazi War on Cancer.* Princeton, NJ: Princeton University Press.

Schäfke, W. 1984. *Blauer Dunst: Vier Jahrhunderte Tabak in Köln.* Köln, Germany: Druck und Verlagshaus Wienand.

Schairer, E., and E. Schöniger. 1943. "Lungenkrebs und Tabakverbrauch." *Zeitschrift für Krebsforschung* 54:261–269.

Schulze, A., and U. Mons. 2006. "The evolution of educational inequalities in smoking: A changing relationship and a cross-over effect among German birth cohorts of 1921–1970." *Addiction* 101:1051–1056.

Schweiger, P. 2010. *Rauchzeichen: Chronik der Tabakforschung in Forchheim von 1927 bis 2006.* Karlsruhe, Germany: Schweiger.

Seyfarth, C. 1924. "Lungenkarzinome in Leipzig." *Deutshe Medizinische Wochenschrift* 50:1497–1499.

Solsten, E. 1996. *A Country Study: Germany.* Library of Congress Call Number DD17. G475. Washington, DC: Federal Research Division, Library of Congress. Available at http://lcweb2.loc.gov/frd/cs/detoc.html.

US Economic Cooperation Administration. 1949. *Third Report to Congress of the Economic Cooperation Administration.* Washington, DC: US Government Printing Office.

Weigel, A. 1993. "Tabakanbau und Entwicklung der Tabaktrockenschuppen in Hatzenbühl." In *Arbeitskreis für Hausforschung: Jahrbuch für Hausforschung, Band 41.* Hausforschung und Wirtschaftsgeschichte in Rheinland-Pfalz. Bericht Über die Tagung des Arbeitskreises für Hausforschung in Sobernheim/Nahe vom 24–28. September 1990. Marburg, Germany: Jonas Verlag für Kunst und Literatur.

Weiss, C. M., and H. W. Herbert. 1854. *History of the French Protestant Refugees, Volume 1 from the Revocation of the Edict of Nantes to Our Own Days.* New York: Stringer & Townswend.

Westphal, C., and G. Doblhammer. 2012. "The diffusion of smoking in East and West Germany: Smoking patterns by birth year." Discussion paper No. 30. Rostock, Germany: Rostock Center for the Study of Demographic Change.

7

Smoking in Spain

ANA I. GIL LACRUZ

INTRODUCTION

When traders from the Americas introduced tobacco to Spain in the 16th century, the Spanish monarchy quickly recognized the potential of the new industry to generate substantial revenues. Hungry for the potential profits, the government established a royal monopoly in 1636 (Comín-Comín and Martín-Aceña, 1999). The royal monopoly controlled and taxed all tobacco products sold in Spain until 1886, when the government granted the monopoly to the Bank of Spain and a private management company named Compañía Arrendataria de Tabacos. These enterprises jointly managed the state-sponsored tobacco monopoly from 1886 to 1945, including the years of the Spanish Civil War and the early part of Franco's dictatorship. In 1945, Franco's regime granted the monopoly to a private company named Tabacalera, which ran the monopoly until 1998.

It is likely that the operation of Spain's tobacco industry as a monopoly affected patterns of smoking in the country not only because the monopoly set prices but also because it influenced whether and how vigorously the Spanish government warned its citizens about the health risks of smoking. As noted repeatedly in this book, since before the 1950s, the scientific community had been accumulating ever more convincing evidence that people damage their health by smoking. However, perhaps because Franco's regime heavily censored its domestic and foreign press, such information rarely appeared in print or broadcast media in Spain (one exception was the Spanish version of *Reader's Digest*). In addition, the Spanish academic community published no scientific papers in Spanish about the health risks of smoking. Whether by coincidence or not, it was in 1975—as Franco's regime was collapsing—that researchers finally published the first scientific evidence of the health consequences of smoking in Spanish (World Health Organization, 1975). Three years later, the Spanish Constitution granted autonomous communities the authority to legislate matters of public health, including regulatory authority over the sale and consumption of tobacco. Still, during the first decade of democracy, both central and regional authorities did not systematically distribute health information (Pascual and Viçens, 2004). There is a general perception that this inactivity came about because the

Spanish government was politically entangled with the industry and directly benefited from its monopolistic revenues.

It was only in 1986, when Spain joined the European Union (EU), that the central Spanish government began to actively regulate the sale and consumption of tobacco. As a condition of EU membership, Spain agreed to adopt a wide range of EU regulations that increased taxes generally and on tobacco in particular. The regulations also restricted how and to whom firms could market tobacco. For example, in 1989, Spain banned firms from advertising cigarettes on television to comply with the EU Directive "Television Without Frontiers." In 1986, the central government adopted the EU's general value added tax (VAT) of 12 percent. In 1992, the government increased the VAT to 16 percent, introduced an ad valorem tax and a minimum excise duty on tobacco, required firms to print health warnings on cigarette packs, and mandated that cigarettes be manufactured so that they contain no more than 15 mg of tar per cigarette.

In 1999, after the Spanish government had rescinded Tabacalera's monopoly, the industry merged with the French tobacco monopoly, SEITA, to form the Altadis Group. However, the government continued to protect the domestic tobacco industry by mandating that firms pay an extra duty on imported tobacco. In 2007, the government eliminated the extra duties.

The end of the monopoly brought new, and often less expensive, cigarette brands to the Spanish market. Adjusted for purchasing power parity, in 2004, the average price of cigarettes in Spain was approximately 85 percent of the EU cigarette price (López-Nicolás, 2004). These prices are low relative to other European countries, in part, because of how Spain levies taxes. As in other European countries, Spanish taxes represent approximately 80 percent of the final cigarette price. However, relative to those countries, Spain levies a lower minimum excise duty and a higher ad valorem tax (European Commission, 2010; Eurostat, 2010; Pinilla, 2004).[1] Consequently, changes in the retail price more directly reflect changes in the manufacturer's price. Perhaps as a result, the fiscal structure induced firms to operate Spanish factories that produced low-cost cigarette brands that helped them maintain a large market share (López-Nicolás and Viudes de Velasco, 2010).

After Spain's EU entry, the Spanish government also began regulating to whom firms could sell tobacco and where people could smoke. In fact, regional governments sometimes adopted tobacco control policies that were stricter than those of the central government. For example, in 1989, the central government banned the sale of tobacco products to anyone younger than 16 years. However, in 1991, the Spanish autonomous community of Catalonia passed a law that prohibited firms from selling tobacco products to anyone younger than 18 years. Regulation of smoking in public places started much later but increased over time. The central government banned smoking in schools and hospitals in 1998; in all workplaces, and all public places apart from some bars and hospitality establishments, in 2006; and in all public places, including previously exempted places, in 2011.

From a political perspective, research is needed to better understand the motivation of the Spanish governments to implement these tobacco control policies because evidence suggests that a majority of the electorate does not support them. In 2005, only 18 percent of smokers, 36 percent of ex-smokers, and 51 percent of nonsmokers thought that banning smoking in public places was a "good" or "very good" idea. Public opinion worsened further after the law was implemented. In 2008, these percentages fell to 12, 21, and 20 percent for smokers, ex-smokers, and nonsmokers, respectively. Some observers suggest that the public does not support these policies because Spanish society generally fails to abide by them (Centro de Investigaciones Sociológicas, 2005, 2008). Although the public increasingly accepts and complies with the 2011 ban, evidence suggests it does so only because authorities are enforcing the ban more strictly. Still, most people ignore the law (Organicaión de Consumidores y Usuarios, 2011). The incidence of smoking in Spanish bars (93 percent) is one of the highest in the EU (European Commission, 2010).

Researchers have suggested that the Spanish governments are implementing new tobacco control policies for fiscal reasons. A study by López-Nicolás (2004) found that the amount spent to treat people who suffer from one or more of six illnesses attributed to smoking accounts for nearly 80 percent of tobacco tax revenues. If this is accurate, it seems implausible that the remaining 20 percent of the public revenue can cover other direct costs plus external costs associated with tobacco use.

Given this national context, in this chapter, we present and discuss the smoking patterns from a life-course perspective for seven cohorts of Spanish men and women, born between 1922 and 1991.

SMOKING PREVALENCE RATES IN HISTORICAL PERSPECTIVE

Figure 7.1 plots smoking prevalence rates by gender and birth cohort (defined by age in 2011) over time. In each subfigure, we selectively mark the year or range of years that important events occurred. We mark the Spanish Civil War (1936–1939), the Franco regime (1939–1975), the adoption of laws to ban sex discrimination in labor markets (1961; for women only), Spain's accession into the EU (1986), and the opening of the tobacco industry to competition (1998). Although not flagged, more recent events—such as cigarette price wars in 2010 and 2011, the implementation of smoking bans in 2006 and 2011, and the economic downturn during the same period—likely affected smoking patterns as well.

Our data reveal smoking patterns that are broadly consistent with those presented in earlier studies that have used similar data and methods (e.g., Fernández et al., 2003).[2] One of the striking patterns is that, despite the substantial economic and political upheavals in Spain, the life-course smoking for Spanish men remained remarkably constant for the four oldest cohorts. Figure 7.1a indicates that men ages 50–89 years smoked in the same way over the course of their lives, despite the fact that the oldest cohort experienced a brutal civil war and the Franco dictatorship, whereas the younger cohorts experienced rapid economic growth and substantial social and informational changes after the end of the Franco regime. At the peak of their smoking prevalence, more than 65 percent of men in each cohort smoked. The smoking prevalence rate dropped dramatically for the three youngest cohorts that came of age after Spain's 1986 EU accession.

Figure 7.1 also reveals dramatic changes in women's smoking behavior over successive cohorts. Among the oldest two cohorts who were 70–89 years old in 2011, practically nobody smoked. Smoking prevalence rose dramatically among the cohorts that came of age at the end of—and just after—the Franco regime. Across all cohorts of women, smoking prevalence was highest in the cohort that was 40–49 years old

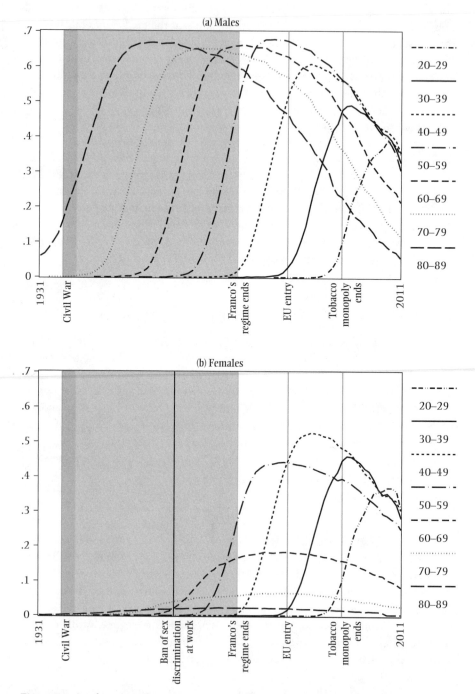

Figure 7.1 Smoking prevalence rates over the life course by gender and birth cohort.
SOURCE: Spanish National Health Survey (SNHS). 1995, 1997, 2001, 2003, 2006, 2011.
Madrid: Instituto Nacional de Estadística.

in 2011. Peak female smoking prevalence falls in all younger cohorts, and in the two youngest cohorts, men and women smoke at almost the same rate. It is notable that the smoking prevalence rates of men and women converged over time because smoking prevalence among men was falling more rapidly than it was among women.

To provide an economic context for these smoking patterns, in Figure 7.2, we plot the trend in per capita gross domestic product (GDP) and cigarette prices over the period of study. Throughout the years the oldest cohorts were growing up, per capita GDP in Spain stagnated—and even fell—during, and just after, the Spanish Civil War. Economic conditions stabilized but did not improve much when the war ended, in part because Franco's totalitarian government initially restricted trade and foreign firms' access to Spain's markets (León-Aguinaga, 2012). The Spanish economy began to grow again in 1953 when Spain signed the Pact of Madrid with the United States. That mutual defense agreement led the United States to invest more than $1 billion in Spain between 1953 and 1959, and during those years Spain's GDP grew 5 percent per annum. Nonetheless, the EU held that the Spanish economy did not qualify Spain as a member country at that time. Instead, Spain joined the International Monetary Fund, the World Bank, and the Organization for European Economic Co-operation—the precursor to the Organization for Economic Cooperation and Development. With help from these organizations, Spain abandoned its closed

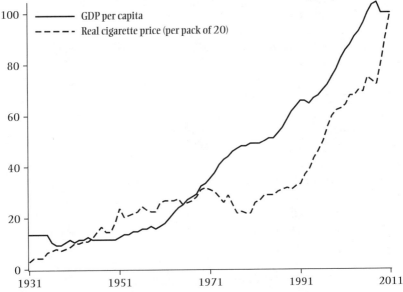

Figure 7.2 Economic development and cigarette prices (2011 = 100).
SOURCES: GDP, Instituto Nacional de Estadística. 2014. "Base de datos sobre la Contabilidad Nacional." Madrid: Instituto Nacional de Estadística. Cigarette prices, Castañeda, J. 1945. *El Consumo de Tabaco en España y sus Factores*. Madrid: Instituto de Estudios Políticos; Comín-Comín, F., and P. Martín-Aceña. 1999. *Tabacalera y el Estanco del Tabaco en España 1636–1998*. Madrid: Fundación Tabacalera; Tabacalera. 1992. *Series históricas de consumo de tabaco elaborado, 1957–1991*. Madrid: Tabacalera; Spanish Market Commission (http://www.cmtabacos.es/wwwcmt/paginas/EN/mercadosEstadisticas.tmpl).

economy. In 1959, it implemented its Stabilization Plan to end inflation and invited foreign investment. These changes led to what is known as the "Spanish miracle"—a period of sustained industrialization, foreign investment, and economic growth that lasted until the oil price shocks of the early 1970s. Between 1959 and 1974, other than Japan, no country's economy grew faster than that of Spain (Puig-Raposo and Álvaro-Moya, 2004). However, the energy crisis of 1973 hit Spain harder than other European countries, a fact that helped to further delay Spain's EU entry. Eventually, the German ultimatum during the Council of Stuttgart in June 1983—which linked the future financing of the EU with its enlargement—led to the Accession Treaty in June 1985 that made Spain an EU member. Thereafter, Spanish economic activity began to rise again due to expectations for economic integration with the other EU countries (Pérez-Fernández, 2005).

Figure 7.2 also shows that real cigarette prices increased dramatically during the study period and, until the end of Franco's regime, often increased at a rate that differed from the trend in per capita GDP. Between 1935 and 1970, the real price of cigarettes rose almost 40 percent, at a rate that exceeded the growth of per capita GDP until approximately 1961. This increase in price coincides with the start of the Spanish Civil War, during which tobacco use was essential among soldiers, and it continued after the war when the tobacco industry was modernized so that it could offer (more expensive) cigarettes of higher quality. The real price of cigarettes fell again in Spain during the 1970s while per capita GDP steadily grew and, consequently, cigarettes became relatively more affordable. From the mid-1980s until 1992, the real cigarette price increased at approximately the same rate as per capita GDP. Starting in 1992, the real price increased faster than per capita GDP, in part because of the tobacco taxes introduced in that year, and continued to do so until 1998, when the Spanish government ended the tobacco monopoly. For almost a decade after this, per capita GDP and cigarette prices grew again at approximately the same rate, but prices escalated sharply when the recent recession hit. Researchers have used this substantial variation in price to estimate models of smoking behavior. For example, using Spanish data from 1957 to 1997, López-Nicolás (2002) showed that changes in cigarette price do not predict whether a person starts smoking, but they do predict whether a smoker quits.

Overall, however, the trends in economic conditions and cigarette prices are not always consistent with the observed smoking patterns of men and women. For example, smoking among men was consistently very popular before the 1990s, when GDP per capita was relatively low and cigarettes were often expensive. The smoking patterns are even more complicated for women, whose behavior appears to change sharply after Franco's death. As we discuss in the next section, it is plausible that these patterns can be explained by the changing social norms that accompanied economic development, as well as the spread of information on the health risks of smoking.

In Figure 7.3, we plot cohort smoking trajectories on an age scale to highlight the similarities and differences in each cohort's smoking behavior when they are at the same point in their life course. This figure reveals a pattern not easy to observe when the trajectories are plotted on the calendar scale. It shows that initiation behavior was strikingly similar among the oldest three cohorts of Spanish men. The first boys in these cohorts began to smoke at approximately age 10 years, and of those who would ever start, most had done so by approximately age 20 years. By contrast, the

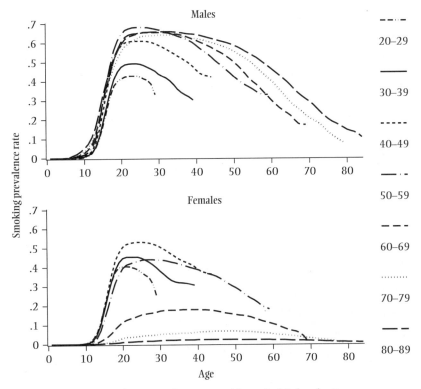

Figure 7.3 Change in smoking prevalence rate with age by birth cohort.
SOURCE: Spanish National Health Survey (SNHS). 1995, 1997, 2001, 2003, 2006, 2011.
Madrid: Instituto Nacional de Estadística.

youngest two cohorts started smoking when they were slightly older, but similar to
the older cohorts, practically all of the eventual smokers in the youngest cohorts had
already started by age 20 years. By plotting the trajectories on a chronological age
scale, we also reveal that the similarity in the smoking trajectories of older cohorts
of Spanish men is limited only to the age of smoking initiation. After reaching a
peak prevalence of 60–68 percent at approximately age 20 years, these male Spanish
smokers systematically quit at different rates as they age. In general, at every age,
fewer men in older cohorts quit than do men of the same age in younger cohorts.
Like Figure 7.1, Figure 7.3 shows that few women smoked in the two oldest generations. Furthermore, cohorts of women who were in their 30s and 40s in 2011 were
the cohorts with the highest smoking prevalence rates. But for all women older than
50 years in 2011, the peak smoking rate largely persists over their remaining lives;
thus, once these women started smoking, they were not likely to quit.

COHORT AND GENDER DIFFERENCES

To further highlight gender differences, in Table 7.1, we report the six summary
measures of smoking behavior described in Chapter 1. This table clearly shows that
older cohorts of Spanish men and women differed greatly in whether, when, and
how they smoked, and that those differences have faded among younger generations.

Table 7.1. SUMMARY INDICATORS OF SMOKING BY GENDER AND BIRTH COHORT

Gender/ cohort	Sample size	Peak prevalence rate	Cigarettes per day	Years smoking	Average age at		
					peak	start	quit
MALES							
80–89	3392	0.67	15	52	31	17	61
70–79	4717	0.65	17	41	35	17	53
60–69	5158	0.66	21	35	29	17	47
50–59	6136	0.68	22	28	26	17	39
40–49	7322	0.61	21	20	24	17	33
30–39	5876	0.49	16	12	24	17	27
20–29	2488	0.39	15	7	22	16	22
FEMALES							
80–89	6237	0.02	13	38	47	29	58
70–79	7203	0.07	13	34	50	27	53
60–69	6815	0.18	14	31	39	22	46
50–59	7239	0.44	16	27	28	18	38
40–49	8178	0.53	14	20	25	17	32
30–39	6468	0.46	14	12	23	17	27
20–29	2519	0.37	12	7	23	16	21

SOURCE: Spanish National Health Survey (SNHS). 1995, 1997, 2001, 2003, 2006, 2011. Madrid: Instituto Nacional de Estadística.

In the oldest cohort, the gender difference between the peak smoking prevalence was 65 percentage points. In the youngest cohort, the peak prevalence rate for men and women is almost equal. Furthermore, the smoking prevalence rate of young cohorts of Spanish women peaked at almost exactly the same age as young cohorts of Spanish men. Whereas older cohorts of Spanish women started smoking later than their male counterparts (29 vs. 17 years old for the oldest cohort), in younger cohorts, female and male smokers started at essentially the same average age. Interestingly, among those who chose to smoke, men and women quit smoking at almost the same average age. Finally, the average female smoker consumes fewer cigarettes than the average male smoker, although the difference ranges only between two and seven cigarettes per day.

Figure 7.4 illustrates these trends graphically by plotting, for each cohort, the ratio of each smoking indicator for men relative to the corresponding indicator for women, with a ratio of 1 indicating that men and women in a given cohort have similar smoking behavior. It is readily apparent that younger cohorts of Spanish women have achieved "equality" with younger cohorts of Spanish men with respect to smoking prevalence (where the size of convergence is most dramatic), the duration of the smoking habit, the age of smoking initiation, and the age at peak smoking prevalence. Along all these dimensions, current generations of women and men smoke in

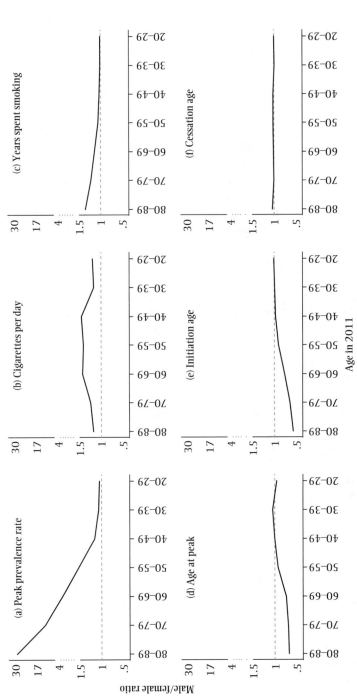

Figure 7.4 Male/female ratios of smoking indicators by birth cohort.

SOURCE: Spanish National Health Survey (SNHS). 1995, 1997, 2001, 2003, 2006, 2011. Madrid: Instituto Nacional de Estadística.

almost identical ways. As noted previously, across all cohorts, women and men who smoke also quit at approximately the same age. Finally, with respect to the number of cigarettes smoked on average, Spanish men have always been and continue to be somewhat heavier smokers than women—a difference that has been sustained across generations.

The gender difference in smoking patterns among cohorts who lived through Franco's regime is not surprising. During the 1930s, the economic and working conditions of most workers were poor, but they were especially oppressive for women. The average working woman earned approximately half of the salary of the average working man. Furthermore, social norms about living arrangements meant that few single women lived independently. Women typically lived with their parents until they married and with their husbands after that. Although feminist groups succeeded in lobbying the Republican government of 1931 to reform many laws (women secured the right to vote, to divorce under certain conditions, and certain forms of maternity leave), the Franco regime either ignored or rescinded those rights after the Civil War (Eiroa San Francisco and Sanmartí Roset, 2011). Those events also eviscerated the small but growing movement for women's rights led by women in the middle and professional classes (Keene, 1999). Franco's regime replaced that movement with the Sección Feminina of the Falange—a group that espoused a more conservative role for women in Spanish society (Enders, 1999). In general, the Franco regime limited women's educational and professional opportunities (Santos, 1994). Throughout its duration, most Spanish women did not work, received less education than men, and stayed at home to raise children. In addition, women could neither own a passport nor exercise property rights. Some limited change concerning the social attitudes about gender roles became evident in the 1960s, when the women's liberation movement began to revive and achieved the passage of laws banning sex discrimination in the labor market. But it was only when Spain ratified its constitution in 1978 that it formally recognized women's rights. And as social norms have changed, so have smoking rates.

After Franco's death, and as industrialization spread throughout Spain, demand for labor rose sharply, especially in urban areas. As a result, a large share of the population moved from the rural areas to the cities,[3] and women increasingly entered the labor force. Between 1950 and 1972, the fraction of Spanish women who worked did not exceed 24.4 percent.[4] From 1972 to 2010, the labor force participation rate of women age 25–59 years rose continuously from 30.5 to 84.4 percent. The economic liberalization also reawakened groups that began to lobby for further social change (Laraña, 1993; Morcillo-Gómez, 1999). Thus, the cohorts of women who came of age after Franco's death in 1975—whose smoking behavior we observe to converge with that of men—acquired more education and entered new and more highly paid occupations (Cebrián-Villar, 2001).

As mentioned previously, the end of the Franco dictatorship also influenced patterns of smoking in Spain because it allowed information on the health risks of smoking to spread in the country. In principle, this development should have resulted in lower smoking rates for both men and women. However, note that, starting in the 1970s, the tobacco industry also began to aggressively market cigarettes to women. It appears that tobacco companies anticipated that the end of Franco's regime might cause women's roles in Spanish society to change, and they began to advertise cigarettes in ways that sought to equate cigarette smoking with positive images of emancipation, success, and gender equality (Amos and Haglund, 2000; Fernández et al., 2004; Schiaffino et al., 2003). An example of such strategic efforts is the large increase in television advertisements for blond tobacco and "light" cigarettes (Shafey et al., 2004).

CONCLUSION

During Spain's long history with tobacco, a wide array of economic, political, social, and regulatory forces shaped who, when, and how Spaniards smoked. In the period we study, from 1927 to 2011, the market for tobacco evolved from a state-sponsored monopoly to a competitive sector. Spain experienced a brutal civil war, a dictatorship, the establishment of a modern democracy, and dramatic changes to its economy and social norms. Spain's entry into the EU in 1986 led to the introduction of tobacco control policies that limited when, where, and how firms could market cigarettes, as well as who could buy them and where they could be smoked.

The patterns of life-course smoking behavior seem to vary systematically with these forces. Three striking patterns stand out. First, among older cohorts, almost all Spanish men and almost no Spanish women smoked. Second, Spanish women took up smoking as they gained control over more economic resources and as social norms changed. The emancipation of Spanish women began in 1961 with the passage of anti-sex discrimination laws, market liberalization, and sustained economic growth that opened employment opportunities for them. These changes accelerated with the end of the Franco regime in 1975 and have solidified with the entry of Spain into the EU. Events marking that emancipation are associated with, first, an increasing and then a decreasing smoking prevalence among Spanish women. Third, smoking patterns of Spanish men and women have converged so that, among younger cohorts of Spaniards, life-course smoking patterns have no gendered pattern.

The rather perverse equality that younger cohorts of Spanish women have achieved with Spanish men has broader public health implications. Because there are essentially no gender differences in the smoking behavior of the youngest cohorts, one expects that these cohorts will likely experience similar health consequences of smoking. Because most of the more severe consequences do not surface until people are in their mid to late 60s, the trends portend a convergence in the rate and incidence of smoking-related illnesses of Spanish men and women (Fernández et al., 2001).

NOTES

1. The excise tax is even lower on loose tobacco than on cigarettes; thus, smokers—especially among young people—typically roll their own cigarettes (López-Nicholas and Viudes de Valesco, 2010).

2. We use the same survey as this study but show slightly different patterns. This is likely because we use larger samples (more survey waves) and a more sophisticated method to correct for differential mortality of smokers and nonsmokers (Lillard et al., 2014).

3. Whereas in 1960, only 49.5 percent of the population was living in rural areas, by 2001, this share had increased to 76.4 percent (Instituto Nacional de Estadística, 2004).
4. Data on labor force participation rates of women are scarce before 1972. These figures are drawn from the Instituto de la Mujer (1990).

REFERENCES

Amos, A., and M. Haglund. 2000. "From social taboo to "torch of freedom": The marketing of cigarettes to women." *Tobacco Control* 9:3–8.

Castañeda, J. 1945. *El Consumo de Tabaco en España y sus Factores*. Madrid: Instituto de Estudios Políticos.

Cebrián-Villar, M. 2001. "Las Fuentes del Crecimiento Económico Español 1964–1973." *Revista de Historia Económica* 19:277–301.

Centro de Investigaciones Sociológicas (CIS). 2005. "Tabaquismo y Nueva Normativa Anti-Tabaco. Estudio No. 2627." Madrid: CIS. Available at http://www.cis.es/cis.

Centro de Investigaciones Sociológicas (CIS). 2008. "Estudio sobre Hábitos Relacionados con el Tabaco. Estudio No. 2751." Madrid: CIS. Available at http://www.cis.es/cis.

Comín-Comín, F., and P. Martín-Aceña. 1999. *Tabacalera y el Estanco del Tabaco en España 1636-1998*. Madrid: Fundación Tabacalera.

Eiroa San Francisco, M., and J. Sanmartí Roset. 2011. "Also in the newspapers: Spanish women in defense of the 2nd Republic." *Observatorio Journal* 5:25–44.

Enders, V. L. 1999. "Problematic portraits: The ambiguous historical role of the Sección Femenina of the Falange." In *Constructing Spanish Womanhood: Female Identity in Modern Spain*, edited by V. L. Enders and P. B. Radcliff, pp 375–397. Albany: State University of New York Press.

European Commission. 2010. *Eurobarometer—Tobacco*. Brussels: European Commission.

Eurostat. 2010. "Price levels for food, beverages and tobacco across the European market differ significantly—Issue number 30/2010." Available at http://ec.europa.eu/eurostat/web/products-statistics-in-focus/-/KS-SF-10-030.

Fernández, E., S. Gallus, A. Schiaffino, A. López-Nicolás, C. La Vecchia, H. Barros, et al. 2004. "Price and consumption of tobacco in Spain over the period 1965–2000." *European Journal of Cancer Prevention* 13:207–211.

Fernández, E., A. Schiaffino, J. M. Borras, O. Shafey, J. R. Villalbi, and C. La Vecchia. 2003. "Prevalence of cigarette smoking by birth cohort among males and females in Spain, 1910–1990." *European Journal of Cancer Prevention* 12:57–62.

Fernández, E., A. Schiaffino, and M. Peris. 2001. "Tabaquismo en mujeres: Un problema de salud emergente." *Enfermedades Emergentes* 3:184–190.

Instituto de la Mujer. 1990. *La Mujer in España: Situación social*. Madrid: Ministerio de Asuntos Sociales.

Instituto Nacional de Estadística. 2004. "Tendencias demográficas durante el siglo XX en España." Madrid: Instituto Nacional de Estadística. Available at http://www.ine.es.

Instituto Nacional de Estadística. 2014. "Base de datos sobre la Contabilidad Nacional." Madrid: Instituto Nacional de Estadística. Available at http://www.ine.es.

Keene, J. 1999. "Into the clear air of the plaza: Spanish women achieve the vote in 1931." In *Constructing Spanish Womanhood: Female Identity in Modern Spain*, edited by V. L. Enders and P. B. Radcliff, pp 325–347. Albany: State University of New York Press.

Laraña, E. 1993. "Modelos de interpretación y cuestiones de método en el estudio de las migraciones Españolas." *Política y Sociedad* 12:121–137.

León-Aguinaga, P. 2012. "La historiografía Española y las relaciones con los Estados Unidos de América: Las consecuencias del Pacto de Madrid y la Transición." *Cuadernos de Historia Contemporánea* 34:357–370.

Lillard, D. R., R. Christopoulou, and A. I. Gil Lacruz. 2014. "Re: Validation of a method for reconstructing historical rates of smoking prevalence." *American Journal of Epidemiology* 180(6):656–658.

López-Nicolás, A. 2002. "How important are tobacco prices in the propensity to start and quit smoking? An analysis of smoking histories from the Spanish National Health Survey." *Health Economics* 11:521–535.

López-Nicolás, A. 2004. "Tabaquismo y economía pública." In *Manual de Tabaquísmo*, edited by J. Jiménez-Ruiz, K. O. Fagerström, and J. L. Díaz-Maroto. Madrid: Aula Médica Edicciones.

López-Nicolás, A., and A. Viudes de Velasco. 2010. "Posibilidades y limitaciones de las políticas fiscales como instrumentos de salud: Los impuestos sobre consumos nocivos. Informe SESPAS 2010." *Gaceta Sanitaria* 24:85–89.

Morcillo-Gómez, A. 1999. "Shaping true Catholic womanhood: Francoist educational discourse on Women." In *Constructing Spanish Womanhood: Female Identity in Modern Spain*, edited by V. L. Enders and P. B. Radcliff, pp 51–69. Albany: State University of New York Press.

Organicaión de Consumidores y Usuarios. 2011, April. "La Nueva Ley del Tabaco. Encuesta a la Población Española de 18 a 75 años." Available at http://www.cnpt.es.

Pascual, F., and S. Viçens. 2004. "Aspectos históricos, económicos y sociales del tabaco." *Adicciones* 16:13–25.

Pérez-Fernández, P. 2005. "La integración económica de España en la Union Europea (1986–1995)." *ICE* 826:107–114.

Pinilla, J. 2004. "Oportunidades y Obstáculos en la Batalla contra el Tabaquismo en España." Invited presentation at the Spanish National Conference of Health Economics. Available at http://www.fgcasal.org/aes/docs/Pinilla.pdf.

Puig-Raposo, N., and A. Álvaro-Moya. 2004. "La guerra fría y los empresarios Españoles: La articulación de los intereses económicos de Estados Unidos en España, 1950–1975." *Revista de Historia Econoómica* 22:387–424.

Santos, J. 1994. "Los orígenes sociales de la democracia en España." *Ayer* 15:165–188.

Schiaffino, A., E. Fernández, C. Borrell, E. Salto, M. Gracia, and J. M. Borras. 2003. "Gender and educational differences in smoking initiation rates in Spain from 1948 to 1992." *European Journal of Public Health* 13:56–60.

Shafey, O., E. Fernández, M. Thun, A. Schiaffino, S. Dolwick, and V. Cokkinides. 2004. "Cigarette advertising and female smoking prevalence in Spain, 1982–1997." *Cancer* 100:1744–1749.

Spanish National Health Survey (SNHS). 1995, 1997, 2001, 2003, 2006, 2011. Madrid: Instituto Nacional de Estadística. Available at http://www.ine.es/jaxi/menu.do?type=pcaxis&path=%2Ft15/p419&file=inebase&L=1.

Tabacalera. 1992. *Series históricas de consumo de tabaco elaborado, 1957–1991.* Madrid: Tabacalera.

World Health Organization. 1975. "Los efectos del tabaco sobre la salud." *Revista de Sanidad e Higiene Pública* 49:203.

PART III

Eastern Europe and Asia

China, Russia, Ukraine, and Turkey

8

Smoking in China

FENG LIU

INTRODUCTION

New World tobacco was introduced to China in approximately 1550 as part of a globalized process that began with the arrival of European traders in the 1520s. It was the participants in those early transregional trade networks (local dockhands, port-based merchants, and traders who traveled inland over long distances) who helped to transform tobacco from an exotic import to a local Chinese product consumed everywhere. Within 100 years of tobacco's arrival, smoking long pipes became a cultural practice widely shared across spatial, class, and gender lines. Despite the efforts of the early Qing state to ban it,[1] many among the Qing elite were already dedicated smokers when the Manchus took Beijing in 1644. Over time, tobacco became essential to the rituals of hospitality and to all social encounters, in part because people believed that it could prevent or treat a host of ailments—purported health benefits that were popularized in medical books. As more people consumed tobacco, more farmers cultivated it. The continuing increase in demand and the relatively low production and transportations costs made tobacco a highly commercialized agricultural product that circulated widely through market networks stretching across the empire (Benedict, 2011).

Demand for particular forms of tobacco shifted as China interacted more with European and other Western cultures. At first, snuff was more popular than pipes, but people increasingly identified it as vulgar. In the early 19th century, water pipe tobacco became quite popular among the elite, and over the course of the century, it began to reach a broader market, including women and the rural gentry (Weining, 2005). In Republican China, however, the emerging urban intelligentsia and the new entrepreneurial class came to regard water pipes and snuff as "old-fashioned." Their preferences and those of "traditional" Chinese consumers shifted to cigarettes (Fang, 1989).

In part, preferences shifted because Western firms promoted machine-rolled cigarettes to millions of Chinese smokers. Those firms introduced new forms of advertising and mass marketing, hired native place-based Chinese trading companies, and commissioned agents and merchant firms with rich experience in the tobacco business (Ma, 2008). As Chinese entrepreneurs established local companies, they competed with the international suppliers on the basis of both product differentiation and price. Some Chinese-owned businesses, such as the Nanyang Brothers Tobacco Company, marketed their cigarette as a "national product" and not a "Western" commodity, even though the raw material, industrial machinery, and technical know-how were all imported. These businesses sold cigarettes at prices low enough to be within reach of consumers at the lower end of the socioeconomic ladder.

Manufactured cigarettes were among the few factory-produced goods consumed everywhere in Republican China. By the 1930s, the ready-made cigarette had become a mass consumer commodity, smoked not only by the modern urban population but also by peasants (Zhang, 2006). Of course, people smoked both factory-produced cigarettes and inexpensive generic cigarettes produced by foreign firms and by smaller Chinese companies, hand-rollers, and counterfeiters. After 1925, local hand-rolling workshops popped up everywhere and made inexpensive "brand-name" cigarettes available to Chinese consumers not only in large cities but also in small towns and villages. Rural residents and poor urban consumers increasingly bought these cheaper cigarettes. By 1935, hand-rolled cigarettes accounted for 25 percent of all cigarettes sold (Shao, 2013).

Foreign businesses lost access to the Chinese market altogether when the People's Republic of China was founded. From then on, the government imposed a quota of goods to produce to all manufacturers and farmers. They received rewards for meeting the quota, and exceeding the quota was rarely beneficial. It was not until Deng Xiaoping announced the "Open Door Policy" in the 1970s that China rejoined the global market. With that policy shift, cigarette sales multiplied. Annual domestic cigarette consumption rose by four times during a period of 30 years, from approximately 0.5 trillion cigarettes in 1978 to more than 2 trillion in 2006 (Peto et al., 2009). Importantly, this increase took place while China sustained a quota system and protected its tobacco industry. Two administrations were established to regulate tobacco production and trade. One was the State Tobacco Administration (STMA), responsible for policy setups, such as the allocation of tobacco and cigarette production quotas among provinces and the pricing of tobacco leaf. The second was the China National Tobacco Company (CNTC), the only legitimate buyer of tobacco leaf in China (Hu et al., 2010). By imposing high tariff rates on imported cigarettes (at 65 percent), China made it extremely difficult for foreign brands to make a profit and guaranteed the monopoly power of the CNTC.

While protected, the national industry modernized its production. By introducing Western machinery (including entire production lines), China saw a dramatic increase in not only cigarette output—from 852 billion in 1981 to 1736 billion in 1993—but also cigarette quality (Zhou, 2000). Due to a change in the quota system adopted in 1992, production of higher quality cigarettes was stimulated. For example, the share in total output of filter-tip cigarettes rose from 5.8 percent in 1982 to 93.5 percent in 1996, which resulted in excess supply of more expensive cigarettes and shortage of cheap cigarettes (Wang, 2009). In response, the CNTC set a rule requiring local tobacco companies to produce a certain amount of low-level cigarettes annually and subsidized them for the relatively low profit margin.

In 2001, China entered the World Trade Organization (WTO). Contrary to most people's belief, entering the WTO did not bring a dramatic change in national cigarette production. Although in 2003 the tariff on cigarette imports declined to 25 percent, in

2005, foreign brands shared only 3 percent of the Chinese market (Peto et al., 2009). The unexpectedly low profits to some extent aided the building of an underground black market for cigarettes in China. To meet the high demand in the black market, production of counterfeit cigarettes soared. Based on 2007 statistics, the estimated counterfeit cigarette production in mainland China was between 93 and 186 billion annually, accounting for up to 3.3 percent of the total (legal and illegal) global cigarette market (Lampe et al., 2012). To control the illegal production and trade of cigarettes, the Chinese government has a set of general and specific laws and regulations, such as Section 140 (Chapter 3) of the Chinese Criminal Law of 1997, which deems the production and trade of counterfeit goods punishable, and the Chinese Law of Tobacco Exclusive Sale, with specific fining clauses on legal traders who sell counterfeit tobacco products.

Currently, China is the largest tobacco producer in the world, providing almost one-third of the global supply. In 2005, it produced 2.435 million tons of tobacco leaf using less than 1 percent of the country's agricultural land. The gross value of flue cured tobacco (the most commonly planted tobacco in China) was 23.23 billion renminbi (RMB) in that same year, contributing 1 or 2 percent to the Chinese agricultural economy (Hu et al., 2010). Twenty-four of the 31 provinces in mainland China, including approximately 4 million farm households or approximately 2 percent of all farmers, grow tobacco. Among them, Yunnan, Guizhou, Henan, and Sichuan have become the four largest producers.

Given the scale of production and the public ownership of the tobacco industry, it is not surprising that the Chinese government has given low priority to anti-smoking policy. At times, public movements played a more important role for tobacco control than the law or regulations. For example, in 1987, China held its first "No Smoking Day," and in 1979 it approved a public notice for the State Council titled "On the Hazards of Smoking and Tobacco Control Advocacy" (Fang et al., 2009). In 2005, China ratified the WHO Framework Convention on Tobacco Control (FCTC). This treaty aims to regulate tobacco companies' actions in party countries using strategies such as forbidding smoking in public; professional help for quitting smoking; health warnings on packages; bans on tobacco advertising, promotion, and sponsorship; and increasing tobacco taxes and prices.

Although China has enforced many of these regulations, enforcement has been inefficient. For example, the implementation guidelines in Article 11 of the FCTC recommend that health warnings on cigarette packages should cover 50 percent (and not less than 30 percent) of the pack surface. But Chinese regulations only require a line to mark one-third of the display area, while the warning text itself covers substantially less than one-third of the display area with tiny characters, making the warning even more unnoticeable (Wan et al., 2012). Another example is that, according to the WHO FCTC's requirement, party countries should adopt price and tax policies to reduce tobacco consumption. Although China did adopt a new tobacco tax structure with the intention to increase retail prices by 3.4 percent, this price increase has not yet passed on to the consumer (Qian et al., 2010; Li et al., 2012). One reason for this is that smokers respond by substituting more expensive for less expensive cigarette brands (Li et al., 2010). Because of this high price elasticity of demand, tobacco companies mainly absorb the tax increase. Thus, it is merely a profit transfer from producers to local and state governments and does not play a significant role in controlling tobacco consumption.

Today, more cigarettes are smoked in China than in any other country in the world. The Chinese smoke one of every three cigarettes smoked globally.[2] China is distinct not only in the sheer volume of consumption but also in very stark differences in patterns of consumption between men and women. For reasons still not fully understood, recent younger cohorts of Chinese women are much less likely to smoke both relative to men and relative to women in the cohorts of their mothers and grandmothers. For example, in 1996, the National Prevalence Survey showed that 63 percent of men and only 4 percent of women older than ages 15–69 years had ever regularly smoked. By 2002, the fraction of male ever-smokers had increased to 66 percent, and the fraction of female ever-smokers had decreased to 3.1 percent (Peto et al., 2009).

Next, we document, in detail, smoking patterns for seven generations of Chinese men and women born during 1920–1989, and we discuss those patterns in light of the aforementioned national context.

SMOKING PREVALENCE RATES IN HISTORICAL PERSPECTIVE

In Figure 8.1, we plot life-course smoking prevalence rates by gender and birth cohort (defined by age in 2009), which are generally consistent with previously published estimates. For example, Weng et al. (1987) and Yang et al. (1999) present cross-sectional smoking prevalence rates for 1984 and 1996, respectively. Because they provide rates by age group, we can compare them to the smoking rates of the equivalent age groups from our data, as a validation exercise. For instance, those who we observe in 2009 to be 80–89 years old (i.e., born between 1920 and 1929) were 55–64 years old in 1984 and 67–76 years old in 1996. Figure 4 of Yang et al. (1999) shows that approximately 43 percent of males in that cohort were smokers in 1984 and approximately 35 percent of that cohort were smokers in 1996. These percentages match our estimates rather well.

In Figure 8.1, we also flag years when noticeable events occurred that might have an impact on smoking behavior. We mark the year when the People's Republic of China was founded (1949); the years of the Cultural Revolution, which was a period of political and economic instability for China (1966–1976); the year of the "Open Door Policy," when China opened its market to the world (1978); and 1994 because that year saw a great flow of information about the health risks of smoking (Yang et al., 2002).

We find some interesting patterns. First, we confirm that smoking in China is a male phenomenon. In every male cohort, the share of smokers at the peak of the smoking trajectory never falls below 50 percent, except in the youngest cohort that may not have yet reached its peak smoking prevalence rate. Smoking prevalence increases across successive generations of men who came of age before the 1978 market reform, it peaks at more than 60 percent for men who came of age immediately after the market reform (i.e., those born during 1950–1959), and it declines across all generations thereafter. This decline is more noticeable for the cohort of men who reached adulthood after information about the smoking health hazards began to spread more widely. In contrast to men, in no cohort of women did smoking prevalence exceed 10 percent, and every successive cohort of women smoked less.

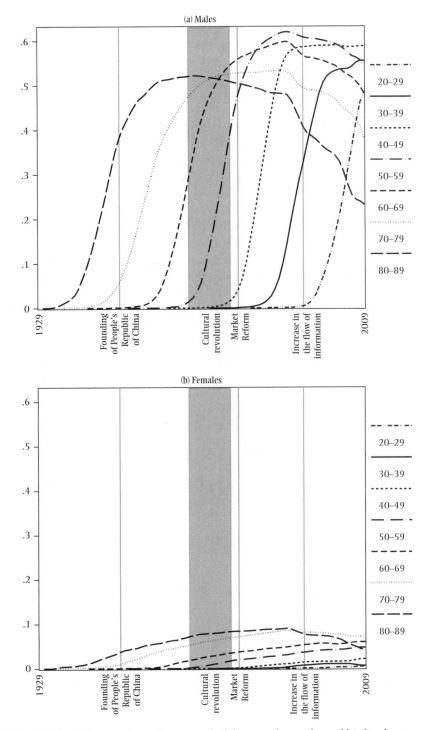

Figure 8.1 Smoking prevalence rates over the life course by gender and birth cohort.
SOURCE: China Health and Nutrition Survey (CHNS). 1991, 1993, 1997, 2000, 2004, 2006, 2009. Chapel Hill, NC/Beijing: Carolina Population Center, University of North Carolina/ National Institute of Nutrition and Food Safety, Chinese Center for Disease Control and Prevention.

The intergenerational pattern of smoking among Chinese women runs counter to the stylized patterns suggested in the "cigarette epidemic" model of Thun et al. (2012). Those authors argue that, as a country develops economically, the prevalence of smoking among women will first increase and then decline, lagging that of men by a few decades. Clearly, the Chinese experience does not follow this model. In our data, smoking prevalence among women peaks three generations earlier than smoking prevalence of men. As we explain in the next section, this pattern likely relates to Chinese cultural norms and customs.

To provide more economic context for the smoking patterns, in Figure 8.2, we plot trends in cigarette prices and real gross domestic product (GDP) per capita for the period 1950–2009, for which data are available. Throughout this period, the Communist party led the Chinese government. The variation in the price data reflects both changes in cigarette taxes imposed by the government and changes that result from market forces. Both the price of cigarettes and per capita GDP rose dramatically during the period, with most of the increase occurring after the economic reforms in the late 1970s. Before 1978, there was less year-to-year variation in cigarette price because these were officially set by the central government. After 1978, prices increased at roughly the same rate as the GDP but slowed down around 1996. Between 1997 and 2000, they fell sharply, and they remained almost unchanged from 2000 to 2009. Song and Zheng (2012) suggest that the government actively forced cigarette manufacturers to not raise prices when higher taxes were levied. Given that, at the same time, GDP per capita kept rising, cigarettes became more affordable. Still, it is during this period that smoking rates among men have fallen the most, which suggests that the spread of anti-smoking information might have played a larger role than economic factors.

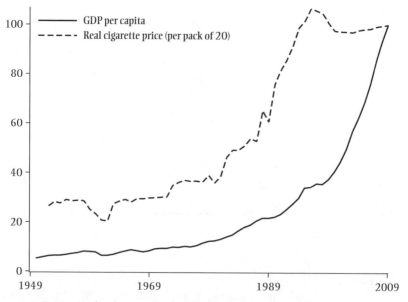

Figure 8.2 Economic development and cigarette prices (2009 = 100).
SOURCES: GDP, Conference Board Total Economy Database; Prices, *China Statistical Yearbook*.

In Figure 8.3, we plot smoking prevalence rates on an age scale to more easily compare smoking patterns of different cohorts when members of each cohort were the same chronological age. This figure shows that men in the oldest cohort were less likely to smoke than similarly aged men in all but the youngest three of the later cohorts. At the same time, men in the oldest cohorts started to smoke at older ages than did men in later cohorts. Interestingly, the average age of initiation has steadily fallen over time—a point that becomes more apparent in Table 8.1. Figure 8.3 also shows that the smoking trajectories are generally flat, and they are only slightly flatter for men in the oldest two cohorts, which suggests that men in those cohorts were less likely to quit smoking as they aged than were similarly aged men in younger cohorts. Unlike male cohorts, older cohorts of women had a larger share of smokers than did younger cohorts at every age. However, as with men, once women start smoking, they generally do not quit. This high persistence of the smoking habit in China has been documented in previous research. Reports in 2005 and 2010 indicated that approximately 74 and 84 percent of smokers, respectively, did not want to quit or never thought about quitting (China Ministry of Health, 2010).

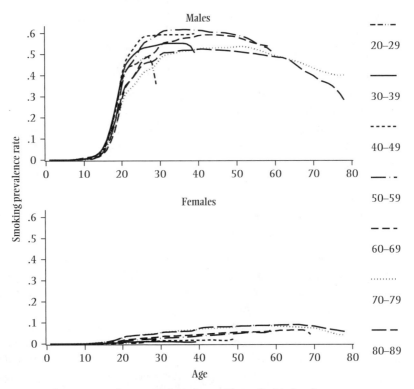

Figure 8.3 Change in smoking prevalence rate with age by birth cohort.
SOURCE: China Health and Nutrition Survey (CHNS). 1991, 1993, 1997, 2000, 2004, 2006, 2009. Chapel Hill, NC/Beijing: Carolina Population Center, University of North Carolina/National Institute of Nutrition and Food Safety, Chinese Center for Disease Control and Prevention.

Table 8.1. SUMMARY INDICATORS OF SMOKING BY GENDER AND BIRTH COHORT

Gender/ cohort	Sample size	Peak prevalence rate	Cigarettes per day	Years smoking	Average age at		
					peak	start	quit
MALES							
80–89	1340	0.52	14	49	42	23	69
70–79	2803	0.53	15	42	53	24	63
60–69	4119	0.60	17	34	45	23	56
50–59	5841	0.62	18	27	36	22	47
40–49	5084	0.59	17	19	37	20	38
30–39	4043	0.56	15	11	35	19	29
20–29	1852	0.49	13	5	24	18	21
FEMALES							
80–89	1568	0.09	10	40	65	33	72
70–79	3183	0.08	10	35	55	32	64
60–69	4242	0.06	12	29	64	29	56
50–59	6394	0.05	12	24	55	27	48
40–49	5699	0.02	12	16	44	24	
30–39	4076	0.01	13	11	31	19	36
20–29	1742	0.00	5	11	25	16	

NOTE: Average quitting age is blank for women in the 20–29 and 40–49 years cohorts because these cohorts never quit smoking.

SOURCE: China Health and Nutrition Survey (CHNS). 1991, 1993, 1997, 2000, 2004, 2006, 2009. Chapel Hill, NC/Beijing: Carolina Population Center, University of North Carolina/National Institute of Nutrition and Food Safety, Chinese Center for Disease Control and Prevention.

COHORT AND GENDER DIFFERENCES

To reveal more cohort and gender differences masked by the Figures 8.1 and 8.3, in Table 8.1 we report, for each gender and cohort, the six summary measures of smoking behavior described in Chapter 1 (i.e., smoking duration, the number of cigarettes smoked per day, the age of initiation, the age of cessation, the age when the cohort reached its peak smoking prevalence, and the peak smoking rate). Table 8.1 more clearly shows the bell-shaped pattern of peak smoking prevalence across successive cohorts of men and the consistently declining rate of peak smoking prevalence among successive cohorts of women. Among men, both the smoking prevalence rate and average cigarette consumption were highest in the middle-aged cohorts, but for women the corresponding pattern is different. The oldest cohort of women had the highest smoking rates, but the highest number of cigarettes smoked per day was in a younger cohort. For example, whereas among 80- to 89-year-old women smoking was more popular, 30- to 39-year-old women smoked more heavily.[3]

Table 8.1 also shows that over successive cohorts of all women and of men since the 70- to 79-year-olds, the average smoker starts at increasingly younger ages. The average age of initiation among men and women fell from 23 and 33 years, respectively, in the oldest cohort to 18 and 16 years in the youngest cohort. It is notable that, even though not many women smoke in the youngest cohort, those women who do smoke start at younger ages than male smokers in that cohort. Another noticeable pattern is that, on average, women in the youngest cohort have smoking histories more than twice as long as those of their male counterparts. The 20- to 29-year-old women are more likely to become persistent smokers than are men in the same birth cohort, who nonetheless smoke more heavily during their relatively short smoking period.

Gender differences in smoking patterns are more obvious in Figure 8.4, which plots male/female ratios of the six smoking indicators presented in Table 8.1 by birth cohort. Figure 8.4a shows that the ratio of peak prevalence rates of men and women increases progressively across generations, reaching the impressively high value of 123 for the youngest cohort. As reported in Table 8.1, this number results from a maximum prevalence rate of 0.4 percent for women and 49 percent for men. Figures 8.4b, 8.4c, and 8.4e confirm that among women in all but the youngest cohort the smoking prevalence rate was approximately 30 percent lower than among their male counterparts, had shorted smoking histories, and started smoking later. The youngest cohort presented a different picture: Women aged 20–29 years smoked approximately 60 percent less cigarettes than their male counterparts but spent more years smoking, with a younger initiation age. Finally, Figure 8.4f shows that women of all cohorts quit smoking at older ages than their male counterparts.

To understand these gender differences in smoking behavior, one should be familiar with China's social norms regarding offering gifts and the role of women in society. Giving gifts is a long-existing cultural phenomenon in China, especially prevalent during Mid-Autumn and the Chinese New Year festivals. Use of propriety and proper etiquette are strongly emphasized in Confucianism and are seen as pivotal in maintaining harmony among social hierarchical relationships (Rich and Xiao, 2012). Cigarettes are among the most common gifts that people offer each other, perhaps because they are easy to buy and easy to carry around. Accepting a cigarette can symbolize a person's willingness to engage in a future business partnership (Wank, 2000). A 2008 Internet survey in China conducted by the think tank Research Center for Health Development showed that 52 percent of respondents have offered cigarettes to others; 61 percent agreed that offering cigarettes is an effective way to develop and maintain relationships; and 51 percent agreed that cigarettes are appropriate gifts for families, friends, and relatives during the holidays (Rich and Xiao, 2012). Thus, to some extent, this ritualized "gifting" culture unfortunately helped increase cigarette consumption in China.

In addition to smoking participation, offering cigarettes as gifts also promotes the persistence of the smoking habit because it entails a continuing exposure to cigarettes. The 2008 Internet survey also indicated that 80 percent of respondents believed that it was rude to refuse cigarettes offered by others (Rich and Xiao, 2012). Moreover, in a prospective cohort study collecting data from 11,583 self-reporting Chinese adolescents, the ability to refuse an offered cigarette strongly predicted future smoking status (Grenard et al., 2006).

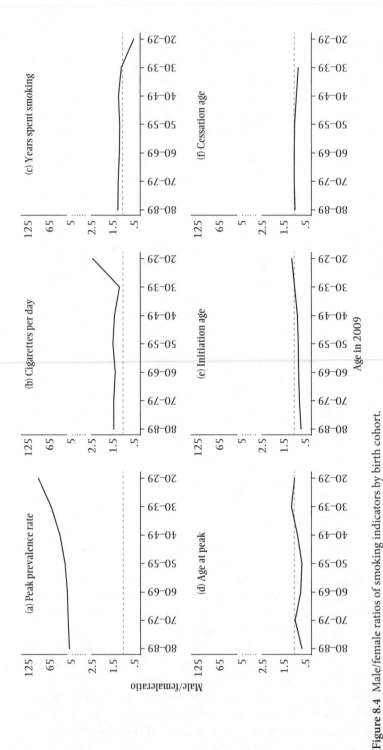

Figure 8.4 Male/female ratios of smoking indicators by birth cohort.
SOURCE: China Health and Nutrition Survey (CHNS). 1991, 1993, 1997, 2000, 2004, 2006, 2009. Chapel Hill, NC/Beijing: Carolina Population Center, University of North Carolina/National Institute of Nutrition and Food Safety, Chinese Center for Disease Control and Prevention.

This gifting culture also relates to the large range of cigarette prices in China, which start at 1 RMB ($0.14) and increase to more than 220 RMB ($33) per pack (Xiao and Kohrman, 2008). People typically offer cigarettes of different quality in different situations: A cigarette given to a boss or business partner would likely have a higher price than that shared with a neighbor or gate guard (Rich and Xiao, 2012). Being aware of this, some foreign firms deliberately promote their brands as luxury brands. Research suggests that people who smoke foreign brands in China are more image conscious than those who regularly consume Chinese brands, and they discriminate against the cheap foreign brands that are perceived to be inferior (Chu et al., 2011).

Although the use of cigarettes as gifts is very common, it obviously has much lower influence on smoking rates among women compared to men. The powerful social norms regarding women's role in society offer an explanation for this. Before the 20th century, it was generally considered uncouth or unchaste for women to smoke in public. In the first decade of the 20th century, respectable women could smoke, but it was something they did at home. Chinese intellectuals began to promote the idea that public smoking was a sign of promiscuity and that if women of child-bearing age smoked, they would cause the Chinese people to become extinct. The May Fourth Movement of 1919 (a protest against the imperial government after the Treaty of Versailles) added a nationalist flavor to this line of reasoning (Benedict, 2011). That movement predisposed the Chinese public to accept the notion that women who smoked were selfish, pleasure-seeking, and self-indulgent consumers of a foreign product that, by undermining their reproductive capacities, threatened the health and well-being of the nation. These campaigns had some success up to the early Republican years, when the so-called "new women" began boldly smoking cigarettes in public. However, this shift in attitudes was short-lived. In the 1930s and through the 1949 revolutionary era, female smoking became increasingly associated with loose morals, foreign decadence, and bourgeois extravagance, and it echoed the previous idea of threatening reproduction and signaling insufficient national loyalty. As a result, in Mao's China, most women did not smoke, and this norm persisted over time, despite several counteracting forces.

An example of a factor that promoted smoking among women, running counter to social norms, was the voucher policy from 1960 to 1980. During that time, the Chinese had to use vouchers to purchase food and other life necessities, including cigarettes. Vouchers for buying cigarettes were handed out for free to every adult. Although a significantly larger percentage of women initiated smoking cigarettes during the period than men (Fang et al., 2009), overall smoking rates among women remained low and decreasing.

Cigarette suppliers have also tried to alter the cultural perceptions. They have advertised cigarettes with images that portray female smokers as elegant, romantic, sexually attractive, sociable, emancipated, feminine, and rebellious. However, the smoking patterns we observe in our data suggest that, so far, those efforts have not been successful.

CONCLUSION

China has a long history of tobacco production and consumption, which can be dated back to the 1550s. Today, it has the largest population of smokers and is the largest tobacco producer in the world. However, during the past two decades, information on the hazards of smoking has spread more widely, and average smoking prevalence has been steadily decreasing.

Interestingly, smoking in China has always been—and increasingly is—a male phenomenon. Smoking prevalence is much higher in all cohorts of men relative to women, and this difference has widened across generations. The age at smoking initiation is higher for women than men, except for the two most recent cohorts of adults. Especially for women ages 20–29 years in 2009, our data suggest that they started smoking at a younger age than their male counterparts, and they also smoke more persistently than men.

In 2005, China ratified the WHO Framework Convention on Tobacco Control, but the progress in anti-smoking policy has been generally slow. As this process accelerates and the rules regulating tobacco production and cigarette consumption become stricter, smoking prevalence should decline more significantly.

NOTES

1. In 1638, one imperial edict in China declared that the possession, use, or sale of tobacco was a capital offense.
2. The 2002 National Smoking Prevalence Survey showed that there were approximately 300 million reported current smokers in that year (China Ministry of Health, 2006).
3. Earlier studies documented the changing intensity of cigarette use over time using aggregate data. According to these studies, the average daily cigarette consumption among Chinese men increased from 4 to 10 cigarettes from 1972 to 1992, but due to a steep rise in the late 1990s, it increased to 15 cigarettes (Yang et al., 2008; Peto et al., 2009). Similarly, the share of smokers who consume more than 20 cigarettes per day doubled between 1998 and 2003, exceeding 50% (Qian et al., 2010).

REFERENCES

Benedict, C. 2011. *Golden-Silk Smoke: A History of Tobacco in China, 1550–2010.* Berkeley: University of California Press.

China Health and Nutrition Survey (CHNS). 1991, 1993, 1997, 2000, 2004, 2006, 2009. Chapel Hill, NC/Beijing: Carolina Population Center, University of North Carolina/National Institute of Nutrition and Food Safety, Chinese Center for Disease Control and Prevention. Available at http://www.cpc.unc.edu/projects/china.

China Ministry of Health. 2006. "China smoking and health report 2006." Beijing: China Ministry of Health.

China Ministry of Health, Center for Disease Control and Prevention (CDC). 2010. "Gats China Report." Beijing: China CDC.

Chu, A., N. Jiang, and S. A. Glantz. 2011. "Transnational tobacco industry promotion of the cigarette gifting custom in China." *Tobacco Control* 20(4):e3.

Fang, H., and J. A. Rizzo. 2009. "Did cigarette vouchers increase female smokers in China?" *American Journal of Preventive Medicine* 37:s126–s130.

Fang, X. 1989. "On the Shanghai modern national cigarette industry" (in Chinese). *Shanghai Economic Research* 6:15.

Grenard, J. L., Q. Guo, G. K. Jasuja, J. B. Unger, C. P. Chou, P. E. Gallaher, et al. 2006. "Influences affecting adolescent smoking behavior in China." *Nicotine and Tobacco Research* 8:245–255.

Hu, T., Z. Mao, J. Shi, and W. Chen. 2010. "The role of taxation in tobacco control and its potential economic impact in China." *Tobacco Control* 19:58–64.

Lampe, K., M. K. Kurti, A. Shen, and G. A. Antopoulous. 2012. "The changing role of China in the global illegal cigarette trade." *International Criminal Justice Review* 22:43–67.

Li, Q., A. Hyland, G. T. Fong, Y. Jiang, and T. Elton-Marshall. 2010. "Use of less expensive cigarettes in six cities in China: Findings from the International Tobacco Control (ITC) China Survey." *Tobacco Control* 19:i63–i68.

Li, Q., T. Hu, Z. Mao, R. J. O'Connor, G. T. Fong, C. Wu, J. et al. 2012. "When a tax increase fails as a tobacco control policy: The ITC China project evaluation of the 2009 cigarette tax increase in China." *Tobacco Control* 21:381.

Ma, A. 2008. *The Influence of BAT Business Activities on Shandong* (in Chinese). Qingdao: Ocean University of China.

Peto, R., Z. M. Chen, and J. Boreham. 2009. "Tobacco: The growing epidemic in China." *Cardiovascular Disease Prevention and Control* 4:61–70.

Qian, J., M. Cai, J. Gao, S. Tang, L. Xu, and J. A. Critchley. 2010. "Trends in smoking and quitting in China from 1993 to 2003: National Health Service Survey data." *Bulletin of the World Health Organization* 88:769–776.

Rich, Z. C., and S. Xiao. 2012. "Tobacco as a social currency: Cigarette gifting and sharing in China." *Nicotine & Tobacco Research* 14:258–263.

Shao, Y. 2013. "Development of old system of Chinese tobacco industry and its modern fate" (in Chinese). *Chinese Tobacco Science* 12:6.

Song, G., and R. Zheng. 2012. "Price, tax and cigarette smoking: Simulations of China's tobacco tax policy." *Frontiers of Economics in China* 7:604–626.

Thun, M., R. Peto, J. Boreham, and A. D. Lopez. 2012. "Stages of the cigarette epidemic on entering its second century." *Tobacco Control* 21:96–101.

Wan, X., S. Ma, J. Hoek, J. Yang, L. Wu, J. Zhou, et al. 2012. "Conflict of interest and FCTC implementation in China." *Tobacco Control* 21:412–415.

Wang, J. 2009. "Global-market building as state building: China's entry into the WTO and market reforms of China's tobacco industry." *Theory and Society* 38: 165–194.

Wank, D. 2000. "Cigarettes and domination in Chinese business networks: Institutional change during the market transition. In *The Consumer Revolution in Urban China*, edited by D. S. Davis, pp 268–286. Berkeley: University of California Press.

Weining, T. 2005. "Smoking custom in China and tobacco spreading way during Ming and Oing Dynasty" (in Chinese). *Journal of Chinese Historical Geography*. 17:97–106.

Weng, X. Z., Z. G. Hong, and D. Y. Chen. 1987. "Smoking prevalence in Chinese aged 15 and above." *Chinese Medical Journal* 100:886–892.

Xiao, S., and M. Kohrman. 2008. "Anthropology in China's health promotion and tobacco." *Lancet* 372:1617–1618.

Yang, G., L. Fan, J. Tan, G. Qi, Y. Zhang, J. M. Samet, et al. 1999. "Smoking in China: Findings from the 1996 National Prevalence Survey." *Journal of the American Medical Association* 282:1247–1253.

Yang, G., L. Kong, W. Zhao, X. Wan, Y. Zhai, L. C. Chen, et al. 2008. "Emergence of chronic non-communicable diseases in China." *Lancet* 372:1697–1705.

Yang G. H., J. M. Ma, N. Liu, and L. N. Zhou. 2002. "Smoking and passive smoking in Chinese." *Chinese Journal of Epidemiology* 26:77–83.

Zhang, H. 2006. *The Tobacco Industry in Henan From 1912 to 1937* (in Chinese). Henan, China: Henan University.

Zhou, H. 2000. "Fiscal decentralization and the development of the tobacco industry in China." *China Economic Review* 11:114–133.

9

Smoking in Russia and Ukraine Before, During, and After the Soviet Union

DEAN R. LILLARD AND ZLATA DOROFEEVA

INTRODUCTION

Of all the countries included in this book, the Russian Federation and Ukraine, both individually and collectively, provide what are arguably the most interesting contexts for studying similarities and differences in smoking patterns of successive generations in and across countries. The smoking patterns of people living in the Russian Federation and Ukraine have been shaped by historical, political, and tobacco-related events common among cohorts growing up when the two countries belonged to the Union of Soviet Socialist Republics (USSR), as well as country-specific events and developments that occurred after they separated in 1992. These events have been dramatic, tragic, and consequential.

Events include the establishment of a society under the USSR in which the economy was largely directed by the central government, an organization that led to social and economic disasters, including the widespread famine that Stalin's government caused when it forced collectivization on Soviet agriculture. As in other countries, World War II also disrupted economic and social life, in addition to decimating the male population. In the subsequent period, the USSR economy grew and then stagnated again. Political events such as the Sino-Soviet split in 1960 disrupted tobacco markets for many years.

Some of these events (e.g., the famine induced by forced collectivization) affected the social and economic well-being of Ukrainians to a much greater extent than they affected people living in Russia. To capture the shared history and the differing environments in the two countries, we briefly describe the pre-USSR period and then introduce the context in the USSR that older Ukrainians and Russians shared up to 1991. Starting in 1992, the Russian Federation and Ukraine operated as independent nations whose economic and social policies potentially diverged. Here again, it is interesting to compare and contrast smoking patterns to search for evidence of lingering similarities and growing differences as the two countries follow different tobacco control policies and experience different economic conditions. We discuss post-USSR developments for Russia and Ukraine in separate sections. Finally, we also present patterns of smoking behavior of residents of those countries in separate sections.

Pre-USSR Period

Tobacco first arrived in Russia in the mid-16th century, but historians point to Peter the Great as the person who established the large-scale commerce that supplied the growing demand for tobacco because previous rulers opposed the consumption of tobacco (Frederiksen, 1943). In 1634, Czar Mikhail Romanov had made it illegal for residents of Russia (foreign and native) to possess, buy, or sell tobacco (Frederiksen, 1943). The edict stipulated that the state could execute violators and confiscate their property. Although the ban reinforced a decree that the Orthodox Church had previously issued, people still consumed tobacco. After 10 years of failed enforcement efforts, Alexei Romanov, son and successor of Czar Mikhail, established a state tobacco monopoly in 1646. He reasoned that, in addition to providing revenue to the government, it would be easier to control consumption. However, within 3 years, after continuing opposition and intense pressure from the powerful patriarch Nikon, Czar Alexei rescinded the monopoly and again prohibited consumption (Bogoslovski, 1941). The prohibition lasted until the early 18th century when Peter the Great could not resist the revenue potential of a domestic tobacco industry. He established the domestic cultivation of tobacco and actively promoted smoking (Frederiksen, 1943). In 1716, he invited a Holland master to establish a tobacco plantation and factory in the small Ukrainian town of Akhtyrsk. High transportation costs and low-quality tobacco caused the domestic tobacco industry to decline, but tobacco consumption continued to rise.

As in other countries, after the invention of the cigarette-rolling machine in 1881, the Russian tobacco industry began to mass produce cigarettes. An early design of cigarettes called *papirosa* became widespread. Relative to pipes or cigars, papirosas were easier to smoke. The production of papirosas quickly became one of the most profitable sectors of the tobacco industry. By the end of the 19th century, the Russian tobacco industry finally bore fruit. In mid-century, there were four large tobacco factories operating in Moscow (Osipova, 2007). Merchants advertised tobacco widely in newspapers and magazines, and through the 20th century, the tobacco industry continued to develop.

During the period spanning the 19th and 20th centuries, the tobacco industry actively sought to develop a market for cigarettes among women. The industry used pictures of women with modern hairstyles and dresses, smoking papirosas, to try to create the image in the minds of women that smoking signaled independence. Before that time, the industry ignored women as potential consumers of tobacco, in part because the Orthodox Church had successfully cultivated the social view that women who smoked were immoral (Levin, 2009). This view not only dominated social norms in 19th-century Russian and Ukrainian society but also persisted well into the 20th century after the USSR was established (Kelly, 2009; Starks, 2009).

USSR

The 1917 Bolshevik revolution altered the Russian tobacco industry. After the revolution, the Bolsheviks nationalized tobacco factories, halted all tobacco exports, and, in 1918, monopolized tobacco agriculture (Osipova, 2007). Because the government shut down private shops that sold tobacco, it became difficult to buy tobacco. The Bolshevik government quickly prohibited the barter trading that naturally arose. By the end of the 1920s, the market for tobacco was in severe disequilibrium. Demand continued to be high, but supply was severely limited.

The domestic tobacco industry began to recover during the first "pyatiletka"—the famous 5-year plan of state production that ran from 1928 to 1932. The USSR rapidly increased exports, mainly to Finland, whose imports of USSR leaf tobacco quintupled from 63,395 pounds in 1922 to 300,383 pounds in 1933 (Hutson, 1937). In the latter half of the 1930s, the Soviet tobacco industry launched a new brand, "Belomorkanal," that quickly gained popularity. It remained popular for decades and is still sold in Russia today (Gorchakova, 2009). However, the turmoil of World War II disrupted the tobacco industry. Almost all production halted because most tobacco factories were in war zones. Because tobacco helped battlefield performance, the Soviet government attached strategic importance to the delivery of tobacco to soldiers. The USSR provided cigarette papers and strong leaf tobacco (mahorka) with rations to soldiers in World War II (US War Department, 1943).

In contrast to common perceptions, tobacco was advertised in the USSR. Although there is evidence that British firms bought advertising as early as 1944, most credible evidence indicates that domestic firms started advertising in 1947 (Markham, 1964). A 1947 *New York Times* article reported that, although the government had banned commercial radio advertising in 1935, Radio Moscow again began to air commercial advertising ("Russians Pleased by Radio 'Spot Ads,'" 1947). According to Gruliow (1962), cited by Markham (1964), the content of the tobacco advertising in the USSR was similar to that of advertising in other countries.

The USSR tobacco market was again disrupted in 1960 when the country stopped importing tobacco from China because China and the USSR split politically. To replace the lost Chinese tobacco, the USSR imported up to 75 percent of all tobacco grown in Bulgaria (Neuburger, 2009). Despite continuing imports of Bulgarian tobacco, the USSR tobacco industry did not return to its pre-war level of production until 1965.

The Soviet tobacco industry introduced innovations some years after they were introduced in other countries. Filtered cigarettes were introduced in the United States in the late 1950s. The Soviets introduced filtered cigarettes in 1965 and light cigarettes in the late 1970s and early 1980s (Gorchakova, 2009). The industry also bought Western technology and contracted with Western firms to modernize production processes.

Soviet citizens traded cigarettes on illegal contraband markets—often at prices much higher than the official state-set cigarette price. Because the price of foreign cigarettes on this contraband market was so high, mostly wealthier smokers bought foreign brands such as Marlboro, Winston, and Kent cigarettes. The USSR also tried to satisfy demand by importing cigarettes—usually from Bulgaria. Until 1991, between 70 and 90 percent of imported cigarettes came from Bulgaria (Neuburger, 2009).

An anti-smoking element from the early history of Russia and Ukraine existed after the Bolshevik revolution, but that movement was as ineffective in the USSR as it had been in czarist Russia or Ukraine. In 1920, Nickolay Semashko, the first "People's Commissar of Health," with the permission of Lenin, attempted but failed to pass a smoking ban (Starks, 2009). He did, however, convince the government to stop issuing tobacco to soldiers, but this policy was soon abandoned. As mentioned previously, tobacco was issued as part of regular rations to troops in World War II. Although the Ministry of Health recognized the health risks of smoking, the Soviet government launched no widespread anti-tobacco campaign. It did print and distribute anti-smoking posters in two periods—from the late 1920s until 1934 and from 1967 through the 1970s. In the intervening years, from 1935 to 1966, the government produced and distributed only a handful of posters (Fox, 2009a, 2009b).

In the 1970s and early 1980s, the Soviet government began to introduce tobacco control policies, and it implemented some health awareness policies. The government banned smoking on all flights of 3 hours or less in 1973 and extended it to flights of 4 hours or less in 1977. Despite the bans, anecdotal reports suggest that the government did not enforce it (Deber, 1981). The government proposed a general public awareness campaign about the dangers of smoking in 1977 and required the industry to test a warning label. It did so in 1978 on a small batch of Iava cigarettes, and later the government gradually required that the label be printed on cigarette packages of all brands (Deber, 1981). In 1980, the government issued further regulations that sought to increase anti-smoking campaigns, establish smoke-free workplaces, and limit youth access to tobacco.

The substantial potential for government revenues from tobacco likely influenced the evolution of the industry. The lure of revenue helped build opposition to tobacco control attempts in the 1920s and 1930s. In addition, after the election of Mikhail Gorbachev as General Secretary of the Communist Party of the Soviet Union in 1985, he introduced *perestroika*—the political movement that applied market-like reforms to increase the efficiency of the socialist regime. As part of the perestroika reforms, Gorbachev sought the assistance of Western firms to upgrade and modernize production capacity in the tobacco industry.

In December 1991, Ukraine, Russia, and Belarus signed the Commonwealth of Independent States (CIS) treaty and officially ended the USSR. From that date onward, residents of those countries faced market conditions and regulatory environments that increasingly diverged from each other.

Russia Post-USSR

The establishment of the Russian Federation led to rapid changes in the market conditions and tobacco control regulations that both potential and regular smokers faced. In 1992, the Russian Federation fully opened its markets to firms based in other countries. In the period immediately after the breakup of the Soviet Union, from 1993 to 1997, the Russian cigarette market was characterized by high levels of contraband cigarette sales and by "shadow" production of cigarettes (Joossens et al., 2000). The cigarettes sold, even brands available in other countries, had significantly more tar than the same brands sold in the United States (Kholmogorova and Prokhorov, 1994). In 1995, the Russian government first levied excise taxes on all imported cigarettes. Because Western firms were investing heavily in former republics of the USSR, the production of cigarettes increased dramatically from 1995 onward (Gilmore, 2004). At the same time, firms increased advertising on television, billboards, magazines, and newspapers, targeting youth, women, and especially urban residents (Gilmore and McKee, 2004, 2005).

The new Russian government began to more actively try to control the consumption and marketing of tobacco. The government regulated tobacco advertising in 1993 and 1995, restricting its content and when it aired and mandated warnings, but both attempts were ineffective. In 1996, tobacco advertising on television and radio was finally banned (Demin, 2001). The government passed more significant legislation in 2001 when it banned youth smoking, smoking in public transportation and other public places, and required that firms print warning labels on cigarette packs. A watershed event occurred in 2008 when the Russian government accepted the World Health Organization's Framework Convention on Tobacco Control (FCTC). To comply with the FCTC, the government passed new regulations in 2010 to enlarge the mandated health warnings on cigarette packs and, in 2012, required that firms include graphic images as part of the mandated health warnings. In February 2013, President Vladimir Putin signed a law establishing 100% smoke-free environments and making it illegal for companies to give away free tobacco products and sponsor events. In addition, if tobacco companies lobby legislators in writing, the law requires that the companies post the letters for the public to read. Starting in 2014, tobacco companies operating in Russia are no longer allowed to advertise tobacco products with point-of-sale displays.

Ukraine Post-USSR

Both during and after the dissolution of the USSR, conditions in Russia and Ukraine differed. For example, during and after Stalin's forced collectivization of agriculture, millions of Ukrainians starved to death. In addition, Gorbachev's policies of perestroika and *glasnost* ("openness") were implemented later in Ukraine than in other Soviet republics because Volodymyr Shcherbytsky, a conservative Communist appointed by Brezhnev and the First Secretary of the Ukrainian Communist Party, delayed implementing the reforms.

When Ukraine gained independence, its government began to regulate tobacco markets and consumption. In 1992, the government prohibited tobacco advertising in all forms, but, as in Russia, the law included no enforcement mechanism, so the advertising ban was largely ignored. A 1996 law prohibited tobacco advertising on national and cable television and radio, in publications targeted at youth age 17 years or younger, in public transportation, on billboards located within 300 meters of children's or educational facilities, and at social/cultural events with large attendance. The 1996 law also required that printed advertising contain a health warning. The government expanded the size of the health warnings in 2003 (from 5 to 15 percent of the pack's surface area) and, in the same legislation, restricted how tobacco companies could promote themselves when they sponsored public events. The government also made it illegal for companies to display a product's brand name.

At approximately the same time, in 1997, the Ukrainian government began to establish smoke-free public places—starting with a ban on smoking in health care facilities. Over time, it expanded the public areas where people were not allowed to smoke. The government prohibited smoking in buildings and on the premises of preschools, educational institutions, health protection institutions, and sport competition venues in 2002. In 2005, it expanded this list to include smoking bans at workplaces and in public places, except for specially designated smoking areas. The 2005 law required that owners of all public places establish smoke-free areas in at least 50 percent of the public space (Law of Ukraine No. 2899-IV, 2005).

In 1998, the government made it illegal for youth younger than 18 years to buy or sell tobacco. However, because the law applied to individuals, it was practically unenforceable. To reduce enforcement costs, in 2002, the government instead made it illegal for firms to sell tobacco to anyone younger than 18 years.

As mentioned previously, during this time, international tobacco companies were investing heavily in the production and promotion of tobacco in both Russia and the Ukraine. They also heavily lobbied government officials to weaken tobacco control legislation that was proposed and passed (Demin, 2001).

SMOKING IN THE RUSSIAN FEDERATION

Smoking Prevalence Rates in Historical Perspective

In Figure 9.1, we plot the life-course smoking trajectories of men and women in 10-year birth cohorts who were alive across the major events of 20th-century Russia. The men and women in the oldest cohorts were 80–89 years old in 2010. Born after the Bolshevik revolution, they came of age just before and during World War II. Their life experiences differ sharply from the men and women who were 20–29 years old in 2010. That generation came of age in the newly independent Russia.

As in all chapters, Figure 9.1a plots smoking prevalence rates of men. Figure 9.1b plots the smoking prevalence rates of corresponding cohorts of women. In both panels, we mark the start and end years during which Russians fought in World War II (WWII) because the Soviet government issued tobacco to its troops. We also mark 1970 as the start of efforts to modernize cigarette production in the USSR. We mark 1978 as the date when warning labels appeared widely on domestic brands of cigarettes, and it was at approximately this time that the USSR began to establish public health campaigns about the dangers of smoking. We mark 1985, the date when Mikhail Gorbachev was elected General Secretary of the Communist Party, because he introduced market reforms and invited foreign cigarette companies into the USSR markets, thus opening the way for their heavy investment in both production and marketing of cigarettes in all former republics of the USSR. We mark 1992 as the year the Russian Federation was independently established and 1998 as the year of financial crisis. Finally, we mark 2008 because Russia accepted the FCTC in that year.[1]

Russian men's smoking prevalence was more or less constant across the oldest four cohorts and increased slightly among men aged 40–49 years in 2010, who reached adulthood as Gorbachev came to power. In other countries, the prevalence of smoking was highest among men in the oldest cohort and then steadily declined in subsequent cohorts. However, the rate of men's smoking prevalence in Russia only began to decline among men who grew up as the USSR was dissolving. Many things were changing during this time. Not only were the youngest two cohorts exposed

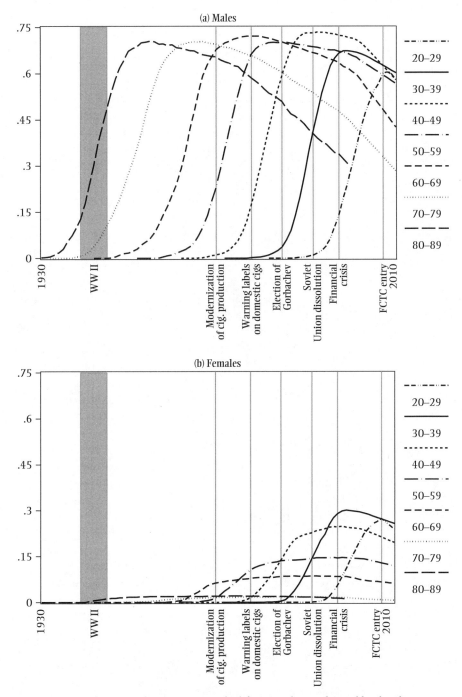

Figure 9.1 Smoking prevalence rates over the life course by gender and birth cohort.
SOURCE: Russian Longitudinal Monitoring Survey (RLMS). 1995, 1996, 1998, 2000–2010.
Moscow/Chapel Hill, NC: National Research University Higher School of Economics/
ZAO "Demoscope"/CPC.

to more information than were cohorts that preceded them but also they grew up during periods of financial crisis. As noted previously, in the late 1970s, the USSR restarted its public health campaigns, and the newly independent Russian government stepped up those efforts in the 1990s.

During the 20th century, the rate of smoking prevalence among women increased from practically zero in the oldest two cohorts to approximately 30 percent in the youngest cohort. It was women in cohorts born after World War II who first began to smoke. The rate of smoking prevalence started to accelerate among the cohort of women coming of age in the 1970s, when the USSR began to upgrade its tobacco industry, and then increased dramatically among women in the cohort that came of age after 1985—that is, during the period of Gorbachev's perestroika and the foreign investment of international cigarette firms.

The other notable pattern in women's life-course smoking trajectories during this transition is that they are not hump-shaped. Notice that, prior to the cohort of women age 30–39 years in 2010, smoking trajectories of women increased and then stayed flat because the vast majority of smokers in those cohorts never quit. Over successive cohorts, the trajectories gradually take on the shape of trajectories one observes in other countries.[2] Consistent with the pattern one observes for men, smoking was most prevalent among women in the cohort that came of age after Russia became independent, and then it began to decline as the barriers between Russia and the rest of the world eased.

The smoking prevalence rates shown here seem to be at odds with rates reported in Gilmore (2005), but in fact they likely reflect the difference in rates estimated from cross-sectional and longitudinal data. Gilmore reports rates from more than 20 studies that use cross-sectional surveys, many administered in Moscow. Across all the surveys, the smoking prevalence rate for men (women) ranges from 45 percent (10 percent) in the 1980s to 64 percent (30 percent) in 1996. Because in the cross section, the population includes older people who have already quit and young people who have not yet begun, one cannot directly compare these rates to the ones we report. Unlike Gilmore, Perlman et al. (2007) measure smoking behavior with retrospectively reported data and produce smoking rates that are largely consistent with our results (e.g., they report that the smoking rate of Russian men who were 35–44 years old in 2000 is 69.6 percent—an estimate that is very close to the smoking rates we report in 2000 for men who were 40–49 and 50–59 years old in 2010).

To connect the observed smoking patterns with the economic context in which they took place, we present, in Figure 9.2, trends in per capita gross domestic product (GDP) and the real cigarette price from 1930 to 2010. The GDP data are from Bolt and van Zanden (2013). They report, and we use, per capita GDP of the USSR until 1991 and the per capita GDP of Russia from 1992 to 2010. We compute the real cigarette price in terms of minutes of work in each year.[3] We plot the GDP per capita and the cigarette price series relative to the 2010 value of each series observed in Russia.

Figure 9.2 shows that before World War II, the real price of cigarettes fell from close to 8000 times its 2010 level to approximately 300 times the 2010 price and continued to fall until 1956. Although these real prices seem excessively high, they are in line with historical information. During the 1930s, the Soviet government collectivized agricultural production. This process generally disrupted agricultural

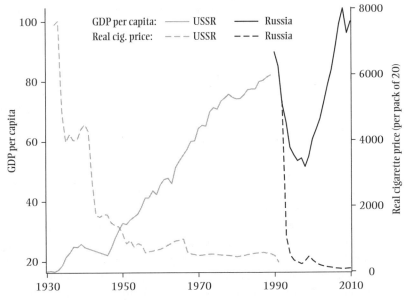

Figure 9.2 Economic development and cigarette prices (2010 = 100).
SOURCES: GDP, Bolt, J., and J. L. van Zanden. 2013. "The first update of the Maddison Project; Re-estimating growth before 1820." Maddison Project Working Paper 4. Prices, 1992–2010 Russian Federation State Statistical Agency; 1937–1991, State Committee of the USSR official price lists.

markets. At the same time, the government levied new taxes. Bokarev (2009) cites official government documents from the Soviet archives to report that the tax rate on factory-produced tobacco, papirosi, and makhorka increased from 1930 to 1931 by between 71 and 250 percent (more in villages than in cities). Moreover, these were official prices. The black market price in cities for makhorka was four times the official price (Bokarev, 2009).

Here, we have adjusted prices to be in terms of hours of work (for workers paid the average monthly wage who work 160 hours per month), and we plot them over time relative to their 2010 value. In 1932, the average worker had to work approximately 7.4 hours to buy a pack of 20 cigarettes (20 g of tobacco). However, prices declined rapidly as the turmoil of the forced collectivization subsided. By 1939, the average worker had to work approximately 4 hours to buy a pack of 20 cigarettes; by 1943, the price fell to 1.7 hours, and by 1950 it fell further to 1.2 hours of work. When we define these prices in terms of the number of hours that a 2010 worker (earning the mean monthly wage) had to work, unsurprisingly they become very large. By 2010, cigarettes in Russia were cheap and plentiful. Thus, relative to the 2010 cost, the real price of cigarettes was huge in the early years of our sample period.

With the dissolution of the USSR, prices increased, but wages did not immediately adjust. As a result, the real cigarette price spiked in 1992 to more than 6000 times the 2010 level. As nominal wages increased, prices returned to their pre-dissolution downward trend and increased only briefly during the financial crisis of 1998. As noted previously, as part of his perestroika reforms, Gorbachev invited foreign cigarette manufacturers to help revitalize the Soviet tobacco factories. They clearly succeeded. Between 1994 and 2005, the real price of cigarettes fell dramatically. Although not shown here, in those years, per capita cigarette consumption doubled.

Figure 9.2 also documents the steady increase in per capita GDP from the end of World War II until 1989. The dissolution of the USSR disrupted production and the Russian economy in general. However, the 1998 currency reform, coupled with dramatic increases in the price of oil, sparked a dramatic rise in per capita GDP that lasted until the 2000s.

The trends of increasing per capita GDP and rapidly falling cigarette prices in Figure 9.2 may help to explain the smoking patterns shown in Figure 9.1. Average incomes were mostly rising and the real price of cigarettes was (mostly) falling during the 1970s and 1980s even as the Soviet government started to educate its citizens about the health risks associated with smoking. The patterns in smoking prevalence suggest that the extra information was not enough to convince people to not smoke as their incomes rose in both absolute and relative terms. But there is also evidence that economic factors do not explain everything. Consider the pattern of smoking among men and women in the cohort that was in its prime smoking initiation years when the USSR dissolved—the cohort that was 30–39 years old in 2010. The USSR's dissolution caused per capita GDP to drop sharply and caused the real price of cigarettes to (briefly) spike. Whereas men in the transition cohort and the next younger cohort did smoke less than the previous generation, women in the transition cohort smoked more. Furthermore, although the rate of smoking prevalence decreased somewhat in the next cohort of Russian women—those who grew up after 1992—the rate is not much lower. The failure of the female smoking prevalence rate to decline much in the post-USSR Russia is consistent with the targeting of advertising at female smokers noted previously (Gilmore and McKee, 2004, 2005).[4] More broadly, culture and social norms may also explain observed patterns in gendered smoking behavior.

Cohort and Gender Differences

In Figure 9.3, we line up each cohort's smoking prevalence rate by chronological age so one can compare similarities and differences in smoking behavior of different cohorts when members were the same age. Strikingly, Russian men of different cohorts smoked in similar ways at similar ages except for men in the oldest cohort. Men in the oldest five cohorts started and quit smoking at approximately the same rate at the same ages. Men in the youngest two cohorts started smoking at approximately the same ages as men in other cohorts, but unlike those men, they started quitting sooner.

Figure 9.3 also shows that the age of initiation is steadily declining across successive cohorts of Russian women. The long right-hand tail of the trajectory in all but the youngest two cohorts shows again that, once they start, they seldom quit. This pattern began to change in the youngest three cohorts. Women in these cohorts are quitting sooner and at higher rates than women in the older cohorts.

To delve deeper in the smoking patterns, in Table 9.1, we present our six summary measures of smoking behavior. The data show that the peak smoking prevalence rate for the older cohorts of men is relatively constant between 70 and 73 percent

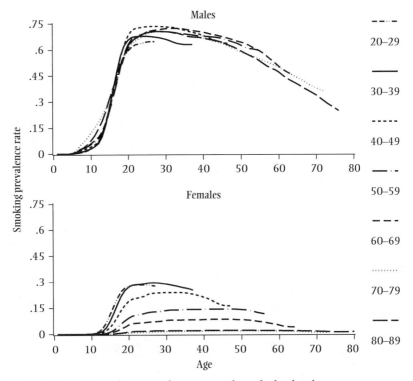

Figure 9.3 Change in smoking prevalence rate with age by birth cohort.
SOURCE: Russian Longitudinal Monitoring Survey (RLMS). 1995, 1996, 1998, 2000–2010. Moscow/Chapel Hill, NC: National Research University Higher School of Economics/ZAO "Demoscope"/CPC.

before declining in the younger two cohorts. Although men in the oldest cohort smoked at approximately the same rate as men in the next four cohorts, they smoked fewer cigarettes on average. Smoking intensity was highest among men in the four middle cohorts—those aged 30–69 years in 2010. On the average day, smokers in those cohorts consumed 17 or 18 cigarettes.

Women's peak rate of smoking prevalence increased from 2 percent in the oldest cohort aged 80–89 years in 2010 to 30 percent in the cohort aged 30–39 years in 2010, and it decreased slightly to 27 percent in the youngest cohort. Interestingly, although the smoking prevalence rate varied tremendously across various cohorts, consumption was similar. In each cohort, the average female smoker consumed between 10 and 12 cigarettes per day.

In the oldest five cohorts, men reached their peak smoking prevalence rate when the average smoker was between 28 and 31 years of age. We do not discuss the two youngest cohorts because all members of those cohorts were not old enough by 2010 to have reached their peak smoking prevalence. Among women, except for the oldest cohort, each successive cohort reached its peak smoking prevalence rate at increasingly younger ages. Among men, the average age of smoking initiation was almost constant among the six oldest cohorts of men at approximately 17 years of age. It then fell in the youngest two cohorts. Among women, the average smoker in the

Table 9.1. SUMMARY INDICATORS OF SMOKING BY GENDER AND BIRTH COHORT

Gender/ cohort	Sample size	Peak prevalence rate	Cigarettes per day	Years smoking	Average age at		
					peak	start	quit
MALES							
80–89	2,082	0.71	13	44	28	17	50
70–79	4,381	0.70	16	42	31	16	48
60–69	4,661	0.72	18	33	31	18	44
50–59	7,636	0.70	18	20	29	17	38
40–49	7,618	0.73	17	23	28	17	34
30–39	7,351	0.67	17	15	25	16	27
20–29	7,588	0.60	14	8	23	16	20
FEMALES							
80–89	4,633	0.02	10	40	49	26	56
70–79	8,277	0.02	10	31	49	28	50
60–69	6,716	0.09	11	26	47	25	42
50–59	10,139	0.15	11	18	43	23	37
40–49	8,921	0.25	12	18	33	20	31
30–39	8,293	0.30	10	12	24	18	26
20–29	8,086	0.27	10	7	22	16	20

SOURCE: National Research University Higher School of Economics/ZAO
"Demoscope"/Carolina Population Center (CPC), University of North Carolina. 1995,
1996, 1998, 2000–2010. "The Russian Longitudinal Monitoring Survey—Higher School
of Economics." Moscow/Chapel Hill, NC: National Research University Higher School
of Economics/ZAO "Demoscope"/CPC.

oldest three cohorts initiated smoking when she was between 25 and 28 years old.
Starting with the cohort age 70–79 years in 2010, the average female smoker in every
successive cohort took up smoking at increasingly younger ages. By the youngest
cohort, men and women were starting at the same age.

As in other countries discussed so far, conditional on being a smoker, the average age of quitting was more broadly similar for men and women. If anything,
female smokers in the oldest cohorts are waiting longer to quit than their male
counterparts.

Figure 9.4 more starkly highlights the convergence in smoking behavior of
Russian men and women in peak smoking rates, age at peak, age at initiation, and
age at cessation. It also highlights how smoking behavior of men and women differs.
In all cohorts, even in the youngest ones, more men smoke, men smoke more cigarettes, and men smoke longer than women. The prevalence rates of men and women
are converging, even as the prevalence rate of younger cohorts of men is declining, because the smoking prevalence rate of women is rising faster among younger
cohorts than the rate is declining in the corresponding cohorts of men.

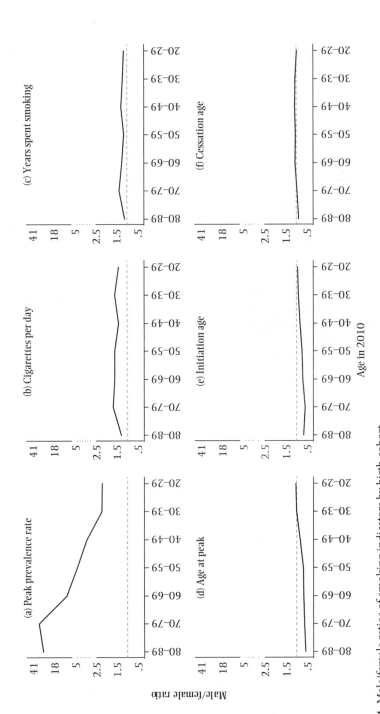

Figure 9.4 Male/female ratios of smoking indicators by birth cohort.

SOURCE: Russian Longitudinal Monitoring Survey (RLMS). 1995, 1996, 1998, 2000–2010. Moscow/Chapel Hill, NC: National Research University Higher School of Economics/ZAO "Demoscope"/CPC.

As previously noted, this convergence in smoking patterns between genders may arise in part because, after 1991, Western tobacco companies targeted their marketing efforts at women to tap into the relatively large pool of potential smokers (Lunze and Migliorini, 2013). However, it may also be related to women's access to formal work and changing social norms on gender roles. In the USSR, the proportion of women working increased rapidly during the first half of the 20th century from approximately 25 percent in 1922 to just over 50 percent in 1974 (Lapidus, 1975). In part, this increase occurred because the share of men declined in the population after World War I, the purges of Stalin, and World War II. Lapidus notes that, in 1959, 63.4 percent of the people ages 35 years or older were female. The increase in female labor force participation was driven mostly by economic need but also by a drive for equality. Despite the Marxist rhetoric about equality between the sexes, however, and although constitutionally women were granted equal rights and equal access to and participation in all aspects of society, in reality women were underrepresented in higher paying occupations and in positions of authority (Lapidus, 1975). In addition, although more women were attending university and entering traditionally male occupations, they earned less than men. For example, in the 1980s, women constituted a majority of people employed in health care (75 percent), as physicians and economists (66 percent), and in education (75 percent), but these women earned less on average than did the average USSR worker (Zickel, 1991). As the USSR stagnated, women's labor force participation also stagnated. The labor force participation rate of women ages 20–29 years, which had increased from an already high 80 percent in 1959 to 88 percent in 1974, declined to 73 percent by 1991, when the country dissolved. Thereafter, it steadily declined, and by 2012, only 53 percent of Russian women ages 20–29 years worked.[5]

SMOKING IN UKRAINE

Smoking Prevalence Rates in Historical Perspective

In Figure 9.5, we plot smoking prevalence rates for cohorts of men and women in Ukraine who were 20–79 years old in 2007.[6] Again, we mark notable events on the timeline to remind readers of events that may have affected smoking patterns. We plot mostly the same events as in Figure 9.1 because those events, which occurred in the USSR, likely had similar influence on Ukraine and Russia. We mark 1999, 7 years after Ukraine became independent, because in that year the Ukrainian government more than doubled the excise tax on cigarettes.

The smoking trajectories of Ukrainian men in Figure 9.5 show a pattern that is similar with the pattern observed among Russian men. Namely, over successive cohorts, more, not fewer, Ukrainian men smoked. The rate of smoking prevalence increased from approximately 60 percent of men in the oldest three cohorts to 70 percent in the next two cohorts, those aged 40–49 and 30–39 years in 2007. The rate declined to approximately 60 percent in the next cohort that was aged 20–29 years in 2007. Practically none of the Ukrainian women who smoked were in the oldest three cohorts. The rate of smoking prevalence increased thereafter to reach 20 percent in the youngest two cohorts.[7] These levels are more or less similar to levels reported by Gilmore et al. (2001), who use cross-sectional data from a 2000 survey in Ukraine.

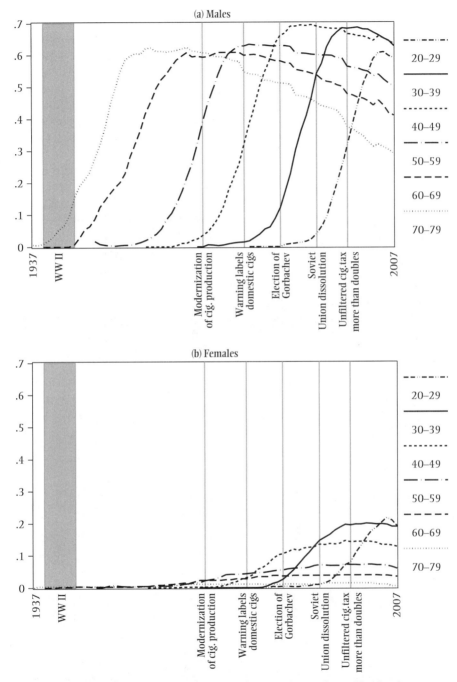

Figure 9.5 Smoking prevalence rates over the life course by gender and birth cohort.
SOURCE: Ukrainian Longitudinal Monitoring Survey (ULMS). 2003, 2007. Bonn, Germany: Institute for the Study of Labor, International Data Service Center.

They report smoking prevalence rates of 61.5, 66.8, and 42.5 percent among men who, in 2000, were aged 18–29, 30–49, and 50 years or older, respectively, and rates of 23.6, 12.6, and 2.0 percent among women in the same age groups, respectively. Although those authors use more broadly defined age categories and cross-sectional data, the general levels of smoking prevalence match well with those reported in Figure 9.5.

To understand the economic context in which these patterns formed, in Figure 9.6, we present trends in GDP per capita for the period from 1990 to 2010 and in real cigarette price from 1995 to 2007. As we did for Russia, we compute the real cigarette price in terms of minutes of work in each year.[8] The value for each year in both series is plotted relative to their 2007 value.

One of the difficulties in compiling data for Ukraine is that there exists a robust market for smuggled cigarettes. Researchers at the International Center of Political Studies estimate that, in 1996, 25 billion black market cigarettes were smuggled into Ukraine and that most of them were international brands. During the 1998 currency crisis, smuggling disappeared. After the currency stabilized in 1999 and 2000, the black market for cigarettes arose again, but most of the cigarettes were smuggled from Russia or Moldova (Alcohol and Drug Information Centre (ADIC–Ukraine), n.d.). Here, we report prices that were for legal cigarettes.

Figure 9.6 shows that both prices and per capita GDP in Ukraine followed patterns similar to those in the Russian Federation. While real cigarette price was dropping after Ukraine gained its independence, it peaked at more than 600 times its 2007 level during the currency crisis and fell dramatically and quickly once the crisis

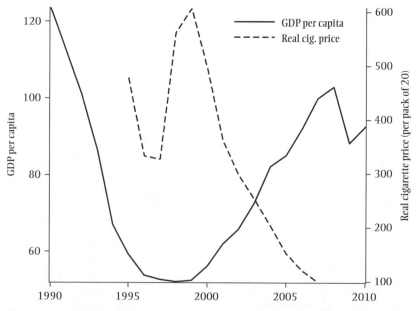

Figure 9.6 Economic development and cigarette prices (2007 = 100).
SOURCES: GDP, Bolt, J., and J. L. van Zanden. 2013. "The first update of the Maddison Project; Re-estimating growth before 1820." Maddison Project Working Paper 4; Prices, Alcohol and Drug Information Center, Ukraine (www.adic.org.ua; accessed 2008).

was resolved. Immediately after the dissolution of the USSR, from 1990 through the end of the 1990s, per capita GDP fell sharply—to less than 60 percent of its 2007 value—but it started to grow again in 1999. The similar economic changes that Russia and Ukraine experienced during the study period are consistent with the similarities in the smoking dynamics in the two countries.

Not shown in Figure 9.6, because we could not find a full data time series, is the relative difference in per capita GDP in Russia and Ukraine when both were still part of the USSR. However, available evidence suggests that the per capita GDP in the Ukraine was much lower than the per capita GDP in Russia.[9] This difference may explain why the pattern of smoking in the Ukraine is similar to the pattern in Russia but the levels of peak smoking prevalence are uniformly lower in practically all cohorts of men and women.

Cohort and Gender Differences

In Figure 9.7, we line up each cohort's smoking prevalence rate by chronological age to compare similarities and differences in smoking behavior when members of each cohort were the same age. The figure shows that the oldest and youngest cohorts of men started smoking at similar ages, and the middle cohorts started at slightly older but also similar ages. The figure also confirms the pattern noted previously—that

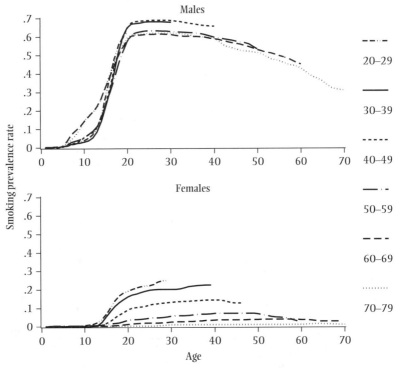

Figure 9.7 Change in smoking prevalence rate with age by birth cohort.
SOURCE: Ukrainian Longitudinal Monitoring Survey (ULMS). 2003, 2007. Bonn, Germany: Institute for the Study of Labor, International Data Service Center.

the rate of women's smoking prevalence increased continuously across successive cohorts from almost zero in the oldest cohort to 20 percent in the youngest cohorts.

In Table 9.2, we present our six summary measures of smoking behavior. This table reveals that older cohorts of men and women reached their peak rate of smoking prevalence when they were older compared to all successive cohorts. Smoking intensity was highest among the middle cohorts of men and generally declined among women. The increase in smoking prevalence of men in all but the youngest cohort and the increase in smoking prevalence overall are consistent with evidence from legal cigarette sales reported by Peng and Ross (2009). They find that, although official cigarette prices increased between 1997 and 2007, tobacco advertising and legal sales both increased. They present evidence suggesting that rising incomes help explain the increase. The average age of men's initiation was more or less constant, whereas for women it fell steadily and approached the average initiation age of men. The oldest two cohorts of men reached their peak smoking prevalence when the average man was approximately 32 years old. Later cohorts of men reached their peak smoking prevalence 3–6 years sooner. Among women, the age at which cohorts reached their peak smoking prevalence rate fell steadily from 58 and 55 years for the oldest and second oldest cohorts, respectively, to 28 years for the cohort of women who turned 30–39 years old in 2007. People in the youngest cohorts were not old enough in 2007 to have reached their peak rate. One observes no consistent pattern in the age at which smokers quit in each cohort. In the oldest cohorts, women smoked longer than men. In the younger cohorts, men smoked longer than women.

Table 9.2. SUMMARY INDICATORS OF SMOKING BY GENDER AND BIRTH COHORT

Gender/ cohort	Sample size	Peak prevalence rate	Cigarettes per day	Years smoking	Average age at		
					peak	start	quit
MALES							
70–79	236	0.62	16	43	32	16	47
60–69	461	0.61	19	43	32	16	48
50–59	583	0.63	20	35	26	17	42
40–49	604	0.70	18	27	29	17	36
30–39	507	0.69	18	18	27	17	29
20–29	599	0.61	15	9	22	16	21
FEMALES							
70–79	328	0.01	20	36	58	34	65
60–69	747	0.04	11	34	55	28	52
50–59	835	0.07	12	26	44	25	42
40v49	775	0.15	10	21	35	22	29
30–39	599	0.20	11	15	28	19	27
20–29	689	0.22	9	7	22	17	21

SOURCE: Ukrainian Longitudinal Monitoring Survey (ULMS). 2003, 2007. Bonn, Germany: Institute for the Study of Labor, International Data Service Center.

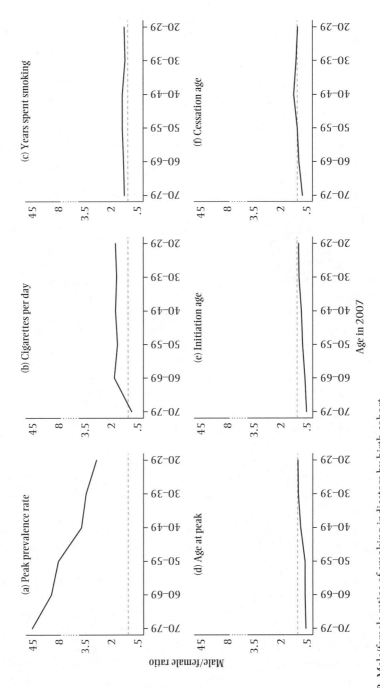

Figure 9.8 Male/female ratios of smoking indicators by birth cohort.

SOURCE: Ukrainian Longitudinal Monitoring Survey (ULMS). 2003, 2007. Bonn, Germany: Institute for the Study of Labor, International Data Service Center.

Finally, in Figure 9.8, we plot the ratio of each statistic in Table 9.2 for men relative to women, by cohort. In all six panels, any deviation above 1 indicates that the value of the indicator was higher for men than it was for women (and vice versa). Figure 9.8 more clearly shows that although younger cohorts of Ukrainian men and women are smoking in more similar ways, some differences persist. In the youngest cohort, Ukrainian men and women start at approximately the same age, reach their peak smoking prevalence at approximately the same age, and quit at approximately the same age. However, fewer Ukrainian women smoke in each cohort, they smoke fewer cigarettes on average, and they still smoke slightly fewer years than do men of the same age.

In contrast to Russian women, it appears that the prevalence and intensity of smoking among young Ukrainian women are not converging toward the levels of Ukrainian men. However, as noted previously, younger cohorts of women are smoking more than women in older cohorts. Thus, it is still unclear whether Ukrainian men and women are going to converge in all aspects of smoking behavior, as they are in Russia and in other countries, or whether they will forge a different path. As for Russia, feminism and female labor force participation rates stalled in the Ukraine before and during the dissolution of the USSR. Marsh (1996) and Zhurzhenko (2004) both note that in many ways, the situation for women in Ukraine has regressed more than it has in Russia. In both countries, however, there are social forces at work that reinforce roles for women that discourage them from working and from achieving full equality with men. In this particular case, the emphasis on those "traditional" roles may partly explain why women in both countries are not smoking like men.

CONCLUSION

Smoking behavior of Russians and Ukrainians evolved in the context of economic, social, and political conditions of the Soviet Union and the turmoil engendered by the transition from a centrally planned economy to one in which market forces generally operate. The pattern of smoking of men, when they were living in the USSR, does not neatly fit in the common narrative that claims that smoking is a luxury good. Among older cohorts of both Russians and Ukrainians, a majority of men smoked, even those with lower incomes. At the same time, few women smoked. However, evidence indicates that decisions to smoke do respond to economic factors. As Russia and Ukraine developed economically, first as part of the Soviet Union and later independently, the rate of smoking of Russian men stayed relatively constant and increased only slightly after the election of Gorbachev, whereas rates of smoking among Ukrainian men followed the same pattern but increased more dramatically when Gorbachev came to power. Also in both countries, more women started smoking as incomes rose and as Western cigarette companies began to operate in Russia. The multinational tobacco companies actively promoted smoking and actively sought to weaken tobacco control policies. Although women's smoking prevalence rose in both countries, the life-course smoking patterns of younger Ukrainian women differ from those of younger Russian women. Because we are describing smoking patterns of broadly defined birth cohorts, we have not been able to search for patterns relative to the changes in tobacco control policies that have (mostly) occurred only recently. It is possible—even likely—that a multivariate analysis will reveal whether and how

those policies and changing social norms might have contributed to differences in smoking behavior of men and women of different ages. That analysis remains to be done.

NOTES

1. The Appendix lists websites and sources that review more of the history of tobacco-related events in the USSR and Russia.
2. These patterns match well those presented in Roberts et al. (2012).
3. See Kravis (1951). The data sources and method used in the compilation of the price series are described in the Appendix.
4. Other evidence suggests that women have suffered greater psychological stress than men and that this may also explain the persistence of smoking among women during the transition (Hinote et al., 2009).
5. See the Organization for Economic Cooperation and Development labor force statistics by sex and age (available at http://stats.oecd.org/Index.aspx?DataSetCode=LFS_SEXAGE_I_R; accessed March 20, 2013) and the US Bureau of Labor Statistics report No. 1040, "Women in the Labor Force: A Databook" (February 2013; available at http://www.bls.gov/cps/wlf-databook-2012.pdf; accessed November 16, 2013).
6. The Ukrainian surveys interview individuals who are 75 years old or younger. Thus, Ukraine is the only country in our sample for which we do not plot a smoking trajectory for the 80- to 89-year-old cohort.
7. These patterns match well those presented in Roberts et al. (2012) and are broadly similar to those presented in Andreeva and Krasovksy (2007). We find a lower rate for women than they report, but results are not directly comparable because age groupings do not match perfectly.
8. In the Appendix, we list data sources and describe the methods we used to compute the cigarette price.
9. Bolt and van Zanden (2013) report per capita GDP for each region in 1973 and from 1992 onward. In 1973, per capita GDP was 76 percent of the level in Russia. In 1992 and in all subsequent years, it was 50 percent or less—in part because of the oil and gas wealth that Russia developed after its independence.

REFERENCES

Alcohol and Drug Information Centre (ADIC–Ukraine). n.d. Available at http://adic.org.ua/adic/reports/econ/ch-1/1-2.htm; accessed October 23, 2008.

Andreeva, T. I., and Krasovsky, K. S. 2007. "Changes in smoking prevalence in Ukraine in 2001–5." *Tobacco Control* 16:202–206.

Bogoslovski, M. M. 1941. *Petr I: Pervoe Zagranicnoe Putesliestvie (March 9, 1697–August 25, 1698) Vol. II.* Moscow: Ogiz-Sotsekgiz.

Bokarev, I. U. P. 2009. "Tobacco production in Russia: The transition to Communism." In *Tobacco in Russian History and Culture: From the Seventeenth Century to the Present,* edited by M. Romaniello and T. Starks, pp 132–147. New York: Routledge.

Bolt, J., and J. L. van Zanden. 2013. "The first update of the Maddison Project; Re-estimating growth before 1820." Maddison Project Working Paper 4. Available at http://www.ggdc.net/maddison/maddison-project/home.htm.

Deber, R. A. 1981. "The limits of persuasion: Anti-smoking activities in the USSR." *Canadian Journal of Public Health* 72:118–126.

Demin, A. K. 2001. "Tobacco control policy making in Russia and the role of civil society." *Research for International Tobacco Control.* Available at http://web.idrc.ca/uploads/user-S/11195580731GFHR_AD.pdf

Fox, K. F. 2009a. "'Tobacco is poison': Soviet era anti-smoking posters." In *Tobacco in Russian History and Culture: From the Seventeenth Century to the Present*, edited by M. P. Romaniello and T. Starks, pp 183–224. New York: Routledge.

Fox, K. F. 2009b. "Za Zdorovye! Soviet health posters as social advertising." *Journal of Macromarketing* 29:74–90.

Frederiksen, O. J. 1943. "Virginia tobacco in Russia under Peter the Great." *Slavonic and East European Review* 2:40–56.

Gilmore, A. B. 2005. " Tobacco and transition: Understanding the impact of transition on tobacco use and control in the former Soviet Union." San Francisco: Center for Tobacco Control Research and Education, University of California at San Francisco. Available at http://www.escholarship.org/uc/item/3rw2c04c.

Gilmore, A. B., and M. McKee. 2004. "Moving east: How the transnational tobacco industry gained entry to the emerging markets of the former Soviet Union. Part II: An overview of priorities and tactics used to establish a manufacturing presence." *Tobacco Control* 13:151–160.

Gilmore, A. B., and M. McKee. 2005. "Exploring the impact of foreign direct investment on tobacco consumption in the former Soviet Union." *Tobacco Control* 14:13–21.

Gilmore, A. B., M. McKee, M. Telishevska, and R. Rose. 2001. "Epidemiology of smoking in Ukraine, 2000." *Preventive Medicine* 33:453–461.

Gorchakova, E. 2009. "The Iava Tobacco Factory from the 1960s to the early 1990s: An interview with the former director, Leonid Iakovlevich Sinel'nikov." In *Tobacco in Russian History and Culture: From the Seventeenth Century to the Present*, edited by M. Romaniello and T. Starks, pp 203–247. New York: Routledge.

Gruliow, L. 1962. "Advertising–USSR." In *Collier's Encyclopedia*, Vol. 1, pp 152–153. New York: Collier.

Hinote, B. P., W. C. Cockerham, and P. Abbott. 2009. "Post-communism and female tobacco consumption in the former Soviet states." *Europe-Asia Studies* 61(9):1543–1555.

Hutson, J. B. 1937. "Consumption and production of tobacco in Europe." Technical Bulletin No. 587. Washington, DC: US Department of Agriculture.

Joossens, L., F. J. Chaloupka, D. Merriman, and A. Yurekli. 2000. "Issues in the smuggling of tobacco products." In *Tobacco Control in Developing Countries*, edited by P. Jha and F. Chaloupka, pp 393–406. Oxford: Oxford University Press on behalf of the World Bank and the World Health Organization.

Kelly, C. 2009. " 'The lads indulged themselves, they used to smoke. . .': Tobacco and children's culture in twentieth-century Russia." In *Tobacco in Russian History and Culture: From the Seventeenth Century to the Present*, edited by M. Romaniello and T. Starks, pp 158–182. New York: Routledge.

Kholmogorova, G. T., and A. V. Prokhorov. 1994. "West goes east: The new tobacco situation in Russia." *Tobacco Control* 3:145–147.

Kravis, I. B. 1951. "Techniques of comparing purchasing power among nations." *Monthly Labor Review* 72:195–197.

Lapidus, G. W. 1975. "USSR women at work: Changing patterns." *Industrial Relations* 14:178–195.

Law of Ukraine No. 2899-IV. 2005. "Measures to prevent and reduce the consumption of tobacco products and their harmful influence on the population's health." Passed September 22.

Levin, E. 2009. "Tobacco and health in early modern Russia." In *Tobacco in Russian History and Culture: From the Seventeenth Century to the Present*, edited by M. Romaniello and T. Starks, pp 44–60. New York: Routledge.

Lunze, K., and L. Migliorini. 2013. "Tobacco control in the Russian Federation—A policy analysis." *BioMed Central Public Health* 13:64.

Markham, J. W. 1964. "Is advertising important in the Soviet economy?" *Journal of Marketing* 28:31–37.

Marsh, R. 1996. *Women in Russia and Ukraine*. Cambridge, UK: Cambridge University Press.

Neuburger, M. 2009. "Smokes for big brother." In *Tobacco in Russian History and Culture: From the Seventeenth Century to the Present*, edited by M. Romaniello and T. Starks, pp 225–243. New York: Routledge.

Osipova, A. 2007, January/February. "Smoke of the motherland." *Russian Life* 1690. Available at http://www.russianlife.com/archive/article/params/Number/1690.

Peng, L., and H. Ross. 2009. "The impact of cigarette taxes and advertising on the demand for cigarettes in Ukraine." *Central European Journal of Public Health* 17(2):93–98.

Perlman, F., M. Bobak, A. Gilmore, and M. McKee. 2007. "Trends in the prevalence of smoking in Russia during the transition to a market economy." *Tobacco Control* 16:299–305.

Roberts, B., A. Gilmore, A. Stickley, D. Rotman, V. Prohoda, C. Haerpfer, et al. 2012. "Changes in smoking prevalence in 8 countries of the former Soviet Union between 2001 and 2010." *American Journal of Public Health* 102:1320–1328.

"Russians pleased by radio 'spot ads.'" 1947, June 2. *New York Times*.

Russian Longitudinal Monitoring Survey (RLMS). 1995, 1996, 1998, 2000–2010. Moscow/Chapel Hill, NC: National Research University Higher School of Economics/ZAO "Demoscope"/CPC. Available at http://www.cpc.unc.edu/projects/rlms-hse.

Starks, T. 2009. "Papirosy, smoking, and the anti-cigarette movement." In *Tobacco in Russian History and Culture: From the Seventeenth Century to the Present*, edited by M. Romaniello and T. Starks, pp 132–147. New York: Routledge.

Ukrainian Longitudinal Monitoring Survey (ULMS). 2003, 2007. Bonn, Germany: Institute for the Study of Labor, International Data Service Center. Available at http://idsc.iza.org/?page=27&id=56.

US War Department. 1943. "Morale-building activities in foreign armies." Special Series No. 11. Washington, DC: Military Intelligence Service, Special Service Division, US War Department.

Zhurzhenko, T. 2004. *Strong women, weak state: family politics and nation building in post- Soviet Ukraine*. In *Post-Soviet Women Encountering Transition: Nation-Building, Economic Survival, and Civic Activism*, edited by K. Kuehnast and C. Nechemias. Washington, DC: Woodrow Wilson Center Press with Johns Hopkins University Press.

Zickel, R. E. 1991. *Soviet Union: A country study*. Area Handbook Series, pp 550–595. Washington, DC: Library of Congress Federal Research Division.

10

Smoking in Turkey

ZEYNEP ÖNDER

INTRODUCTION

When merchants introduced tobacco to Turkey at the beginning of the 17th century, they claimed it would cure illnesses that some believed were caused by humidity. Over the ensuing years, Ottoman Empire sultans vacillated between policies that opposed the consumption of tobacco and policies that promoted its production and consumption. Ultimately, as in other countries, the Turkish government could not resist the revenues it could raise by taxing the production and consumption of tobacco. By 1864, the Empire raised 4 percent of its total revenue from tobacco taxes (de Velay, 1978).

The desire for revenue shaped how the government organized the Turkish tobacco industry and how it regulated the sale and consumption of tobacco during the time of the Ottoman Empire and after the Republic of Turkey was established in 1923. From 1862 to 1984, the industry operated as a monopoly. In its early years, the Tobacco Monopoly Administration (Tutun Inhisar Idaresi) controlled tobacco cultivation, trade, cigarette production, and tobacco taxes. After the establishment of the Republic of Turkey, the monopoly became a state-sponsored monopoly. In 1946, the government renamed the monopoly TEKEL (the General Directorate of Tobacco, Tobacco Products, Salt, and Alcohol Enterprises).

The government used TEKEL to subsidize tobacco cultivation and to support tobacco farmers. Every year, TEKEL had to set a (sometimes artificially high) price for tobacco and buy all of the crops that farmers grew but did not sell. Any tobacco that TEKEL did not sell, it stored. Unsurprisingly, it quickly accumulated an excess supply (Food and Agriculture Organization of the United Nations, 2003).

Both the industry and the government sought to increase their revenues by increasing tobacco consumption. For example, in 1935, certain tobacco manufacturers inserted coupons into cigarette packs that people could submit to enter a sweepstakes lottery (Dogruel and Dogruel, 2000). Some of these efforts targeted men. For instance, from 1934 until 1981, the government distributed free cigarettes (10 g of tobacco per day) to military conscripts.[1] Because men must serve in the military at age 20 years or after graduating from college, during this period, every Turkish man received free tobacco for at least 18 months,[2] regardless of whether or not he smoked

(Haber, 2010). Women received no free cigarettes directly. Although they might have gotten some free cigarettes from brothers, boyfriends, or husbands serving in the military, the amounts would likely have been small because military bases were typically far from places of origin and the military did not allow conscripts to leave the base often during the months they served.

Although TEKEL operated as a monopoly, market forces still influenced the decisions its managers made. For example, shifting knowledge about the health risks of smoking forced TEKEL to produce and distribute a filtered cigarette. Since the 1930s, German and, later, British and US scientists amassed increasingly convincing evidence that smoking damages health. In the 1950s, articles published in the English language press alerted smokers to the health risks of smoking and caused US and UK manufacturers to develop and market filtered cigarettes. Turkish smokers began trying to buy foreign filtered cigarettes as information detailing the health risks of smoking reached them. Because TEKEL refused to produce a filtered cigarette, Turkish smokers began to buy foreign-produced filtered cigarettes on the black market. Initially, TEKEL tried to maintain demand for its own unfiltered cigarettes through a misinformation campaign. TEKEL claimed that, because its unfiltered cigarettes were made from high-quality Turkish tobacco, smoking these cigarettes would not harm health. The company also tried to convince Turkish smokers that, by not producing a filtered cigarette, it was maintaining the quality of the cigarettes (Dogruel and Dogruel, 2000). Smokers were not persuaded. They continued to demand increasingly fewer domestically produced unfiltered cigarettes. Finally, in 1958, TEKEL started to produce filtered versions of its cigarette brands (Dogruel and Dogruel, 2000).

In 1984, the government began to dismantle the tobacco monopoly. Initially, the government let TEKEL profit from the demand for foreign-made cigarettes. The government lifted the ban on imported cigarettes but continued to vest in TEKEL the exclusive right to import, price, and distribute both domestic and foreign tobacco products for domestic consumption. In 1986, the government let international and domestic companies other than TEKEL produce tobacco products in Turkey if those companies shared ownership with TEKEL[3] (Council of Ministers, 1986).[4] TEKEL retained the right to sell the products, but the government would not let any firm advertise tobacco products on radio or television or through any other state-owned institution.

As the market opened, Turkish smokers not only encountered new cigarette types and brands but also began to see more advertising. Although it was illegal to advertise tobacco on radio or television, the government did let foreign firms advertise in newspapers and display neon signs at points of sale.[5] In 1985, TEKEL launched a campaign to promote its own brands over the imported brands.[6] In 1991, the government dropped the requirement that firms, domestic and foreign, had to partner with TEKEL if they wanted to manufacture tobacco products in Turkey (Council of Ministers, 1991; Republic of Turkey, 1991). Advertising and the number of available brands increased again because this legislation let foreign and domestic firms price and distribute their products as long as their annual production in Turkey exceeded 2000 tons. In 1992, Philip Morris International and Sabanci Holding jointly established and launched Turkey's first private tobacco company. The Turkish cigarette market continued to expand in subsequent years as other multinational firms, such as R. J. Reynolds and British American Tobacco, established subsidiaries in Turkey. In 2008, TEKEL was fully privatized. Since then, the Turkish tobacco industry has operated with a limited number of firms that compete for consumers.

Turkey's government first implemented tobacco control policies in 1981, expanded coverage in fits and starts through the mid-1990s, and then, starting in the early 2000s, broadened the scope and intensity of the policies. Turkey's 1981 tobacco control legislation required that firms print a label on cigarette packs that warned consumers about the dangers of smoking. Over time, the government mandated increasingly stronger wording that more directly warned consumers about the health risks of smoking. The language evolved from the phrase, "Attention: Affects your health" in 1981 to "Cigarettes are harmful to health" in 1986 and, finally, "Cigarette smoking is dangerous to health" in 1991.[7] Starting in 1986, the tobacco control labeling provisions required that the warning also appear in all print advertising. Also in 1986, the Turkish State Radio and Television Corporation (TRT) began to air 60-second public service announcements that warned about the harmful effects of smoking. The Turkish government first restricted where people could smoke in public in 1991, when it banned smoking in public transportation vehicles. The 1991 legislation attempted to ban all cigarette advertising on television, radio, and billboards. The Grand Assembly passed the bill, but the president vetoed it (Bilir et al., 2009). Five years later, the government banned cigarette advertising in magazines and newspapers and the promotion of cigarettes, mandated the airing of anti-tobacco television programs, and expanded the list of public places where people could not smoke.

It is unclear if these policies had any effect on smoking behavior. Although after 1996 people smoked fewer cigarettes on average, the overall smoking prevalence rate did not change (Bilir and Önder, 2000). Furthermore, contemporaneous changes in other factors make it statistically difficult to identify any causal relationship. However, some analysts suggest that the evidence might be mixed because the broadcasters obeyed the letter but not the spirit of the law. Broadcasters aired anti-tobacco programming only in late-night time slots. Furthermore, the government failed to assign to any particular agency either the responsibility to enforce the law or the authority to collect penalties when firms violated its provisions (Önder, 2002).

In the 2000s, Turkey expanded its tobacco control policies. In 2002, it established the Tobacco and Alcohol Market Regulatory Authority (TAPDK) and gave the agency broad regulatory authority. In 2004, Turkey signed the World Health Organization's Framework Convention on Tobacco Control; in 2005, it strengthened its warning label requirement; and in 2008, it more broadly restricted where people could smoke and to whom and how firms could market tobacco (Law No. 5727). The 2008 law also required that companies present more specific and targeted public education about the health risks of smoking. It did this by requiring that public and private television and radio stations broadcast at least 90 minutes of programs every month about the health consequences of tobacco consumption and specifying when those programs had to air.

During the 2000s, the government also changed how it taxed tobacco. Before 2002, the government generally levied ad valorem taxes at a rate the Cabinet set annually. However, only a portion of the resulting revenue funded anti-tobacco campaigns. The government allocated the rest to other groups. For example, in 2000, the Cabinet earmarked 10 percent of the wholesale price for the defense industry, 15 percent of the retail price for the general education fund, and the "Grazing Ground Fund" and "Military Veterans" each received 2 percent of the retail price. The government also levied taxes on imported tobacco and imported cigarettes in the amounts of $3 per kilogram and $0.40 per pack, respectively. The government earmarked the revenue from imported tobacco and tobacco products for a fund to support domestic tobacco farmers (Önder, 2002). The government also levied a value added tax (VAT) in 1984 that has gradually increased over time (Law No. 6473).[8]

Starting in 2002, the government reformed the structure of its tobacco taxes. It replaced most of the ad valorem taxes with a special consumption tax on all tobacco products. Initially set at 49.5 percent of the retail price, the government raised the rate to 55.3 percent in 2003. In the beginning, it taxed locally grown tobacco at a lower rate than it taxed imported tobacco. However, these tax policies were quickly changed when revenues declined as tobacco companies substituted domestic tobacco for imported tobacco in cigarettes. Under the new policy, firms had to pay an excise tax on cigarettes that sold for less than a given price. On more expensive cigarettes, firms paid an ad valorem tax set to be a certain percentage of the retail price. For example, in late 2008, firms paid 1.55TL per pack of cigarettes that sold for less than 2.67TL per pack and 58 percent of the per-pack retail price of cigarettes that sold for more than 2.67TL per pack. In addition, smokers paid a VAT. On cigarettes that sold for more than 2.67TL, smokers paid a total tax that averaged 73.25 percent of the retail price. On low-priced cigarettes, the combined tax burden was even higher: Smokers paid taxes equal to as much as 103.8 percent of the retail price. In 2014, the excise tax rate on cigarettes was at a maximum of 3.75TL or 65.25 percent of the retail price. In addition, the government collected a specific tax of 0.13TL per pack. Overall, computed as a fraction of the retail price, tobacco taxes increased from 44 percent in 1994 to 82.25 percent in 2014 (Önder, 2002).[9]

The evolution of Turkey's tobacco market from a state-sponsored monopoly to a more competitive industry, the shifting landscape of marketing efforts by private firms, the changing social structures, and evolving government tobacco control policies shaped who smoked, as well as when and how much they smoked. To obtain a clear picture of the smoking patterns in the country, we next present life-course smoking trajectories of seven cohorts of Turkish men and women who were born during the years 1918–1988 and we discuss those trajectories in light of the national context.

SMOKING PREVALENCE RATES IN HISTORICAL PERSPECTIVE

In Figure 10.1, we plot smoking prevalence rates by gender, birth cohort (defined by age in 2008), and calendar year. This figure shows that smoking was, and still is, more prevalent among Turkish men than women. Smoking prevalence increased across successive cohorts of Turkish men in the period after World War II and through the end of the 1970s. In every cohort we track, at least every other Turkish man smoked, and among men ages 50–59 years in 2008, three out of four smoked during the late 1970s and early 1980s. Male smoking prevalence reached its peak in that cohort. Although every other man still smoked in the three successive cohorts, smoking prevalence has been steadily declining.

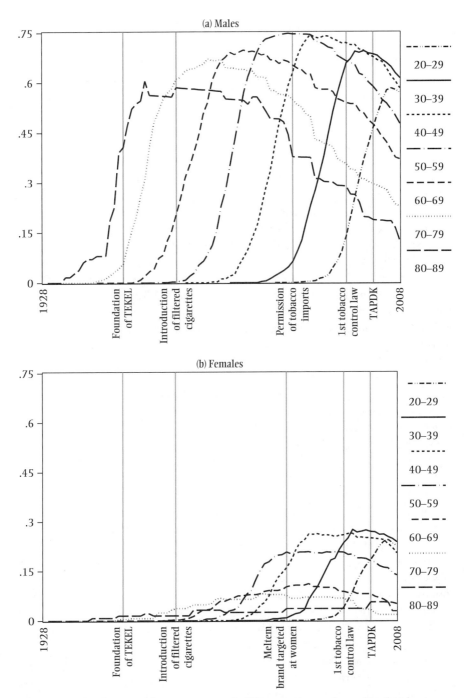

Figure 10.1 Smoking prevalence rates over the life course by gender and birth cohort.
SOURCE: Global Adult Tobacco Survey—Turkey (GATS). 2008. Copenhagen: World Health Organization.

One observes a similar but less clear pattern in the life-course smoking pattern of successive cohorts of Turkish women. For them, smoking prevalence rates were low but rising across successive cohorts as the Turkish economy grew and as the Turkish society began to change. Smoking prevalence was highest among the cohorts of women who came of age in the 1970s, 1980s, and 1990s. As in the case for men, evidence suggests that peak smoking prevalence rates are also declining among younger cohorts of Turkish women: The peak rate is lower for the youngest cohort of Turkish women than it was in the previous cohort. However, the trend is not as obvious or strong as it is among recent cohorts of men. One point of note is that women in the two most recent cohorts are those who were deciding to smoke during an era of increasing tobacco control regulations and more widespread health information.

In Figure 10.1, we also flag selected events in Turkey that could plausibly have affected individuals' decisions to smoke. We list the establishment of the tobacco monopoly TEKEL (1946) because it quickly led to cigarettes being distributed free of charge to every man completing his compulsory military service (usually at approximately age 20 years). We also list the launch of filtered cigarettes in 1958—a time when consumer magazines in the United States and United Kingdom published high-profile stories about health risks of smoking. We mark 1983 (for women) and 1984 (for men) because at approximately that time, the Turkish cigarette industry changed dramatically. In 1983, TEKEL introduced a new menthol-flavored brand, Meltem, targeted at women.[10] In 1984, for the first time since the Republic of Turkey was established, the government let firms import foreign cigarettes. It became immediately apparent that Turkish smokers preferred imported cigarettes. We also mark 1996 because in that year, the Turkish Parliament passed its first major tobacco control legislation. Finally, we mark 2002 because starting in that year, and continuing to the present day, the Turkish government has passed and implemented increasingly binding tobacco control policies. To do so, the government established the TAPDK to specifically regulate tobacco consumption and marketing.

These events seem to be correlated with smoking decisions of different cohorts. For example, smoking prevalence increased among the cohort of men who "came of smoking age" after 1934, when the military began to issue free cigarettes to conscripts. Perhaps because women did not get free cigarettes, their prevalence rates did not change at this time. Women's smoking prevalence began to increase among cohorts coming of age after 1958, when TEKEL first introduced filtered cigarettes. Few women smoked in cohorts growing up before this time, perhaps because the traditions of the Ottoman Empire counted being a nonsmoker—in addition to beauty, honor, and chastity—as one of the preferred characteristics of women (Karakartal, 2003). Among successive cohorts of women growing up after 1960, smoking prevalence increased suddenly and continuously. As we discuss in the next section, this increase is associated with increased rates of migration from rural to urban areas and changes in social norms and the status of women in society.

Although Turkey's tobacco control laws changed in 1996 and 2002, it is unclear from Figure 10.1 if those events are associated with changes in subsequent patterns of life-course smoking. Among cohorts that came of age after the government implemented those laws, men smoke less but women's smoking prevalence is largely unchanged.

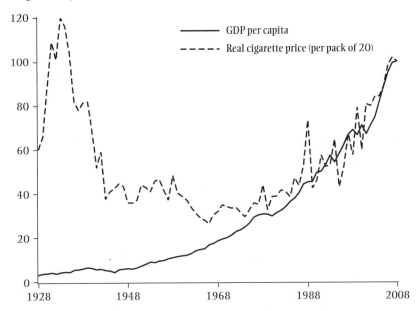

Figure 10.2 Economic development and cigarette taxes (2008 = 100).
SOURCES: GDP, Central Bank of the Republic of Turkey. Prices: 1925–1960, Ilter (1989);
1961–2002, Turkish Institute of Statistics; 2003–2008, Turkish Tobacco and Alcohol
Markets Regulatory Authority.

Because disposable income affects smoking decisions, we show, in Figure 10.2,
trends in inflation-adjusted cigarette prices and per capita gross domestic product
(GDP) between 1925 and 2008. Except for the period of the Great Depression in the
1930s and sporadic periods thereafter, real per capita GDP in Turkey increased faster
than the real price of cigarettes in almost every period, thus making cigarettes progressively more affordable. Beginning in approximately 1965, the real price of cigarettes increased at roughly the same rate that per capita GDP increased. However, in
some years, the cigarette price fluctuated tremendously with general inflation. For
example, general price inflation reached highs of 28 percent in 1992 and 106 percent in 1994. These periods of inflation might have affected cigarette consumption
patterns because the inflation affected the relative prices of traded and nontraded
goods. Starting in 2002, real cigarette prices increased rapidly as the government
levied new tobacco taxes, a development that is consistent with the decline in smoking rates among young men in that same period.

COHORT AND GENDER DIFFERENCES

Figure 10.3 plots the life-course smoking trajectories from a different perspective—on
the scale of chronological age. This perspective allows one to directly compare the
smoking behavior of different cohorts when members were the same age. The difference between the smoking prevalence rate of males and females, evident in Figure
10.1, is even more striking here. In every cohort, men start smoking sooner, and at
every age, more men smoke. Figure 10.3 also shows that, across different cohorts,
smoking behavior of men is more similar than it is for women. Furthermore, it

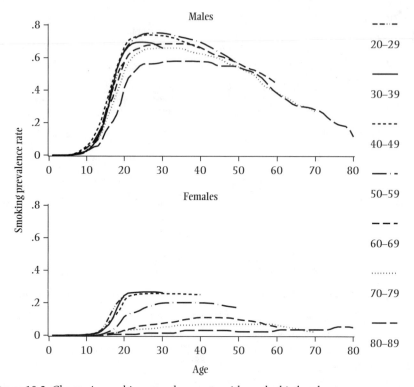

Figure 10.3 Change in smoking prevalence rate with age by birth cohort.
SOURCE: Global Adult Tobacco Survey—Turkey (GATS). 2008. Copenhagen: World
Health Organization.

highlights differences in smoking participation over the middle and later portions of
the life cycle. The hump shape of men's life-course smoking trajectories indicates that
a substantial fraction of men who start smoking subsequently quit. The relatively flat
smoking trajectories of women indicate that, once women choose to smoke, they
seldom quit.

In Table 10.1, we provide details on six aspects of life-course smoking behavior
not easily inferred from the figures. In that table, we show that the peak smoking
prevalence rate of different cohorts of men increased from 61 percent among the
oldest cohorts to a high of 75 percent among men age 50–59 years in 2008. In cohorts
that followed, the peak smoking prevalence rate declined slowly. Among the cohort
of men 30–39 years old in 2008, at most 70 percent smoked at one point. By contrast,
the peak smoking prevalence rate of women has been steadily increasing in younger
cohorts. At its peak, only 6 percent of women smoked in the oldest cohort. The peak
smoking prevalence rate increased more than fourfold, to 28 percent, among the
cohort of women age 30–39 years in 2008.

Table 10.1 also reveals that, cigarette consumption of men follows the same pattern as their peak smoking prevalence; that is, it is higher in the middle-aged cohorts
compared to all other cohorts. In contrast, the average daily consumption of cigarettes among women is roughly constant across cohorts, although we do not have
valid consumption estimates for the oldest two cohorts because smoking rates in

Table 10.1. SUMMARY INDICATORS OF SMOKING BY GENDER AND BIRTH COHORT

Gender/ cohort	Sample size	Peak prevalence rate	Cigarettes per day[a]	Years smoking	Average age at		
					peak	start	quit
MALES							
80–89	57	0.61	13	41	25	21	57
70–79	245	0.67	12	41	31	19	53
60–69	388	0.70	22	37	29	19	49
50–59	640	0.75	24	33	29	18	43
40–49	809	0.74	21	26	24	17	36
30–39	924	0.70	20	18	26	17	29
20–29	543	0.58	16	10	23	16	23
FEMALES							
80–89	72	0.06		27	77	46	64
70–79	277	0.08		29	42	31	56
60–69	420	0.11	12	29	44	28	49
50–59	610	0.21	11	28	34	23	44
40–49	811	0.26	12	23	34	20	36
30–39	967	0.28	10	15	24	19	27
20–29	851	0.24	11	8	22	17	22

[a]The numbers of cigarettes for female cohorts ages 80–89 and 70–79 years are left blank because we observed less than 5 and less than 25 smokers in those cohorts, respectively. These samples yield unreliable and implausibly high cigarette consumption estimates.

SOURCE: Global Adult Tobacco Survey—Turkey (GATS). 2008. Copenhagen: World Health Organization.

these cohorts are very low and our sample of smokers is small. In all cohorts for which we have reliable estimates, female smokers consume approximately 10–12 cigarettes per day.

Table 10.1 also highlights trends in the age at which men and women crossed particular smoking thresholds. In both sexes, more recent cohorts achieved their peak smoking prevalence rate at generally younger ages. The cohort of men aged 70–79 years in 2008 reached its peak smoking prevalence rate at age 31, whereas the cohort age 30–39 years in 2008 reached its peak at age 26. Likewise, the cohort of women ages 70–79 years in 2008 reached its peak smoking prevalence when the average member of the cohort was 42 years old, whereas women in the cohort age 30–39 years in 2008 reached their smoking prevalence peak when the average member was 24 years old.

To more directly compare smoking behavior of men relative to women, we take the gender ratio of the statistics in Table 10.1 and plot them in Figure 10.4. This figure shows more clearly that the peak prevalence rate in 80- to 89-year-old males was more than 10 times higher than the peak prevalence rate in 80- to 89-year-old

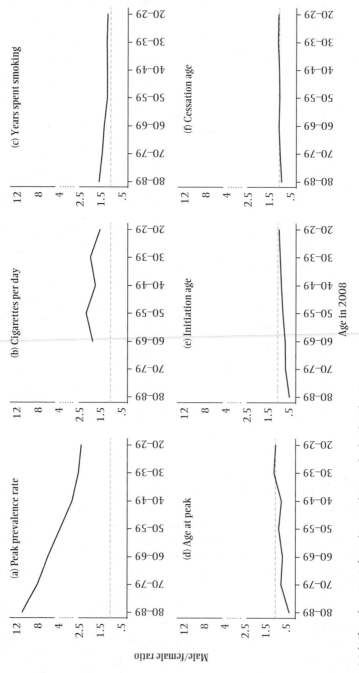

Figure 10.4 Male/female ratios of smoking indicators by birth cohort.
SOURCE: Global Adult Tobacco Survey—Turkey (GATS). 2008. Copenhagen: World Health Organization.

females. Males and females experience cessation at similar ages. Although ages at peak and initiation are similar in the younger cohorts, among older cohorts, the average woman started smoking when she was approximately twice as old as when the average male smoker started. Finally, the average number of cigarettes smoked by men remained significantly higher than the corresponding number smoked by women across all cohorts for which we can obtain valid estimates of cigarette consumption.

The changing gender differences in smoking behavior are consistent with the dramatic increase in urbanization that happened over time, which brought changes to the traditional roles of women in society. During the 1960s, the fraction of the population living in urban areas increased only slightly from 33 percent to 38.5 percent, but starting in approximately 1980, the rate of migration from rural to urban areas increased dramatically, especially among youth. By 2000, the urbanization rate had almost doubled to 64.9 percent. As people moved to cities, fewer people lived in traditional multigenerational extended families. Instead, the nuclear family, without older family members, became more common in urban areas (Kiray, 1984). Whereas in rural areas women worked as unpaid family members, in urban settings they became housewives and increasingly participated formally in the labor force (Ozbay, 1995).

Of course, changes in the traditional gender roles in Turkey also occurred among the population that was not urbanized. Ataturk, founder and leader of the Republic of Turkey until 1938, actively promoted a secular society. Leaders in the 1950s and 1960s followed the same policies, and in 1980, the government formalized them under the new constitution. During this period, women faced increasingly less restrictive social norms, and the government actively encouraged parents to educate their daughters. Thus, rates of women's smoking may also have increased as women generally attained more education, participated more often in the labor market, had more money, and demanded additional legal rights. A landmark year for these changes was 1975—the year that was labeled International Women's Year. That label prompted more Turkish women to compare their situation to what women in other Western countries experienced and led them to demand additional legal rights (Tekeli and Koray, 1991). Although the overall female labor force participation rate declined from 72 percent in 1955 to 34 percent in 1990, much of this occurred because fewer women worked in the agriculture sector; in urban areas, the female labor force participation rate increased (Turkish Industry and Business Association, 2000).

The military government of Turkey that took power in 1980 actively supported the social changes. Of course, the military government not only prohibited political activity but also deliberately acted to reduce the extent to which ideological groups influenced social behavior. However, exactly because the government actively policed such activity, it made sure that the debate on women's role in society took place in the public forum. In these years, women demanded more equal rights and freedom from traditional social roles, and the government responded by introducing secular civil codes and increasing women's formal education (Tekeli, 1990). This modernization process caused a restructuring of intra-household relations and (mostly symbolic) changes in the meaning of and process by which Turkish women construct their identities (Erturk, 1995).

CONCLUSION

During the past 80 years, cigarette consumption in Turkey has spread, peaked, and started to contract. A surprisingly large fraction of Turkish men smoke, and smoking prevalence rates—although they first increased and then somewhat decreased across generations—have remained consistently higher than 58 percent during the period of study. Smoking rates among Turkish women have shown an impressive increase across generations and have fallen only slightly among the youngest cohort. Whereas older cohorts of Turkish women seldom smoked, in our sample approximately 25 percent of the youngest cohort of women smokes. These patterns are correlated with how the tobacco industry is organized and with social norms about the behavior of women, migration patterns, prices, and tobacco control policies. To inform future anti-smoking interventions, more in-depth research is needed to establish the degree to which the correlations suggested by the descriptive patterns are causal or not.

NOTES

1. This information was published in the Turkish newspaper, *Milliyet*, on March 14, 1981.
2. The length of compulsory service varied over time. Until 1934, it was 18 months. Thereafter, it changed to 40 months in 1941, 30 months (1945), 24 months (1950), 20 months (1970), 18 months (1984), 15 months (1992), and 19 months (1993). From 1993 to 2013, the length of compulsory service gradually decreased almost every year to 12 months in 2013 (Millî Savunma Bakanliği, 2014). Duration of service may also vary with the assigned duties of the soldier.
3. According to the law for tobacco and tobacco monopoly (Law No. 1177), the preparation for sale and the sale of tobacco and all tobacco products as well as their imports are under the state monopoly, which is managed by TEKEL (Republic of Turkey, 1969). This statement was repealed with another law (Law No. 3291) published on May 28, 1986.
4. The Council of Ministers did not explicitly specify that TEKEL had the right to set the prices of the jointly produced or imported products. The council also did not specify the minimum fraction of shares TEKEL must own.
5. Information comes from editions of *Milliyet* that were published on February 13, 1984, and October 31, 1987.
6. When it was a monopoly, TEKEL advertised only when it launched a new brand and did not target women or youth (Dagli, 1999). Information comes from an edition of *Milliyet* that was published on November 5, 1985.
7. Information comes from an edition of *Milliyet* that was published on March 10, 1981.
8. Initially, the VAT was 10% (or 9.09% of retail price), and it increased to 12% in January 1993, 15% in November 1993, 17% in December 1999, and 18% in May 2001.
9. Author's calculation.
10. Information comes from an edition of *Milliyet* that was published on March 14, 1983.

REFERENCES

Bilir, N., B. Cakir, E. Dagli, T. Erguder, and Z. Önder. 2009. "Tobacco control in Turkey." Geneva: World Health Organization.

Bilir, N., and Z. Önder. 2000. "Impact of the ban on smoking in public places in Turkey: Proceedings II." Proceedings of the 7th International Conference on System Science in Health Care Budapest, Hungary: pp 220–225.

Council of Ministers. 1986. "Decision No. 86/10911." *Official Gazette*.

Council of Ministers. 1991. "Decision No. 91/1755." *Official Gazette*.

Dagli, E. 1999. "Are low-income countries targets of the tobacco industry?" *International Journal of Tuberculosis and Lung Disease* 3:2113–2118.

de Velay, A. 1978. *Turkiye Maliye Tarihi*. Ankara, Turkey: Maliye Bakanligi Tetkik Kurulu.

Dogruel, A. S., and F. Dogruel. 2000. *Osmanlı'dan Günümüze Tekel*. Istanbul: Tarih Vakfi Yurt Yayinlari.

Erturk, Y. 1995. "Rural women and modernization in southeastern Anatolia." In *Women in Modern Turkish Society: A Reader*, edited by S. Tekeli, pp 141–152. London: Zed Books.

Food and Agriculture Organization of the United Nations (FAO). 2003. *Issues in the Global Tobacco Economy: Selected Case Studies*. Rome: FAO.

Global Adult Tobacco Survey—Turkey (GATS). 2008. Copenhagen: World Health Organization. Available at http://www.euro.who.int/en/health-topics/disease-prevention/tobacco/publications/more-publications-on-tobacco/global-adult-tobacco-survey-turkey.

Haber, S. 2010. "Sigara yasağını ilk defa Osmanlı Devleti uygulamış." Available at http://www.samanyoluhaber.com/gundem/Ilk-defa-Osmalilar-uygulamis/437981.

Ilter, M. 1989. "Tutun and Tutun Mamullerinde Devlet Tekelince Yapilmis Olan Satis Fiat Ayarlamalari." Sale Price Adjustments on Tobacco and Tobacco Products Made by Government Monopoly. unpublished manuscript.

Karakartal, O. 2003. "Kadin ve Sigara." In *Tutun Kitabi*, edited by E. G. Naskali, pp 454–458. Istanbul: Kitabevi Yayinlari.

Kiray, M. B. 1984. "Büyük Kent ve Değişen Aile." In *Türkiye'de Ailenin Değişimi: Toplumbilimsel Incelemeler*, edited by T. Erder, pp 69–78. Ankara, Turkey: Türk Sosyal Bilimler Derneği.

Millî Savunma Bakanliği (MSB). "Askerlik Hizmet Sureleri." Ankara, Turkey: MSB. Available at http://www.asal.msb.gov.tr/er_islemleri/gun.kadar%20askerlik%20hiz.htm. Accessed June 7, 2014.

Önder, Z. 2002. "HNP discussion paper—Economics of tobacco control paper No. 2: Economics of tobacco control in Turkey." Washington, DC: International Bank for Reconstruction and Development/The World Bank.

Ozbay, F. 1995. "Changes in women's activities both inside and outside the home." In *Women in Modern Turkish Society: A Reader*, edited by Sirin Tekeli, pp 89–111. London: Zed Books.

Republic of Turkey. 1969, May 30. "No. 13210." *Official Gazette*.

Republic of Turkey. 1991, May 3. "No. 20860." *Official Gazette*.

Tekeli, S. 1990. "The meaning and limits of feminist ideology in Turkey." In *Women, Family and Social Change in Turkey*, edited by F. Özbay. Bangkok: UNESCO.

Tekeli, S., and M. Koray. 1991. "Devlet-Kadin-Siyaset." In *Türkiye Sosyal Ekonomik Siyasal Araştirmalar Vakfi*. Istanbul: Anadolu Matbaa Tic.

Turkish Industry and Business Association (TUSIAD). 2000. *Kadin Erkek Esitligine Dogru Yuruyus: Egitim, Calisma Yasami ve Siyaset*. Publication No. TUSIAD-T/2000-12/290. Istanbul: TUSIAD.

PART IV

Cross-Country Patterns

11

Smoking by Men in Cross-Country Perspective

PHILIP DECICCA, LOGAN MCLEOD, AND FENG LIU

INTRODUCTION

With the exception of indigenous peoples throughout the Americas, cigarette smoking, as we now know it, was relatively uncommon until the dawn of the 20th century. Spurred by two world wars, smoking prevalence increased dramatically in the first half of the 20th century, particularly among males in then rapidly developing countries such as the United States and United Kingdom (Forey et al., 2013). With this steep increase in male smoking prevalence came increased rates of lung cancer and related disease (Peto et al., 2012). This rise spurred reports in both the United Kingdom and United States warning of the lung cancer risk as well as other deleterious health effects of smoking (Royal College of Physicians of London, 1962; US Department of Health, Education, and Welfare, 1964).

Whereas smoking prevalence and the number of cigarettes smoked have declined in developed countries, smoking remains on the rise in less developed nations. Interestingly, in many of these nations, it is men who lead the way in terms of the timing of smoking initiation and the amount smoked. For example, among US males, who exemplify the experiences of men living in a developed nation, the average number of cigarettes smoked per day increased from 1 to 4 cigarettes per day between 1910 and 1930 and then from 4 to 10 cigarettes between 1930 and 1950 (Peto et al., 2012). One observes a nearly mirror-image pattern among men living in nations whose economies are still developing. Average consumption by Chinese men increased from 1 to 4 cigarettes per day between 1952 and 1972 and then from 4 to 10 cigarettes per day between 1972 and 1992—basically four decades after the same pattern was observed among US men (Gu et al., 2009).

In this chapter, we contribute to this literature by describing cross-country patterns in male smoking behavior over the life course, based on the experiences of the 10 nations covered in this book. We then present evidence that points to factors that may be correlated with this aggregate behavior before providing some concluding thoughts.

CROSS-COUNTRY PATTERNS IN SMOKING BEHAVIOR

As mentioned in Chapter 1, in what follows, we describe cross-country patterns in smoking behavior of men using four important indicators: the peak smoking prevalence, the average number of cigarettes consumed, the average age of smoking initiation, and the average age at cessation—all by 10-year birth cohorts.

We start with Figure 11.1, which describes peak smoking prevalence. Comparing prevalence rates of men in older cohorts with rates of men in younger birth cohorts (i.e., reading from right to left), several interesting patterns emerge. First, with few exceptions, peak smoking prevalence rates tend to fall. The drops are most noticeable for the United States and the United Kingdom, two countries that share a common heritage. Peak smoking prevalence declines among UK residents from more than 80 percent of those aged 80–89 years in 2002 to approximately 45 percent of those aged 20–29 years in this same year—a decrease of approximately 35 percentage points. That is, the peak smoking prevalence of the youngest cohort was approximately half the level of the peak smoking prevalence rate of the oldest cohort. Smoking prevalence rates in the corresponding cohorts in the United States are roughly 65 and 33 percent, respectively, again implying that the peak smoking prevalence of the youngest cohort was almost half that of the peak smoking prevalence rate of the oldest cohort. Although the timing differs, Germany, Spain, Canada, and Australia also exhibit similar, but somewhat less dramatic, declines in peak male smoking prevalence across cohorts. The patterns across cohorts of Canadian and Australian men more closely resemble the patterns observed in the United States and United Kingdom.

By contrast, among cohorts of men in Ukraine, Russia, China, and Turkey, whose economies were in transition and developing during this period, the peak smoking prevalence rate trended higher over successive cohorts up to the cohort that was 40–49 years old. In other words, peak smoking prevalence increased substantially

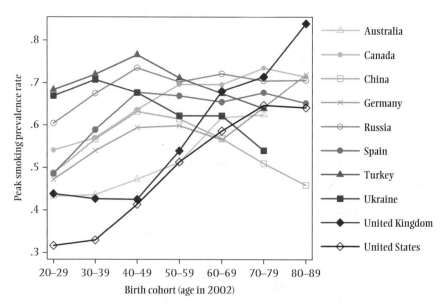

Figure 11.1 Peak smoking prevalence rate by country and cohort.

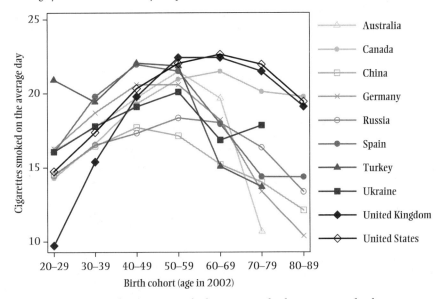

Figure 11.2 Number of cigarettes smoked on average day by country and cohort.

from those aged 80–89 years in 2002 to those aged 40–49 years in 2002. In these countries, male smoking prevalence rates began to decline among men aged 30–39 years, except in Ukraine, where prevalence began to decline only in the youngest cohort of men. This hump-shaped pattern may be the beginning of a steeper decline of the sort evident among US and UK males.

In Figure 11.2, we plot, for each cohort in each country, the number of cigarettes that the average male smoker consumed. One observes a similar pattern in all countries. Across successive cohorts, average consumption follows an inverted U-shaped pattern: It is relatively low in the oldest cohorts, increases in the middle-aged cohorts, and then decreases among the youngest cohorts of men, sometimes dramatically. Several other interesting patterns also emerge. Again, we see a close correspondence between the pattern of average cigarette consumption of men in the United States and the United Kingdom. For example, when they were actively smoking, current and former smokers among US and UK men aged 80–89 years smoked approximately 18 cigarettes per day on average, men aged 60–69 years smoked roughly 23 cigarettes per day, and successively younger cohorts smoked increasingly less cigarettes. The similarity in average cigarette consumption between the two countries begins to diverge among the cohort of men aged 30–39 years. From then on, UK men smoked less than did their US counterparts. In the youngest cohort of men—those aged 20–29 years in 2002—US men smoked approximately 15 cigarettes per day, whereas UK men smoked approximately 10 cigarettes per day—one-third fewer than US males.

Among all countries represented, the UK male experience is unique. Although average cigarette consumption began to decline in all countries among cohorts younger than either the 50- to 59-year-old or 40- to 49-year-old cohorts, the United Kingdom experienced by far the steepest decline. Indeed, in eight of the remaining nine countries, the average number of cigarettes smoked per day by males is nearly

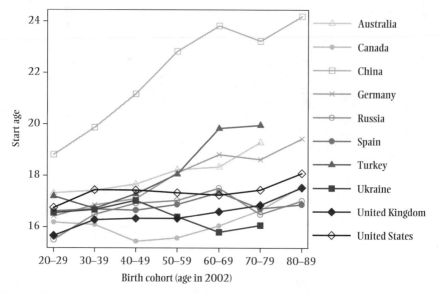

Figure 11.3 Average age of smoking initiation by country and cohort.

identical among those aged 20–29 years in 2002 at roughly 15 cigarettes per day. The only exception is Turkey, where male smokers aged 20–29 years consume more than 20 cigarettes per day—approximately 5 cigarettes per day more than male smokers aged 30–39 years.

Figure 11.3 presents the average age of men's smoking initiation by cohort in the 10 countries. It is striking that, in successively younger cohorts, the cross-country variance in average initiation age declines dramatically. The average age of initiation among men aged 80–89 years in 2002 varied substantially compared to the average age of initiation among men aged 20–29 years in 2002. For example, excluding China, which has a very unique pattern, the average age of initiation ranged from roughly 16 to 20 years in the oldest cohorts. By contrast, in the youngest cohort, the average age of initiation was either 16 or 17 years in 7 of the 9 countries (still excluding China). The age of initiation converged mostly because, over time, new smokers were starting at younger ages in many countries. Turkey, Australia, and Germany experienced very large declines in male age of initiation across successive cohorts, but China experienced the largest decline by far. Among Chinese men who are current or former smokers, the average initiation age was 24 years for the cohort aged 80–89 years in 2002 and 19 years for the cohort aged 20–29 years in 2002. Although Chinese men in the youngest cohort continue to initiate smoking at older ages than their counterparts in other countries, the overall trend across cohorts in all countries is toward a similar average age of initiation.

Finally, Figure 11.4 presents, for all cohorts in all countries, the age at which the average male smoker quit. Note that one can only compare the average age of smoking cessation across countries for a given birth cohort because men in younger cohorts are at different points in their smoking histories (and so may not have yet quit). Because of this issue, Figure 11.4 plots the average age of smoking cessation of each cohort in each country relative to the average age of cessation of the corresponding

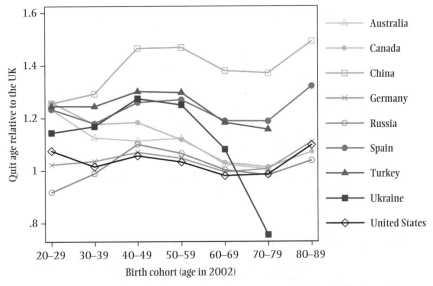

Figure 11.4 Average age of smoking cessation by country and cohort (relative to the United Kingdom).

UK cohort. We label this quit age as the "relative quit age" or "relative quit rate." In general, nearly all cohorts in all countries tended to quit smoking at later ages than similarly aged males in the United Kingdom.

Aside from this general conclusion, we observe two other interesting patterns. First, across all the cohorts in Australia, the United States, Canada, Germany, and Russia, male smokers quit at approximately the same age as UK male smokers. By contrast, male smokers in Turkey, Spain, China, and Ukraine do not. Second, and related to this, male smokers in successively younger cohorts are quitting at an age that is increasingly similar to the age at which UK male smokers quit. Due principally to Turkey, Spain, and China, there is much more variation in relative quit age in the earlier cohorts (i.e., those 70–79 and 80–89 years old in 2002). Indeed, among men in the youngest birth cohort whose members were aged 20–29 years in 2002, the average quit age differs less from the average UK quit age than in all other cohorts. Values range from 1.0 to 1.3 (i.e., an average age equal to or 30 percent older than the corresponding average quit age among UK males). In the youngest cohort, Russian men quit at a slightly younger average age than did men in the 20- to 29-year-old birth cohort in the United Kingdom.

PREDICTORS OF SMOKING BEHAVIOR OF MEN

In this section, we conjecture about possible determinants of the patterns presented previously. Such a discussion is by its nature speculative because we describe patterns across such a long time period within and across so many countries. Although strong evidence suggests that public policies may affect smoking behavior, and although it is possible to link policies to observed patterns, it is much more difficult to "explain" the similarity and differences in patterns because of secular trends over time within countries or at a point in time across nations. Secular trends may be

driven by changing attitudes, norms, beliefs, and other "animal spirits" that are difficult for researchers to observe and quantify. To the extent that such trends exist, and
truly affect smoking patterns, it makes a deep understanding of causality difficult.
We proceed with these caveats in mind.

Our first hypothesis is inspired by Figure 11.1, which shows that, in the more
economically developed countries, peak smoking prevalence markedly declined
between the oldest and youngest birth cohorts. Because this pattern is most prevalent among older cohorts of men in Great Britain, the United States, Russia,
Canada, and Germany, we are led to speculate that it may be partly influenced by
the well-documented surge in smoking prevalence associated with World War II.
Our data show that peak smoking prevalence rate is highest among men in the 80-
to 89-year-old cohort, most of whom were "of age" for World War II, and in the
70- to 79-year-old cohort, whose oldest members were also most likely to have been
involved.

Figure 11.2 also inspires us to conjecture about the striking cross-country similarity of the average daily consumption of cigarettes and the inverted U-shape one
observes across cohorts. The consistency of this pattern across nations suggests that
it is not attributable to policies specific to each country, which were not well syn-
chronized (governments in these countries did not agree on a common tobacco
control framework until 1998), but, rather, to forces common to all countries. In
addition, the pattern peaks in most countries with the cohorts aged 50–59 years in
2002, whose members were roughly teenagers when the United States and United
Kingdom released reports highlighting the deleterious effects of smoking. This pattern is consistent with the hypothesis that fewer members of younger cohorts smoked
because they were some of the first cohorts to learn that smoking harms health. Of
course, an information-based explanation would require that men in nations other
than the United States and United Kingdom also got the information and that it
was new to a large enough segment of the male population. If so, then information
could explain the similarity in within-country patterns—although this inference is
confounded by changes in the composition of smokers over time. For example, if
heavier smokers are more likely to quit (e.g., because they experience deleterious
health effects that lead them to quit) or die from a smoking-related cause, then the
observed within-nation patterns might be driven by changes in the composition of
lighter versus heavier smokers.

Another pattern worth noting is that British male smokers reduced their cigarette
consumption to a much greater degree than did US smokers. As previously shown
in Figure 11.2, whereas US males aged 20–29 years in 2002 smoked 15 cigarettes
per day on average, corresponding British males smoked only 10 cigarettes per day.
This difference is especially interesting when one also observes that the UK smoking
prevalence is more or less constant for the three youngest cohorts and even increases
in the youngest two cohorts, whereas the US smoking prevalence slows down but
continues to fall across these cohorts (see Figure 11.1). Together, the two patterns
suggest that smoking is becoming slightly more popular over time in the United
Kingdom than in the United States but that British smokers tend to be relatively
lighter. This could occur if the new British smokers are less attached to the habit (e.g.,
weekend smokers) or because the US public policy and heavy state cigarette taxes
caused less addicted smokers to quit and, thus, the remaining smokers in the country

smoke on average more cigarettes per day. In any event, the cross-country pattern is striking and worthy of additional study.

As with the patterns in cigarette consumption, the cross-country dynamics in the average age of smoking initiation plotted in Figure 11.3 also lead us to conjecture that the arrival of information about the health risks of smoking might play a role. Because smoking prevalence is decreasing over time as health information is increasing, it could be that the new information available to men in younger birth cohorts successfully dissuaded men from starting to smoke. All else equal, the average initiation age decreases when fewer men start to smoke when they are older and relatively more men start when they are younger. Thus, it is plausible that among the young cohorts that had not yet started to smoke when new information became available, this new information successfully convinced the older men not to smoke. This conjecture may be particularly plausible if one believes that slightly older individuals, as opposed to teenagers, are more likely to get and better able to digest health information.

To close this chapter, we estimate the correlation between the year-by-year smoking prevalence rate of men in each cohort and country and several socioeconomic variables. We do so using multivariate regressions that adjust for age and age-squared and country, time, and cohort fixed effects. Because our set of regressors contains highly correlated variables, we run eight separate ordinary least squares (OLS) regressions, each of which includes a different variable of interest, and we report each of the coefficients in Table 11.1. We find that male smoking prevalence is higher among men who live under more democratic regimes, in more densely populated countries, and in countries with higher average educational attainment among men. Male smoking prevalence is lower when the per capita gross domestic product (GDP), cigarette prices, male labor force participation rates, and fertility rates are higher, and also when a greater share of the population lives in a rural area. Although descriptive in nature, these partial correlations suggest several interesting interpretations.

For instance, consider the finding that male smoking prevalence is higher in countries with a more urbanized population or, alternatively, when population density is greater. It is difficult to interpret this association as anything other than a correlation (or reflection of other factors). It might, for example, reflect local peer effects (e.g., community-level norms), or it could be spurious (e.g., urbanization is a proxy for unobserved wealth associated with increased levels of human capital often observed in urban areas). However, the association is nonetheless interesting and may be worth further investigation.

The correlations in Table 11.1 also suggest that economic growth leads to a lower prevalence of male smoking. Here, we see negative correlations between per capita GDP and male smoking prevalence, as well as aggregate labor force participation and male smoking prevalence, both of which suggest that economic growth reduces smoking participation by males. According to the cigarette "epidemic" model (Lopez et al., 1994), the association of economic development switches from positive to negative as countries enter more advanced stages of smoking diffusion (i.e., as anti-smoking information proliferates and governments adopt anti-smoking policies). Broadly consistent with this hypothesis, Wasserman et al. (1991) and Cheng and Kenkel (2010) found that the income elasticity of cigarette demand in the United

Table 11.1. Correlation of Smoking Prevalence of Men with Selected Variables (Estimates from Linear Regressions)

Variable	Coefficient	Standard error	Observations	R^2
GDP per capita	−0.0136[***]	(0.0008)	3986	0.8537
Democracy	0.0028[***]	(0.0005)	3796	0.8409
Cigarette price	−0.0212[***]	(0.0031)	3045	0.8306
Labor force participation rate	−0.0027[*]	(0.0016)	1804	0.8097
Population density	0.0028[***]	(0.0003)	3071	0.8259
Share of rural population	−0.0056[***]	(0.0005)	3135	0.8238
Educational attainment	0.0250[***]	(0.0031)	3384	0.8335
Fertility rate	−0.0356[***]	(0.0038)	3119	0.8249

NOTES: Each row reports statistics from a separate OLS regression. Data are at the country, birth cohort, and year level of observation. All regressions control for mean cohort age and age-squared, country dummies, year dummies, and birth cohort dummies. GDP per capita is in 1990 International Geary–Khamis dollars, '0,000s (source: Maddison, 2010). Democracy is a scaled measure of regime governance that takes values from −10 to 10 (source: Polity IV Project). Cigarette price is in 2008 US dollars, purchasing power parity adjusted (from various national sources; see country-specific chapters). The labor force participation rate is for males of all ages (source: International Labor Office for Ukraine and China; Organization for Economic Cooperation and Development statistics for all other countries). Population density measures people per square kilometer of land area (source: World Development Indicators). Educational attainment measures average years of total schooling for males (source: Barro and Lee, 2010; missing values interpolated). Fertility rate measures total births per woman (source: World Development Indicators). [*],[**], and [***] indicate statistical significance at the 10, 5, and 1 percent level, respectively.

States changed from positive to negative between the mid-1960s and mid-1980s as more information on the possible deleterious effects of smoking became available. In addition, Christopoulou et al. (2013) reported a similar reversal in the association of male smoking rates and three indicators of economic development in Mexico.

Perhaps somewhat surprisingly, we also find a positive correlation between the level of formal education, measured as the average number of years of schooling for males in a given country, and male smoking prevalence. Because education levels are directly related to economic growth, this finding seems to contradict the notion that economic growth reduces male smoking prevalence. Also, according to the cigarette epidemic model, the association of smoking prevalence with education should resemble the association of smoking prevalence with economic growth; that is, it should switch from positive to negative as countries enter more advanced stages of smoking diffusion. Consistent with this model, Cavelaars et al. (2000) found a positive association in southern Europe and a negative association in northern Europe. However, not all available evidence supports this pattern. For example, Giskes et al. (2005) found that in Italy and the United Kingdom, smoking rates declined faster among the less educated groups, even though both countries were at advanced stages of smoking diffusion. These authors attribute their finding to targeted anti-tobacco policies in these countries.

Finally, we find a negative association between price and cigarette smoking prevalence. Specifically, the relevant estimate in Table 11.1 corresponds to a price elasticity of smoking prevalence of −0.145, which implies that a 10 percent increase in price leads to roughly a 1.5 percent reduction in smoking prevalence. Interestingly, this estimate is similar to recent US estimates that peg this elasticity between −0.1 and −0.3, thus portraying a very inelastic price response (Callison and Kaestner, 2014; DeCicca and McLeod, 2008; Tauras, 2006). By contrast, estimates from more developing countries (e.g., China) suggest a corresponding elasticity in the range of −0.4 to −0.7 (Hu and Mao, 2002; Chen and Xing, 2011). Recall that the estimates we present in Table 11.1 are effectively averages across different country types (i.e., more and less developed) because we pool country-specific data to generate our estimates.

CONCLUSION

This chapter compared the 10-year cohort-specific smoking experiences of males in 10 countries. Although causality is difficult to infer from trends such as these, several interesting patterns emerged. First, similarities in the number of cigarettes smoked each day by US and UK men in older cohorts disappeared and then diverged in younger cohorts. This divergence in average consumption occurred despite, or perhaps because of, a slightly increasing rate of peak smoking prevalence moving from the 40- to 49-year-old to the 20- to 29-year-old cohort in the United Kingdom. As discussed previously, it is difficult to reconcile these patterns, but their discovery points squarely to the need to better understand changes in the composition of cigarette smokers over time. Second, we uncovered interesting and somewhat counterintuitive estimates for the relationship of urbanization and formal education with smoking prevalence. Each of these is worthy of further exploration. Finally, the power of the descriptive smoking epidemic model is confirmed along many dimensions of male smoking. Although interesting, this model only provides an outline of what might happen as an economy develops. The extent to which changes occur needs more rigorous causal analysis in order to be better understood. We believe that this chapter, and the entire compilation, provides sustenance for this important work.

REFERENCES

Barro, R. and J.-W. Lee. April 2010. "A new data set of educational attainment in the world, 1950–2010." *Journal of Development Economics* 104:184–198.

Callison, K., and R. Kaestner. 2014. "Do higher taxes reduce adult smoking? New evidence of the effect of recent cigarette tax increases on adult smoking." *Economic Inquiry* 52:155–172.

Cavelaars, A. E., A. E. Kunst, J. J. Geurts, R. Crialesi, L. Grötvedt, U. Helmert, et al. 2000. "Educational differences in smoking: International comparison." *British Medical Journal* 320:1102–1107.

Chen, Y., and W. Xing. 2011. "Quantity, quality, and regional price variation of cigarettes: Demand analysis based on a household survey in China." *China Economic Review* 22:221–232.

Cheng, K. W., and D. Kenkel. 2010, August 1. "U.S. cigarette demand: 1944–2004." *B. E. Journal of Economic Analysis & Policy* 10.

Christopoulou, R., D. R. Lillard, and J. B. Miyar. 2013. "Smoking behavior of Mexicans: Patterns by birth-cohort, gender, and education." *International Journal of Public Health* 58:335–343.

DeCicca, P., and L. McLeod. 2008. "Cigarette taxes and older adult smoking: Evidence from recent large tax increases." *Journal of Health Economics* 27:918–929.

Forey, B., J. Hamling, A. Thornton, and P. N. Lee. 2013. *International smoking statistics: Web edition*. Sutton, UK: P. N. Lee Statistics and Computing. Available at http://www.pnlee.co.uk/ISS3.htm.

Giskes, K., A. E. Kunst, J. Benach, C. Borrell, G. Costa, E. Dahl, et al. 2005. "Trends in smoking behaviour between 1985 and 2000 in nine European countries by education." *Journal of Epidemiology and Community Health* 59:395–401.

Gu, D., T. N. Kelly, X. Wu, J. Chen, J. M. Samet, J. F. Huang, et al. 2009. "Mortality attributable to smoking in China." *New England Journal of Medicine* 360:150–159.

Hu, T. W., and Z. Mao. 2002. "Effect of cigarette tax on cigarette consumption and the Chinese economy." *Tobacco Control* 11:105–108.

Lopez, A. D., N. E. Collishaw, and T. Piha. 1994. "A descriptive model of the tobacco epidemic in developed countries." *Tobacco Control* 3:242–247.

Maddison Project. n.d. or 2010. Available at http://www.ggdc.net/maddison/maddison-project/home.htm

Peto, R., A. D. Lopez, J. Boreham, and M. Thun. 2012. *Mortality from smoking in developed countries, 1950–2010*. Oxford, UK: Clinical Trial Service Unit and Epidemiological Studies Unit.

Royal College of Physicians of London. 1962. *Smoking and Health: Summary and Report of the Royal College of Physicians of London on Smoking in Relation to Cancer of the Lung and Other Diseases*. London: Pitman.

Tauras, J. 2006. "Smoke-free air laws, cigarette prices and adult cigarette demand." *Economic Inquiry* 44:333–342.

US Department of Health, Education, and Welfare (USDHEW). 1964. *Smoking and Health: Report of the Advisory Committee to the Surgeon General of the Public Health Service*. Public Health Service Publication No. 1103. Rockville, MD: USDHEW.

Wasserman, J., W. G. Manning, J. P. Newhouse, and J. D. Winkler. 1991. "The effects of excise taxes and regulations on cigarette smoking." *Journal of Health Economics* 10:43–64.

12

Smoking by Women in Cross-Country Perspective

REBEKKA CHRISTOPOULOU AND ZEYNEP ÖNDER

INTRODUCTION

Although smoking is generally more widespread in male populations, women also smoke in large numbers. According to the World Health Organization (WHO), nearly 250 million women in the world are daily smokers. In developed countries, smokers comprise approximately 22 percent of the female population, whereas the corresponding share in developing countries is 9 percent.[1] Although in several developed countries smoking among women is currently declining (e.g., Australia, Canada, the United Kingdom, and the United States), in many other countries the habit is still spreading.

Governments should be generally concerned when a high proportion of the population smokes, but they have additional reason to be concerned when women's smoking rates are high because, unlike men, women who smoke directly affect not only their own health but also the health of their current and future children. Apart from the well-known effect of smoking on cancer and cardiac disease, clinical research has shown that smoking among women is associated with adverse endocrine changes (including increases in menstrual problems), reproductive difficulties, complications of pregnancy, low fetal birthweight, higher fetus toxicity, decreased quantity and quality of breastfeeding, and sudden infant death syndrome (Nusbaum et al., 2000). Researchers have also shown that prenatal and postnatal exposure to tobacco smoke may affect children's long-term development; for example, it has been associated with attention deficit disorder and other behavioral problems during childhood (Milberger et al., 1996, 1998; McCrory and Layte, 2012). In fact, many of the previously mentioned associations are demonstratively causal (see the review of evidence in US Department of Health and Human Services, 2014).

To develop policies that ameliorate these many adverse effects, one must first understand what causes women to start and to continue to smoke. However, this task is not straightforward. Studies have shown that the smoking behavior of women differs from that of men in ways that cannot be explained by observable characteristics such as income, age, education, and marital status (Bauer et al., 2007). In other words, there are gender-specific factors that cause women to make different smoking decisions compared to observationally identical men. For example, researchers have found that, all else equal, women are less likely to smoke than men, but once they start smoking, they are less likely to quit and more likely to relapse after an attempt to quit. However, not all evidence supports these patterns (Hersch, 1996; Ward et al., 1997; Osler et al., 1999; Jarvis et al., 2013).

Arguably, several biological, socioeconomic, and cultural determinants of smoking behavior are specific to women. The country-specific chapters of this book discussed many of these determinants. Women have special metabolic responses to nicotine; they often command fewer economic resources that they could use to buy cigarettes; they may face social disapproval if they smoke, especially in traditional societies; or they may simply have different preferences than men, such as a low sensitivity to prices and greater concerns for weight gain, depression, and their family members (Glassman et al., 1990; Waldron, 1991; Williamson et al., 1991; McGee and Williams, 2006). At the same time, women's preferences are influenced by targeted advertisements from the tobacco industry and other social forces, such as feminism (Kaufman and Nichter, 2010).

To evaluate the relative importance of these factors, it is necessary to obtain a clear picture of women's smoking patterns over time and across countries. Although previous studies have documented some of this variation (Waldron et al., 1988; Fiore et al., 1989; Pierce, 1989; Husten et al., 1996; Thun et al., 2012), they examined a narrow time period, a small set of countries, or indicators of smoking behavior that do not fully reflect population exposure to smoking-related health risks (e.g., they examined smoking rates but not cigarette consumption). Throughout this book, we widened the scope of the analysis on all these dimensions. In this chapter, we compare indicators of smoking prevalence, cigarette consumption, age of initiation, and age of cessation across the seven generations of women in the 10 countries of study. We then consider the existing evidence and propose possible hypotheses to explain the observed smoking patterns.

CROSS-COUNTRY PATTERNS IN SMOKING BEHAVIOR

Figure 12.1 plots the peak smoking prevalence rates of each birth cohort (defined by age in 2002) in each country.[2] At first glance, this figure shows no clear patterns because there are significant differences across countries in both the intergenerational evolution and the level of peak prevalence. Of all cohort country groups, at their peak smoking prevalence rate, 40- to 49-year-old Canadian women smoked the most (at 55 percent) and 20- to 29-year-old Chinese women smoked the least (at nearly 0 percent).

Despite the apparent idiosyncratic smoking patterns, there are systematic similarities in Figure 12.1 that are easier to recognize from the perspective of the "cigarette epidemic" model developed by Lopez et al. (1994) and Thun et al. (2012). These authors argue that, as countries develop economically, the prevalence of smoking among women grows to a peak and then declines (lagging that of men by a few decades). In Figure 12.1, one observes such a hump-shaped pattern across cohorts, although the pattern is more evident for some countries than for others. In Australia, Canada, Germany, Russia, Spain, and the United States, the peak smoking prevalence

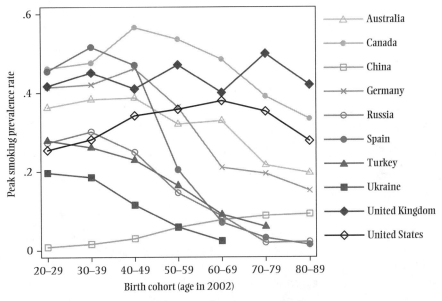

Figure 12.1 Peak smoking prevalence rate by country and cohort.

rate first increases and then decreases across successively younger cohorts. In Turkey and Ukraine, peak smoking prevalence monotonically increases across successive generations, but the increase has already started to slow down among the very young cohorts. In the former group of countries, Spain and Russia reach their peak in the cohort of 30- to 39-year-olds; Canada, Germany, and Australia do so in the cohort of 40- to 49-year-olds; and the United States does so in the cohort of 60- to 69-year-olds. In the latter group, the peak is of course highest for the cohort that is 20–29 years old. Consistent with the cigarette epidemic model, these differences suggest that economically mature countries are at more advanced stages of smoking diffusion relative to newly developed or developing countries.

Across successive cohorts in China and the United Kingdom, however, the cross-cohort pattern of peak smoking prevalence rates does not match the cigarette epidemic story very well. In China, peak smoking prevalence declines across successive generations; that is, it shows symptoms of an advanced stage of smoking diffusion even though China is among the most recently developed countries we study (it started developing quickly after the late 1970s). In the United Kingdom, peak smoking prevalence follows a zigzag course across successive cohorts, and it shows no long-term trend whatsoever. As we discussed in the respective country-specific chapters, it is likely that the female smoking behavior in China and the United Kingdom has been influenced more by cultural and social factors and less so by economic factors. Specifically, in China, smoking became increasingly incompatible with the socially accepted role of women in society, whereas in the United Kingdom, the ups and downs of peak smoking prevalence seem to correspond to the three waves of feminism that emerged during the study period.

Although the peak prevalence rate approximates how popular the smoking habit is, it says nothing about how heavily people smoke. In Figure 12.2, we plot, for each cohort in each country, the number of cigarettes that current and former smokers

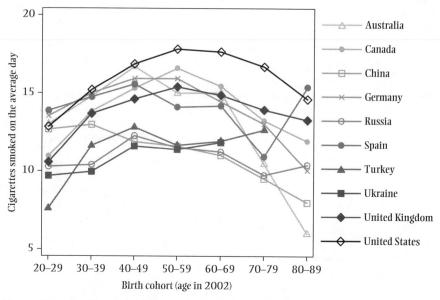

Figure 12.2 Number of cigarettes smoked on average day by country and cohort.

consumed on the average day when they smoked.[3] Interestingly, like smoking prevalence, cigarette consumption also appears to be associated with a country's economic development. Consumption is higher in the advanced economies (highest in almost all US cohorts) and lower in the emerging economies (lowest in almost all Ukrainian cohorts). Moreover, it forms a hump-shaped pattern across successive generations, which seems to be consistently timed across countries; that is, it is generally higher among the middle-aged cohorts and lower among younger and older cohorts. Again, there are exceptions. For example, as discussed in the chapter on China, while smoking prevalence is monotonically falling across successively younger cohorts, average cigarette consumption is monotonically increasing. Thus, although fewer women smoke in China in successively younger cohorts, the ones who do smoke are increasingly heavy smokers.

Of course, the popularity and intensity indicators alone do not fully reflect population exposure to smoking health risks because they miss information on the persistence of the smoking habit. One can deduce such information from the dynamics in smoking initiation and cessation. To this purpose, we respectively plot in Figures 12.3 and 12.4 the average age at which female smokers start and quit smoking by birth cohort and country. Recall that, by construction, quit age increases with cohort age and, therefore, cannot be compared across cohorts. For this reason, in Figure 12.4, we plot the average quit age in every country relative to average quit age in the United Kingdom. The same limitation potentially holds for the age at smoking initiation (i.e., it may increase with cohort age by construction) but to a much lesser extent.[4] Thus, we report data on initiation age in absolute terms.

Figure 12.3 shows that the average start age among female smokers is lower in mature economies (lowest in the United States, United Kingdom, and Canada) and higher in emerging economies (highest in China, Turkey, and Ukraine). In all but a few cases, female smokers in any given generation started to smoke at a younger age

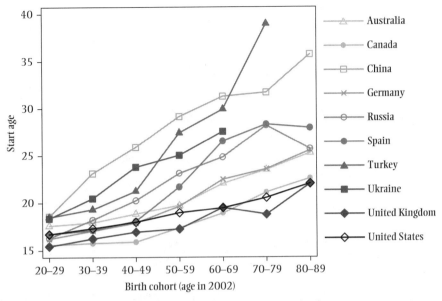

Figure 12.3 Average age of smoking initiation by country and cohort.

than did smokers in the generation that immediately preceded them. Strikingly, the average age of initiation has not only declined across successive cohorts but also converged to a common value. Because older women in developing economies started smoking at much older ages than did those in mature economies, their average age of smoking initiation has fallen more and faster. For example, the average start age was slightly less than 40 years in the cohort of Turkish women age 70–79 years in 2002 and approximately 35 years in the cohort of Chinese women age 80–89 years in 2002. In both countries, it declined below 20 years in the 20- to 29-year-old cohorts (although the decline was much faster in Turkey). By contrast, the average start age in the United Kingdom declined by only 5 years, from 21 (80- to 89-year-old cohort) to 16 years (20- to 29-year-old cohort).

Finally, Figure 12.4 shows that, unlike the three previous indicators of smoking behavior, the average quit age does not follow a consistent pattern across more and less developed countries. The absence of a consistent pattern arises mostly because quit behavior of female smokers in Russia differs from quit behavior in other developing economies. Specifically, women who smoke in China and Turkey wait the longest to quit relative to both women smokers in the United Kingdom and smokers in other countries. Although one would expect a similar pattern among Russian women, our data show that they quit much earlier. In fact, apart from Russia, in no other country do female smokers quit before female smokers in the United Kingdom.

Taken together, the patterns in Figures 12.3 and 12.4 lead us to conclude that in the economically mature countries (especially in the English-speaking countries we study), female smokers start smoking when they are relatively young but also quit smoking when they are young. By contrast, in less developed countries, female smokers start smoking at older ages but also quit much later. Russia is an interesting exception to this pattern because Russian female smokers start smoking at older ages and quit smoking when they are relatively young.

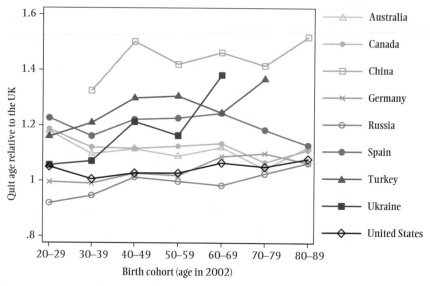

Figure 12.4 Average age of smoking cessation by country and cohort (relative to the United Kingdom).

PREDICTORS OF SMOKING BEHAVIOR OF WOMEN

The systematic patterns across age cohorts that we just documented clearly suggest that economic development could play an important role in the determination of female smoking patterns. Apart from the authors of the cigarette epidemic model, other researchers have also suggested such a role (e.g., Schaap et al., 2009). They all acknowledge that economic development may have diverse effects on smoking outcomes both over time and across demographic groups. As economies develop, individuals and firms access more resources and, therefore, the demand for and supply of cigarettes increases. However, a host of other political, social, cultural, and technological changes take place concurrently, each of which may reinforce or counteract the income effect on smoking.

First, economic development in modern history is linked with industrialization, which in turn is linked with urbanization and waged work. In urbanized societies, more women formally participate in the labor force and thereby get command over economic resources. Also, more women live in small households (as opposed to large rural households that encompass the extended family) and enjoy urban anonymity; thus, they face less familial and social pressure against their smoking. In addition, economies typically prosper in democratic regimes, where laws establish women's rights and information flows freely. In these regimes, women tend to have easier access to cigarettes and face less social disapproval when they smoke, but they are also more exposed to information about the health risks of smoking (given that such information exists). Economic development also weakens dependencies between governments and specific industries, including the tobacco industry. Thus, governments can afford to oppose the industry's interests by increasing cigarette taxes. At the same time, they can afford to spend more on education (expanding their system to include more women) and on tobacco control policies (increasing awareness about the health effects of smoking in general and on women in particular).

To provide some simple evidence about how such factors relate to the female smoking rates in our set of countries, in Table 12.1 we report a set of correlation coefficients. Specifically, we regress the female smoking prevalence rate of each cohort in each year in all 10 countries against country-specific time-series indicators, each of which represents some aspect of the national context in which women were taking their smoking decisions. The set includes gross domestic product (GDP) per capita as a measure of development and a number of variables that co-vary with development—namely, an index of democracy, cigarette prices, female labor force participation, two measures of urbanization (population density and the share of rural population), female educational attainment, and total births per woman.[5] Because these variables significantly co-vary, we run separate regressions for each one while also controlling for age, age-squared, as well as country, year, and cohort fixed effects.

We find that a greater proportion of women smoke in years when GDP per capita, democracy levels, women's participation in the labor force, and average years of

Table 12.1. Correlation of Smoking Prevalence of Women with Selected Variables (Estimates from Linear Regressions)

Variable	Coefficient	Standard error	Observations	R^2
GDP per capita	0.0035***	(0.0006)	3986	0.6879
Democracy	0.0030***	(0.0004)	3794	0.6875
Cigarette price	−0.0044*	(0.0024)	3045	0.6842
Labor force participation rate	0.0015**	(0.0008)	1804	0.6984
Population density	0.0003	(0.0002)	3071	0.6869
Share of rural population	−0.0020***	(0.0004)	3135	0.6877
Educational attainment	0.0175***	(0.0029)	3384	0.6948
Fertility rate	−0.0150***	(0.0030)	3119	0.6883

NOTES: Each row reports statistics from a separate ordinary least squares regression. Data are at the country, birth cohort, and year level of observation. All regressions control for mean cohort age and age-squared, country dummies, year dummies, and birth cohort dummies. GDP per capita is in 1990 International Geary–Khamis dollars '0,000s (source: Maddison, 2010). Democracy is a scaled measure of regime governance that takes values from −10 to 10 (source: Polity IV Project). Cigarette price is in 2008 US dollars, purchasing power parity adjusted (from various national sources; see country-specific chapters). The labor force participation rate is for females of all ages (source: International Labor Office for Ukraine and China; Organization for Economic Cooperation and Development statistics for all other countries). Population density measures people per square kilometer of land area (source: World Development Indicators). Educational attainment measures average years of total schooling for females (source: Barro and Lee, 2010; missing values interpolated). Fertility rate measures total births per woman (source: World Development Indicators). *, **, and *** indicate statistical significance at the 10, 5, and 1 percent level, respectively.

schooling are higher, and fewer women smoke in years when cigarette prices, the share of rural population, and fertility rates are higher. These results find support in previously published evidence. For example, Steckley et al. (2003) and Schaap et al. (2009) find a positive (unconditional) correlation of GDP with smoking rates among women, especially among women who are more educated.[6] Previous studies also report a positive correlation between female smoking and educational attainment in less developed countries (e.g., in southern Europe; Cavelaars et al., 2000) where cigarette diffusion is still at early stages, whereas in more developed countries, higher education is generally associated with a lower risk of smoking among women. It is possible that the less developed countries in our sample drive the negative correlation we find in our results. Finally, previous studies also report a positive correlation between female smoking and urbanization. For example, Pomerleau et al. (2004) found that living in larger urban areas was the strongest predictor of smoking among women in countries of the former Soviet Union. They interpret their finding to reflect that urban women have higher exposure to Western influences and to aggressive advertising campaigns by Western tobacco companies. Similar evidence is also reported in Missouri Department of Health (1995), Pudule et al. (1999), and Idris et al. (2007).

Interestingly, the correlation between smoking and fertility may arise via different channels. Lower fertility may be correlated with higher smoking because they are both consequences of changes in social norms about gender roles. That is, as women become emancipated, they are both more likely to smoke and more likely to use birth control. However, the negative correlation may also arise because smoking affects women's ability to conceive, carry, and deliver healthy children. Both effects work in the same direction.

Finally, the negative correlation between smoking rates and cigarette prices is according to theory. This correlation corresponds to a price elasticity of smoking of -0.07—an estimate that falls at the very low end of the range of elasticities reported in other studies (although most studies report price elasticity of cigarette consumption rather than that of smoking prevalence or participation). For US women, Chaloupka (1990) finds a positive price elasticity of cigarette demand that ranges from 0.852 to 1.41, but all other US estimates are negative and range from -0.118 to -0.510 (Lewit and Coate, 1982; Hersch, 2000; Stehr, 2007). Studies from other countries also find comparable results. Mao et al. (2003) report a price elasticity of cigarette consumption in China of -0.69, Lee et al. (2004) report a price elasticity of smoking intensity in Taiwan of -0.14, and Oglobin and Brock (2003) report a price elasticity of smoking prevalence among Russian women of -0.628.

Two potential predictors of female smoking are missing from Table 12.1 because we lack the necessary data: (1) anti-smoking publications and campaigns and (2) cigarette advertising. Both transmit information that likely affects how women assess the cost and utility of smoking. For example, cigarette advertisements that target women may convince women that they will benefit if they smoke because the advertising emphasizes that being slim is important and that smoking helps with weight control. Similarly, anti-smoking publications and campaigns inform women that smoking negatively affects not only their own health but also their childbearing prospects and their children's health. Although there are no available time-series indicators we can use to capture these informational forces,[7] in the country-specific chapters, we reported key dates when these forces likely started (e.g., with publications of research articles on the smoking health effects and/or official government publications) or ended (e.g., through regulatory advertisement bans in certain media). In all the countries we study, pro-smoking information generally precedes anti-smoking information, but after a period of overlap timed immediately after the 1950s—when scientists began to demonstrate the health effects of smoking—the latter eventually dominates. We conjecture that these informational shifts may be the leading predictors of the hump-shaped pattern in cigarette consumption that is common across most countries in our sample.

CONCLUSION

In summary, we find that the variation of smoking prevalence across countries and cohorts is generally consistent with the predictions of the cigarette epidemic model. Our descriptive analysis shows that smoking diffusion among women in advanced economies is wider but unfolds earlier relative to emerging economies. Our correlation analysis shows that more women smoke as countries become richer and more democratic; as more women participate in education and in formal work; and when cigarette prices, urbanization, and fertility rates are low.

However, unlike the cigarette epidemic model, we do not rely solely on smoking prevalence data. We also show that female smokers in advanced countries consume more cigarettes, initiate smoking, and also quit smoking at younger ages than women in developing countries. Finally, we show that in virtually all countries, the average age at smoking initiation decreases across successive generations, and cigarette consumption is higher among cohorts who came of age after World War II (when most countries started developing) and before the 1970s (when information about the health consequences of smoking started to spread).

In some countries, women's smoking patterns deviate from these patterns. For example, although China and Russia are among the least developed countries in our sample, in China, female smoking prevalence declines monotonically across successive generations, whereas in Russia, women start smoking at relatively old ages but quit smoking while relatively young. In addition, although the United Kingdom is among the most economically advanced countries in our sample, smoking rates of British women show no long-term trend. We interpret these deviations to suggest an important role for social norms and cultural influences, which may be strong enough to dominate over other determinants of smoking behavior.

NOTES

1. See http://www.who.int/tobacco/en/atlas6.pdf.
2. In this figure, as in all subsequent figures, data are missing for some cohorts because we do not plot smoking data for cohorts with fewer than 50 observations or fewer than five smokers. For Ukraine, no data are available for 80- to 89-year-olds.
3. As we note in the Appendix, not all surveys ask ex-smokers to report the number of cigarettes they used to smoke per day when they were smoking regularly. Some surveys collect this information only from current smokers. It follows that we may be mis-estimating cigarette consumption for older cohorts in the corresponding

countries because older cohorts have a higher proportion of ex-smokers relative to younger cohorts. Assuming that people who manage to quit smoking are on average lighter smokers than those who do not, we likely overestimate average consumption for these cohorts.

4. Average start age cannot exceed 29 years in the youngest cohort, 39 years in the second youngest cohort, 49 years in the third youngest cohort, etc. However, our data show that the mean start age is generally lower than cohort age (with the exception of the youngest cohort). Thus, cross-cohort comparability should not be compromised (at least concerning all but the youngest cohort).

5. Note that because most time series are available for the more recent periods in each country, the estimated correlations are based on variation in smoking rates in those periods.

6. By contrast, relying on temporal variation from Mexico, Christopoulou et al. (2013) find a small negative association between per capita GDP and female smoking rates, and only for women with higher than primary education.

7. In unpublished work, Lillard (2014) develops a new information index for the United States that tracks individual exposure to information that advocates for and against smoking. He finds that when exposed to the same anti-smoking information, women are much less likely to start and much more likely to quit smoking than men.

REFERENCES

Barro, R. and J.-W. Lee, April 2010, "A new data set of educational attainment in the world, 1950–2010." *Journal of Development Economics* 104:184–198.

Bauer, T., S. Göhlmann, and M. Sinning. 2007. "Gender differences in smoking behavior." *Health Economics* 16:895–909.

Cavelaars, A. E., A. E. Kunst, J. J. Geurts, R. Crialesi, L. Grötvedt, U. Helmert, et al. 2000. "Educational differences in smoking: International comparison." *British Medical Journal* 320:1102–1107.

Chaloupka, F. J. 1990. "Men, women and addiction: The case of cigarette smoking." NBER Working Paper No. 3267. Cambridge, MA: National Bureau of Economic Research.

Christopoulou, R., D. R. Lillard, and J. B. Miyar. 2013. "Smoking behavior of Mexicans: Patterns by birth-cohort, gender, and education." *International Journal of Public Health* 58:335–343.

Fiore, M. C., T. E. Novotny, J. P. Pierce, E. J. Hatziandreu, K. M. Patel, and R. M. Davis. 1989. "Trends in cigarette smoking in the United States: The changing influence of gender and race." *Journal of the American Medical Association* 261:49–55.

Glassman, A. H., J. E. Helzer, L. S. Covey, L. B. Cottler, F. Stetner, J.E. Tipp, et al. 1990. "Smoking, smoking cessation, and major depression." *Journal of the American Medical Association* 264:1546–1549.

Hersch, J. 1996. "Smoking, seat belts, and other risky consumer behaviors: Differences by gender and race." *Managerial and Decision Economics* 17:471–481.

Hersch, J. 2000. "Gender, income levels, and the demand for cigarettes." *Journal of Risk and Uncertainty* 21:263–282.

Husten, C. G., J. H. Chrismon, and M. N. Reddy. 1996. "Trends and effects of cigarette smoking among girls and women in the United States, 1965–1993." *Journal of the American Medical Women's Association* 51:11–18.

Idris, B. I., K. Giskes, C. Borrell, J. Benach, G. Costa, B. Federico, et al. 2007. "Higher smoking prevalence in urban compared to non-urban areas: Time trends in six European countries." *Health & Place* 13:702–712.

Jarvis, M. J., J. E. Cohen, C. D. Delnevo, and G. A. Giovino. 2013. "Dispelling myths about gender differences in smoking cessation: Population data from the USA, Canada, and Britain." *Tobacco Control* 22:356–360.

Kaufman, N., and M. Nichter. 2010. "The marketing of tobacco to women: Global perspectives." In *Women and the Tobacco Epidemic: Challenges for the 21st Century*, edited by J. M. Samet and S. Y. Soon, pp 69–99. Geneva: World Health Organization.

Lee, J. M., T. S. Hwang, C. Y. Ye, and S. H. Chen. 2004. "The effect of cigarette price increase on cigarette consumption in Taiwan: Evidence from the National Health Interview Surveys on cigarette consumption." *BMC Public Health* 4:61.

Lewit, E. M., and D. Coate. 1982. "The potential for using excise taxes to reduce smoking." *Journal of Health Economics* 1:121–145.

Lillard, D. R. 2014. "Health information and smoking: New (improved) estimates of how information affects behavior." Paper presented at the 5th Biennial Conference of the American Society of Health Economists, University of Southern California, Los Angeles, June 22–25.

Lopez, A. D., N. E. Collishaw, and T. Piha. 1994. "A descriptive model of the cigarette epidemic in developed countries." *Tobacco Control* 3:242–247.

Mao, Z. Z., Y. G. Huan, M. J. Min, J. Samet, and M. Ceraso. 2003. "Adults demand of cigarettes and its influencing factors in China." *Soft Science of Health* 17:19–23.

McCrory, C., and R. Layte. 2012. "Prenatal exposure to maternal smoking and childhood behavioural problems: A quasi-experimental approach." *Journal of Abnormal Child Psychology* 40:1277–1288.

McGee R., and S. Williams. 2006. "Predictors of persistent smoking and quitting among women smokers." *Addictive Behaviors*, 31:1711–1715.

Milberger S., J. Biederman, S. V. Faraone, L. Chen, and J. Jones. 1996. "Is maternal smoking during pregnancy a risk factor for attention deficit hyperactivity disorder in children?" *American Journal of Psychiatry* 153:1138–1142.

Milberger S., J. Biederman, S. V. Faraone, and J. Jones. 1998. "Further evidence of an association between maternal smoking during pregnancy and attention deficit hyperactivity disorder: Findings from a high-risk sample of siblings." *Journal of Clinical Child Psychology* 27:352–358.

Missouri Department of Health. 1995. "Prevalence of smoking by area of residence—Missouri, 1989–1991." *Morbidity and Mortality Weekly Report* 44:494–497.

Nusbaum M. L., M. Gordon, D. Nusbaum, M. A. McCarthy, and D. Vasilakis. 2000. "Smoke alarm: A review of the clinical impact of smoking on women." *Primary Care Update for Ob/Gyns* 7:207–214.

Ogobin, C., and G. Brock. 2003. "Smoking in Russia: The 'Malboro Man' rides but without 'Virgina Slims' for now." *Comparative Economic Studies* 45:87–103.

Osler, M., E. Prescott, N. Godtfredsen, H. O. Hein, and P. Schnohr. 1999. "Gender and determinants of smoking cessation: A longitudinal study." *Preventative Medicine* 29:57–62.

Pierce, J. P. 1989. "International comparisons of trends in cigarette smoking prevalence." *American Journal of Public Health* 79:152–157.

Pomerleau, J., Gilmore, A., McKee, M., Rose, R., and C. W. Haerpfer. 2004. "Determinants of smoking in eight countries of the former Soviet Union: Results from the Living Conditions, Lifestyles and Health Study." *Addiction* 99(12):1577–1585.

Pudule, I., D. Grinberga, K. Kadziauskiene, A. Abaravicius, S. Vaask, A. Robertson, et al. 1999. "Patterns of smoking in the Baltic Republics." *Journal of Epidemiology and Community Health* 53:277–282.

Schaap, M. M., A. E. Kunst, M. Leinsalu, E. Regidor, A. Espelt, O. Ekholm, et al. 2009. "Female ever-smoking, education, emancipation and economic development in 19 European countries." *Social Science & Medicine* 68:1271–1278.

Steckley, S. L., W. B. Pickworth, and H. W. Haverkos. 2003. "Cigarette smoking and cervical cancer. Part II: A geographic variability study." *Biomedicine & Pharmacotherapy* 57:78–83.

Stehr, M. 2007. "The effect of cigarette taxes on smoking among men and women." *Health Economics* 16:1333–1343.

Thun, M., R. Peto, J. Boreham, and A. D. Lopez. 2012. "Stages of the cigarette epidemic on entering its second century." *Tobacco Control* 21:96–101.

US Department of Health and Human Services (USDHHS). 2014. *The Health Consequences of Smoking—50 Years of Progress. A Report of the Surgeon General.* Atlanta, GA: USDHHS, Centers for Disease Control and Prevention, National Center for Chronic Disease Prevention and Health Promotion, Office on Smoking and Health.

Waldron, I. 1991. "Patterns and causes of gender differences in smoking." *Social Science and Medicine* 32:989–1005.

Waldron, I., G. Bratelli, L. Carricker, W. C. Sung, C. Vogeli, and E. Waldman. 1988. "Gender differences in tobacco use in Africa, Asia, the Pacific, and Latin America." *Social Science and Medicine* 27:1269–1275.

Ward, K. D., R. C. Klesges, S. M. Zbikowski, R. E. Bliss, and A. J. Garvey. 1997. "Gender differences in the outcome of an unaided smoking cessation attempt." *Addictive Behaviors* 22:521–533.

Williamson D. F., J. Madans, R. F. Anda, J. C. Kleinman, G. A. Giovino, and T. Byers. 1991. "Smoking cessation and severity of weight gain in a national cohort." *New England Journal of Medicine* 324:739–745.

13

Relative Smoking Patterns of Men and Women in Cross-Country Perspective

DEAN R. LILLARD AND ANA I. GIL LACRUZ

INTRODUCTION

Trends and patterns in the relative smoking behavior of men and women inform our understanding of whether and how the evolution of gender-specific cultural norms and other gender-specific factors might differentially affect smoking decisions of men and women. The authors of previous chapters repeatedly noted that the level and shape of life-course smoking trajectories seem to reflect targeted cigarette advertising, changes in labor force participation rates of women relative to men, changes in women's rights to work and educate themselves, social attitudes about women, their place in society, and what constitutes acceptable or unacceptable behavior—including whether or not it is socially acceptable for women to smoke. Because this chapter focuses on the relative smoking behavior of men and women, we relate that relative behavior to levels of some factors (e.g., per capita gross domestic product (GDP)) and relative differences in other potential influences (e.g., relative schooling of men and women). The levels and evolution of the gender-specific influences, relative to each other, potentially explain and are therefore reflected in the patterns we present.

In the literature on the relative smoking patterns of men and women, researchers often relate observed patterns to the sex-specific smoking diffusion predicted by the so-called "cigarette epidemic" model. Using US data, that model describes a set of stylized patterns of aggregate smoking prevalence and relates them to corresponding patterns of smoking-related mortality (Lopez et al., 1994; Thun et al., 2012). Of note in this context, the model suggests that women's smoking patterns resemble men's smoking patterns (in both level and shape) but only across cohorts separated by a few generations. Although previous chapters in this book documented patterns in some countries that are consistent with this simple description, the observed patterns in other countries (e.g., the United Kingdom and China) are not consistent with it.

A large and quite rich literature, using mostly repeated cross-sectional data, describes how women's smoking patterns differ from those of men. Previous studies confirm our overall finding that a higher fraction of men smoke than women in developed and developing countries throughout the world in a wide range of years and that, in most countries, the rates are converging over time (Waldron et al., 1988; Waldron, 1991; Jané et al., 2002; Pampel, 2006). Studies also show, again using cross-sectional data, that a greater fraction of male immigrants to the United States smoke more than female immigrants to the United States from the same Asian and Latin American countries (Gorman et al., 2014). Here, we offer insights using longitudinal data that follow individuals over the whole course of their lives.

Authors of previous chapters in this volume and others (e.g., Pampel, 2006; Waldron, 1991) review various conjectures the literature offers that might produce differences in the relative smoking behavior of men and women (or that would lead gender-specific smoking behavior to grow more similar over time). One can generally categorize the hypotheses into forces that affect, relative to men, all women in society (e.g., social norms and expectations about proper behavior for women), a subset of women (e.g., women who cigarette firms target with advertising), and individuals (e.g., women who work, earn money, and interact with others in a perhaps new environment outside the home face consumption decisions that revolve around earnings, prices, and the perceived costs and benefits of smoking). Numerous authors suggest that, because social norms have changed together with increasing smoking prevalence of women, those changes might explain the converging patterns of smoking of men and women. Zucker et al. (2005) support this conjecture by finding that nonsmokers are better able to resist gender pressures. At the same time, evidence suggests that, although male and female smokers successfully attempt to quit at the same rate, women are at a much greater risk of relapse than men (Ward et al., 1997).

Finally, individual evaluations of costs and benefits of smoking must also consider whether and how relative smoking patterns relate to differences across cohorts and countries in women's rising incomes, cigarette prices, and an increasing awareness among women of health risks of smoking. In terms of the latter, it is notable that, in addition to gender-specific differences in biological processes that translate smoking into disease (for a review of the evidence, see US Department of Health and Human Services, 2014, especially Chapter 9), women bear children, and compared to men, many women spend a larger amount of time in close proximity to their children. Consequently, it is plausible that women perceive a higher health cost of smoking than do men.

CROSS-COUNTRY PATTERNS IN RELATIVE SMOKING BEHAVIOR OF MEN AND WOMEN

To describe the smoking behavior of men relative to women, we plot four summary measures of each cohort's smoking behavior. For every cohort in all countries we plot, as a scatter, the age at which the average male and female smoker started, the maximum smoking prevalence rate of men and women, the average number of cigarettes men and women smoked each day, and the age at which the average male and female ex-smoker quit. In the four scatterplots, we also draw the 45-degree line, and we do not label the country or cohort associated with any given point. Our goal is to visually reveal whether the (majority of) data points lie on, above, or below the 45-degree line. Where the majority of data points lie indicates whether a given

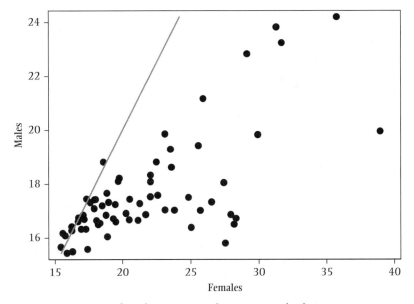

Figure 13.1 Average age of smoking initiation by country and cohort.

smoking indicator is equal between men and women in each cohort and country (most points on the 45-degree line), higher for men relative to women (most points above the 45-degree line), or higher for women relative to men (most points below the 45-degree line).

In Figure 13.1, we plot the average age of smoking initiation of male and female smokers in each cohort for all 10 countries. Because the data points lie below the 45-degree line in Figure 13.1 for most countries and cohorts, it is clear that men started at younger ages than women. However, in a number of cohorts in many countries, men and women began at almost exactly the same age.

Although we do not label the points in Figure 13.1, the points that lie close to the 45-degree line are mostly for younger cohorts. If one refers back to the country-specific chapters, it is clear that, in every country, the average age of smoking initiation of men and women is converging over successively younger cohorts. In Ukraine, Russia, and Turkey, women still start at older ages than men. In Canada and the United Kingdom, women are starting at slightly younger ages than men in their cohort. However, across all countries, there is a clear general trend. In younger cohorts, men and women who smoke start at increasingly similar ages.

Figure 13.2 plots the maximum smoking prevalence rate of men and women in each cohort and country. The figure shows that in every cohort but one, more men smoked at their peak rate of smoking prevalence than did women in the same cohort. The figure also shows the substantial differences in the maximum rate of smoking prevalence of men and women in each cohort within and across countries. As noted in previous chapters, in China, Spain, Russia, Turkey, and Ukraine, the prevalence of smoking among older men is much greater than that for older women. In most but not all countries (e.g., China), men and women in younger cohorts are more likely to smoke at similar rates.

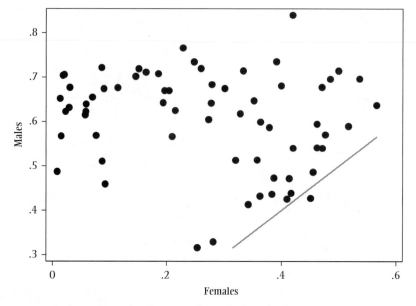

Figure 13.2 Peak smoking prevalence rate by country and cohort.

Figure 13.3 plots the number of cigarettes smoked on average by men and women in each cohort and country. Data points for all but two cohorts lie above the 45-degree line. The pattern indicates that male smokers consumed more cigarettes on average than did female smokers in their cohort. Although we do not label particular cohorts in particular countries, one can verify in the plots in each country-specific chapter that this pattern is stable across cohorts. In contrast to the changes observed for the

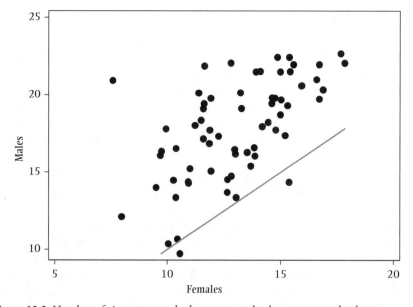

Figure 13.3 Number of cigarettes smoked on average day by country and cohort.

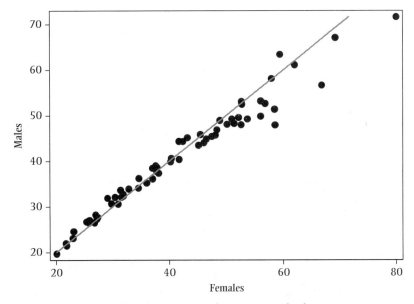

Figure 13.4 Average age of smoking cessation by country and cohort.

age of smoking initiation, women in practically all cohorts continue to smoke fewer cigarettes than do men in their cohorts.

Figure 13.4 plots the average age at which male and female smokers quit smoking in each cohort. A striking majority of data points lie on the 45-degree line. This pattern is striking because these very similar values are the product of widely different cultural, social, and economic conditions in 10 countries during a period that spans up to 80 years. Despite these differences, in almost every country and every cohort, men and women quit at about the same chronological age. Interestingly, the similarity in the men and women's average age of smoking cessation has grown over time. Younger cohorts of male and female smokers increasingly quit at similar ages. Although even the youngest cohort of men in Ukraine, Turkey, and Canada still smoke longer than their female counterparts, in all countries men and women in younger cohorts are more similar in this aspect of smoking behavior than were men and women in previous generations.

PREDICTORS OF RELATIVE SMOKING BEHAVIOR OF MEN AND WOMEN

As discussed previously, the general pattern in most countries is that, over successive cohorts, the smoking prevalence rate of men is declining relative to that of women. In this section, we use the data for our 10 countries to explore whether factors proposed in the literature and in the country-specific chapters correlate with the relative smoking prevalence rate of men and women.

In Table 13.1, we report correlation coefficients with a small set of factors for which we could compile data across all countries and over most years. We relate the relative smoking prevalence rate of men and women to the log of GDP, the degree of democracy, the price of cigarettes, the relative labor force participation rate of

Table 13.1. CORRELATION BETWEEN SMOKING PREVALENCE OF MEN RELATIVE
TO WOMEN AND SELECTED VARIABLES (ESTIMATES FROM LINEAR REGRESSIONS)

Variable	Coefficient	Standard error	Observations	R^2
Log per capita GDP	4.837	(3.489)	3421	0.174
Democracy	−1.367***	(0.218)	3136	0.188
Cigarette price	−0.851*	(0.470)	2675	0.343
Labor force participation rate of men relative to women	6.145***	(0.989)	1689	0.444
Population density	0.176***	(0.043)	2761	0.256
Share of rural population	0.754***	(0.078)	2812	0.268
Ratio of male/female schooling	16.236***	(5.125)	3010	0.135
Fertility rate	−2.201**	(0.611)	2801	0.247

NOTES: Each row reports statistics from a separate ordinary least squares regression.
An observation consists of a birth cohort in a country in a given year. All regressions
control for the ratio of the mean age of men to women for a cohort, country dummies,
year dummies, and birth cohort dummies. The log of GDP per capita is measured in
1990 International Geary–Khamis dollars (source: Maddison, 2010). Democracy is a
scaled measure of regime governance that takes values from −10 to 10 (source: Polity IV
Project). Cigarette price is in 2008 US dollars, purchasing power parity adjusted (from
various national sources; see country-specific chapters). The labor force participation
rate is for men of all ages relative women of all ages (source: International Labor Office
for Ukraine and China; Organization for Economic Cooperation and Development
statistics for all other countries). Population density measures people per square
kilometer of land area (source: World Development Indicators). Ratio of male/female
primary school enrollment is the ratio of the share of males enrolled in primary school
relative to the share of females enrolled in primary school (source: Barro and Lee,
2010; missing values interpolated). Fertility rate measures total births per woman
(source: World Development Indicators). *, **, and *** indicate statistical significance at
the 10, 5, and 1 percent level, respectively.

men and women in each cohort, the population density, the share of the population
in rural areas, the relative schooling of men and women, and the fertility rate of
women. Specifically, we run eight separate regressions, each of which relates the relative smoking prevalence rate of each cohort in each country in each year to one of
the previously mentioned variables. Each regression also controls for the ratio of the
average age of men relative to the average age women in a given cohort plus country,
year, and cohort fixed effects.

We hypothesize that the smoking prevalence rate of men and women will grow
more similar as men's and women's economic and social situations grow more similar over time. Thus, as women work at rates more similar to those of men, get more
similar levels of schooling, and have fewer children, we hypothesize that they will
smoke at rates more similar to those of men. As noted in other chapters, women have
faced social norms that have subjected them to greater social approbation than men.

We hypothesize that economic development, more civil and individual liberties, and movement of the population from rural to urban areas, where women are plausibly less subject to traditional social rules, will lead to women smoking in ways more similar to the way men smoke.

We caution the reader not to infer too much from the results. Each of the reported coefficients is generated using a simple model that excludes a host of individual-specific factors known to determine individual smoking behavior (income, family size, and educational attainment). These correlations are meant to provoke the reader to speculate about these and other omitted variables that might give rise to the strong correlations that the models generate.

To fix how one should read these correlations, keep in mind that the dependent variable—the smoking prevalence rate of men relative to women in a given cohort—ranges from 0 to infinity. For a given cohort, it takes on a value of 0 if no men smoke and some women do. The variable equals 1 if, in a given cohort, the same fraction of men and women smoke. It takes on a value that approaches infinity if more men smoke relative to women. Historically, in every country, this measure has substantially exceeded a value of 1 in older cohorts and has, in most countries (China being the exception), trended toward a value of 1 in successively younger cohorts. Here, positive coefficients indicate that an increase in the level of the explanatory variable is associated with a increase in the rate of men's smoking prevalence relative to that of women. Negative coefficients indicate the opposite.

Results indicate that the log of per capita GDP is uncorrelated with the general average trend toward more similar smoking prevalence rates of men and women. The relative smoking prevalence rate of men and women in each cohort is more similar in countries and years in which the real cigarette price is higher, but the association is statistically insignificant. Authors of previous chapters and other researchers have conjectured, and some evidence suggests, that the price elasticity of cigarette demand differs for men and women (see Chaloupka, 1990). In contrast to this evidence, the sign of the coefficient in our results indicates that, in years when the price of cigarettes is higher, the relative smoking prevalence rate of men and women does not systematically differ from that during years in which the price of cigarettes is lower. However, as noted previously, the models estimated here omit many important determinants of smoking behavior, so one must interpret these results cautiously.

Table 13.1 does present striking and strong statistical associations with several of the measures. In a given cohort, country, and year, women are more likely to smoke at a similar rate as men in countries that have experienced growth in political freedom and when fertility rates are higher. In a given cohort, country, and year, women are less likely to smoke at a similar rate as men when a greater fraction of men work relative to women, when population density is higher, when a greater share of the population live in rural areas, and when men have higher levels of schooling relative to women.

These results are broadly consistent with hypothesized relationships from the literature on gendered smoking patterns detailed in Waldron (1991) and elsewhere and also with statistical evidence in the previous two chapters. DeCicca, McLeod, Liu note in Chapter 11 that the rate of smoking prevalence in a given cohort of men is higher in countries with a more urbanized population, whereas Christopoulou and Önder find in Chapter 12 that the smoking prevalence rate of women is uncorrelated with population density. At the same time, these authors report that in years when a greater share of a country's population lives in rural areas, fewer men in a cohort smoke (Chapter 11) *and* fewer women in a cohort smoke (Chapter 12). Table 13.1 shows that men smoke relatively more than women in years when more of the population lives in rural areas but also when population density is higher. Together, the results in the three summary chapters lead us to wonder about the underlying social and economic factors that would be consistent with the three associations we measure.

The pattern across the other possible correlates of smoking behavior strongly supports conjectures described in Waldron (1991) and elsewhere that women in younger cohorts may be smoking in ways more similar to men because women in those cohorts face more equal economic opportunities (labor markets and higher levels of education), have more time to work because they bear fewer children over their lifetimes (lower fertility rates), and enjoy greater social and political freedom (democracy/polity).

CONCLUSION

The analysis in this chapter helps to identify heterogeneity in smoking behavior that public health officials might use to design policies that reduce the negative impact of smoking behavior among groups for which those costs are highest. The observed patterns confirm that, across all countries, men and women are smoking in increasingly similar ways. Although smoking behavior has not converged uniformly or at the same rate in all countries, we find evidence that their smoking prevalence rates are converging more as men and women participate in the labor force at similar rates, get similar years of schooling, and as women bear fewer children. We also find evidence that men and women smoke at more similar rates as social norms ease, to the extent that those changes are triggered by expansions of democratic institutions and when less people live in rural areas. This evidence indicated that it is possible to explain cross-country and cohort differences in smoking behavior of men and women. What we need are cross-national studies of factors that can explain whether and why men and women consume or do not consume tobacco. That understanding will inform our scientific understanding of health behaviors and the design of public policies that aim to improve the human condition. We eagerly await the future.

REFERENCES

Barro, R. and J.-W. Lee, April 2010, "A new data set of educational attainment in the world, 1950–2010." *Journal of Development Economics* 104:184–198.

Chaloupka, F. 1990. "Men, women, and addiction: The case of cigarette smoking." NBER Working Paper 3267. Cambridge, MA: National Bureau of Economic Research.

Gorman, B. K., J. T. Lariscy, and C. Kaushik. 2014. "Gender, acculturation, and smoking behavior among US Asian and Latino immigrants." *Social Science and Medicine* 106:110–118.

Jané, M., E. Saltó, H. Pardell, R. Tresserras, R. Guayta, J. L. Taberner, et al. 2002. "Prevalencia del tabquismo en Cataluña, 1982–1998: Una perspectiva de género." *Medicina Clínica* 118:81–85.

Lopez, A. D., N. E. Hollinshaw, and T. Piha. 1994. "A descriptive model of the cigarette epidemic in developed countries." *Tobacco Control* 3:242–247.

Maddison Project. n.d. or 2010. Available at http://www.ggdc.net/maddison/maddison-project/home.htm

Pampel, F. C.. 2006. "Global pattern and determinants of sex differences in smoking" *International Journal of Comparative Sociology* 47(6): 466–487.

Thun, M., R. Peto, J. Boreham, and A. D. Lopez. 2012. "Stages of the cigarette epidemic on entering its second century." *Tobacco Control* 21:96–101.

US Department of Health and Human Services (USDHHS). 2014. *The Health Consequences of Smoking—50 Year of Progress. A Report of the Surgeon General.* Atlanta, GA: USDHHS, Centers for Disease Control and Prevention, National Center for Chronic Disease Prevention and Health Promotion, Office on Smoking and Health.

Waldron, I. 1991. "Patterns and causes of gender differences in smoking." *Social Science and Medicine* 32:989–1005.

Waldron, I., G. Bratelli, L. Carriker, W. Sung, C. Vogeli, and E. Waldman. 1988. "Gender differences in tobacco use in Africa, Asia, the Pacific, and Latin America." *Social Science and Medicine* 27:1269–1275.

Ward, K. D., R. C. Klesges, S. M. Zbikowski, R. E. Bliss, and A. J. Garvey. 1997. "Gender differences in the outcome of an unaided smoking cessation attempt." *Addictive Behaviors* 22:521–533.

Zucker, A. N., A. J. Stewart, C. S. Pomerleau, and C. J. Boyd. 2005. "Resisting gendered smoking pressures: Critical consciousness as a correlate of women's smoking status." *Sex Roles* 53:261–272.

PART V

Appendix

14

Description and Sources of Raw Data

DEAN R. LILLARD AND REBEKKA CHRISTOPOULOU

DATA ON SMOKING

As we reference in country-specific chapters, we use data from the Household Income and Labour Dynamics in Australia survey (HILDA, 2007); the British Household Panel Survey (BHPS, 1999, 2002); the Canadian Community Health Survey (CCHS, 2009); the China Health and Nutrition Survey (CHNS, 1991, 1993, 1997, 2000, 2004, 2006, 2009); the German Socio-Economic Panel (SOEP, 2002); the Russian Longitudinal Monitoring Survey (RLMS, 1995, 1996, 1998, 2000–2010); the Spanish National Health Surveys (SNHS, 1995, 1997, 2001, 2003, 2006, 2011); the Turkish administration of the Global Adult Tobacco Survey (GATS, 2008); the Ukrainian Longitudinal Monitoring Survey (ULMS, 2003, 2007); and the Tobacco Use Supplement of Current Population Survey in the US (TUS-CPS, 1967, 1968, 1989, 1992, 1993, 1995, 1996, 1998, 1999, 2001–2003, 2006, 2007). We report the size of the working sample from each database in the table included in each country-specific chapter. Here, we briefly describe the surveys and the retrospective smoking questions they ask. The interested reader can find more details on the websites for each survey, which we also list in this chapter.

Note that the surveys in China, Germany, Russia, Ukraine, and Turkey do not ask former smokers how many cigarettes they smoked when they were smoking regularly. These surveys collect this information only from current smokers. Furthermore, the RLMS and ULMS data on cigarette consumption in Russia and Ukraine include consumption of "papyrosi"—a type of nonfiltered cigarette that is a hollow cardboard tube extended by a thin cigarette paper tube with tobacco.

HILDA

The HILDA is a household-based panel survey that began in 2001 with an initial sample of 7682 households and 13,969 individuals and is administered by the Melbourne Institute of Applied Economic and Social Research (University of Melbourne). The Australian government (through the Department of Social Services) is currently funding the survey for 16 waves. The nationally representative sample is asked about current smoking in each wave. The retrospective smoking questions that we use were asked only in wave 7 of the survey. The exact phrasing of these questions is as follows:

1. Have you smoked at least 100 cigarettes in your entire life?
2. (If ever-smoker:) How old were you when you began to smoke regularly?
3. (If ever-smoker:) And are you still a smoker?
4. (If current smoker:) On average, how many cigarettes do you now smoke per [day/week/month]?
5. (If former smoker:) Think back to the year you last smoked regularly. What year was that?
6. (If former smoker:) And about how many cigarettes per day were you smoking at this time?

For more details, see http://www.melbourneinstitute.com/hilda.

BHPS

The BHPS gathered demographic and smoking data from a nationally representative sample of UK residents during the period 1991–2009. It was a household-based panel survey administered by the Institute for Social and Economic Research, which initially (in 1991) sampled approximately 10,000 individuals aged 16 years or older in 5000 households. The entire original sample and all family members (by blood or marriage) were followed in subsequent annual surveys. Starting with wave 4 (1994), the BHPS began to survey youth aged 11–15 years. Each year, the BHPS asked every household member to report whether they currently smoke and how much they smoke on average. In 1999, the survey asked all current and former smokers to report the age at which they first smoked. In 2002, the survey asked former smokers to report the age at which they quit. In fact, cessation information is also available in the 1999 wave. In 1999, the BHPS also asked former smokers about the amount of time that had elapsed since they had quit. We do not use those data because the survey elicited responses in broad and uninformative categories. Instead, we use the exact quit ages reported on the 2002 survey. In 2009, the BHPS sample was subsumed in the sample of a new study called "Understanding Society," also known as "The UK Household Longitudinal Study." The exact phrasing of the questions we use is as follows:

1. Have you ever smoked a cigarette, a cigar, or a pipe? (1999)
2. Do you smoke cigarettes at all nowadays? (1999, 2002)
3. (If current smoker:) Approximately how many cigarettes a day do you usually smoke, including those you roll yourself? (1999, 2002)
4. Have you ever smoked cigarettes regularly; that is, at least one cigarette a day, or did you smoke them only occasionally? (1999, 2002)
5. (If ever-smoker:) About how many cigarettes did you smoke in a day when you last smoked them regularly? (1999)
6. (If ever-smoker:) How old were you when you (first) started to smoke cigarettes regularly? (1999)
7. (If former smoker:) How old were you when you last stopped smoking? (2002)

For more details, see https://www.iser.essex.ac.uk/bhps.

CCHS

The CCHS is a nationally representative household-based survey conducted annually by Statistics Canada. It gathers both cross-sectional data on health status and the determinants of health, including health behaviors, use of health services, as well as extensive socioeconomic and demographic information. It gathers detailed data on smoking behavior, including both current and retrospective smoking information. The exact phrasing of the retrospective questions that we use is as follows:

1. At the present time do you smoke cigarettes daily, occasionally, or not at all?
2. (If current smoker:) How many cigarettes do you smoke each day now?
3. Have you ever smoked cigarettes daily?
4. (If ever-smoker:) At what age did you begin to smoke cigarettes daily?
5. (If former smoker:) How many cigarettes did you usually smoke each day?
6. (If former smoker:) At what age did you stop smoking (cigarettes) daily?

For more details, see http://www23.statcan.gc.ca/imdb/p2SV.pl?Function=getSurvey& SDDS=3226.

CHNS

The CHNS is a national panel survey that began in 1989 with a sample of approximately 4400 households and a total of 16,000 individuals. Follow-up surveys were administered in 1991, 1993, 1997, 2000, 2004, 2006, and 2009. The survey is conducted in nine provinces (Guangxi, Guizhou, Heilongjiang, Henan, Hubei, Hunan, Jiangsu, Liaoning, and Shandong), and no sampling weights are provided. Designed to examine how the transition of Chinese society is affecting its population, the survey contains detailed information on health, demographic, socioeconomic, and nutrition status. Starting in 1991, CHNS asks respondents to report whether or not they ever smoked, the age at which they started smoking, the number of cigarettes they smoke every day, and, for ex-smokers, how long ago they stopped smoking. The exact phrasing of the questions is as follows:

1. Have you ever smoked cigarettes (including hand-rolled or device-rolled)?
2. (If ever-smoker:) How old were you when you started to smoke? (years)
3. (If ever-smoker:) Do you still smoke cigarettes now?
4. (If current smoker:) How many cigarettes do you smoke per day?
5. (If former smoker:) How long ago did you stop smoking? (months)

For more details, see http://www.cpc.unc.edu/projects/china.

SOEP

The SOEP is a longitudinal survey of households that began in 1984. When analyzed with sample weights, it is nationally representative. The SOEP began with a sample of 6000 households in the western states of Germany representing a disproportionate number of non-German migrant workers. In 1990, 6 months after the Berlin Wall fell and before East and West Germany officially reunited, the SOEP administered its survey to residents living in states in the former East Germany. Those individuals were followed in subsequent years. The SOEP attempts to collect information from all household members aged 16 years or older. Surveys administered in 1998, 1992, 2001, 2002, and 2004 collected data on contemporaneous smoking status. In 2002 and 2012, the SOEP asked all respondents to retrospectively report on lifetime smoking behavior. Because, at the time of data analysis, the 2012 data had not been released, our results are based only on the 2002 wave. The exact phrasing of the questions is as follows:

1. Have you ever smoked before, i.e. have you smoked at least 100 cigarettes or other tobacco products in your life?
2. (If ever-smoker:) How old were you when you began to smoke regularly?
3. (If ever-smoker:) Do you currently smoke, be it cigarettes, a pipe, or cigars?
4. (If current smoker:) How many cigarettes, pipes, or cigars do you smoke per day? Please give the daily average of the previous week.
5. (If former smoker:) When did you give up smoking? Please provide the year and, if possible, the month.

For more details, see http://www.diw.de/en/soep.

RLMS

The RLMS is an annual survey, conducted in Russia, of all individuals from a nationally representative sample of more than 4000 households (approximately 10,000 individual interviews). The RLMS Phase 2 provides 18 waves of data from surveys administered between 1994 and 2012. Interdisciplinary in orientation, the RLMS collects information used by a wide range of social scientists. During each interview, the RLMS collects in-depth data on smoking behavior of each individual aged 13 years or older. In addition to age of initiation and cessation, the smoking data include ever-smoked status, current smoking status, and number of cigarettes smoked. The exact phrasing of the questions is as follows:

1. Do you now smoke?
2. (If current smoker:) Please recall: When did you start smoking? How old were you then?
3. (If current smoker:) What do you mainly smoke? I will list various types of tobacco products and you tell me, please, which you smoke most often. (Papyrosi, Filtered cigarettes, Unfiltered cigarettes, Self-rolled cigarettes, Pipe, Don't know, Refuse to answer)
4. (If current smoker:) About how many individual cigarettes or papyroses do you usually smoke in a day?
5. (If current non-smoker:) Have you ever smoked?
6. (If former smoker:) How many years ago did you quit smoking?

For more details, see http://www.cpc.unc.edu/projects/rlms-hse.

SNHS

The SNHS is a cross-sectional survey similar to the US National Health Interview Surveys. Administered every other year in Spain, it collects data on self-reported health, primary and specialized healthcare, perceptions of life expectancy, life habits, behavior associated with health risk factors, and the use of health services and pre-ventive practices. The SNHS collects detailed information from people aged 16 years or older on cigarette consumption, including frequency, average quantity, and ret-rospective information on initiation and (for former smokers) cessation. The exact phrasing of the questions is as follows:

1. Could you tell me if you currently smoke? (Yes, I smoke daily; Yes, I smoke but not daily; No, I do not currently smoke, but I used to smoke; No, I do not currently smoke, and I have never smoked daily; Do not know; No answer)
2. (If current smoker:) What kind of tobacco product do you currently smoke daily? (Cigarettes; Pipe; Cigars; Do not know; No answer)
3. (If current smoker:) On average, how many units of tobacco product do you currently smoke per day? (Number of cigarettes; Number of pipes; Number of cigars)
4. (If current or former smoker:) At what age did you start smoking?
5. (If former smoker:) How long ago did you stop smoking?
6. (If former smoker:) What kind of tobacco product did you used to smoke daily? (Cigarettes; Pipe; Cigars; Do not know; No answer)
7. (If former smoker:) On average, how many units of product did you used to smoke per day? (Number of cigarettes; Number of pipes; Number of cigars)

For more details, see http://www.ine.es/jaxi/menu.do?type=pcaxis&path=%2Ft15/p419&file=inebase&L=1.

GATS

The GATS is a survey that collects data for tobacco use in countries with the high-est smoking rates. Sixteen countries participate in the GATS project, which was coordinated by the Centers for Disease Control and Preventions (CDC), the World Health Organization, the John Hopkins Bloomberg School of Public Health, and the Research Triangle Institute. CDC contracted with the Turkish Statistical Institute (TSI) to administer the GATS in Turkey. The questionnaire was pretested in August 2008, and the fieldwork was conducted in November of the same year. Questions on both contemporaneous and retrospective smoking behavior were included. The exact phrasing of the questions is as follows:

1. What is your tobacco usage status at present? (Every day, less than every day, none)
2. Have you used tobacco every day in the past?
3. What was your tobacco usage status in the past? (Every day, less than every day, none)
4. (If former or current smoker:) At what age did you first start to use tobacco every day?
5. (If current smoker:) How many tobacco products are you using at present?
6. (If former smoker:) How long ago did you quit using tobacco?

For more details, see http://www.who.int/tobacco/surveillance/en_tfi_gats_tur-key_2009.pdf.

ULMS

The ULMS is a longitudinal panel survey of the Ukraine, similar to the RLMS. The ULMS is a statistically representative sample of the Ukrainian population aged between 15 and 72 years, comprising 4000 households and approximately 8500 individuals. Although the ULMS did not include smoking questions in its early years, we convinced the ULMS group to add those questions to their survey starting in 2003. We only use data from the 2003 and 2007 surveys because no sampling weights were produced for the 2004 wave. The exact phrasing of the questions is as follows:

1. Do you now smoke?
2. (If current smoker:) Please, remember when did you start smoking? How old were you then?
3. (If current smoker:) About how many individual cigarettes or papyrosi do you usually smoke in a day?
4. (If current non-smoker:) Have you ever smoked?
5. (If former smoker:) Please, remember when did you start smoking? How old were you then?
6. (If former smoker:) How many years ago did you quit smoking?

For more detail, see http://idsc.iza.org/?page=27&id=56.

TUS-CPS

The TUS-CPS is a survey of tobacco use sponsored by the National Cancer Institute and Centers for Disease Control and Prevention (CDC) that has been administered as part of the US Census Bureau's Current Population Survey. The TUS-CPS is a key source of national, state, and sub-state level data from US households regarding smoking, use of tobacco products, and tobacco-related norms, attitudes, and policies. It uses a large, nationally representative sample of civilian, non-institutionalized population aged 18 years or older (15 years or older data for 1992–2006). Approximately 64 percent of respondents complete the TUS-CPS by telephone, and 36 percent complete it in person; most data are self-reported (approximately 20 percent are by proxy for a few measures of use). The exact phrasing of the questions we use is as follows:

1. Have you smoked at least 100 cigarettes in your entire life?
2. (If ever-smoker:) How old were you when you first started smoking cigarettes fairly regular?
3. (If current smoker:) On average, how many cigarettes do you now smoke a day?
4. Have you ever smoked cigarettes every day for at least 6 months?
5. (If former smoker:) About how long has it been since you last smoked cigarettes every day?
6. (If former smoker:) When you last smoked every day, on average, how many cigarettes did you smoke daily?
7. (If former smoker:) About how long has it been since you completely stopped smoking cigarettes?

For more detail, see http://appliedresearch.cancer.gov/tus-cps.

DATA ON CIGARETTE PRICES AND TAXES

Cigarette price (and tax) data in this book come from diverse sources that we list here. To the best of our knowledge, we are the first to publish the price data for Turkey for the period 1925–1959. We are also the first to comprehensively compile the official USSR cigarette prices over so many years. For several countries, we imputed the average price of cigarettes in some years. Here, we describe the algorithm we used to do so. At a future date, we will post all data on our project website together with codes we used to impute the prices.

Australia

All prices for Australia are drawn from the *Australian Ministry of Labor Gazette* (various issues).

Canada

The series for the average cigarette price in Canada consists of data that directly measure the average cigarette price and a data series that we impute. All data that we directly use come from Statistics Canada, and all data we use to impute the earlier series are from either Statistics Canada or its predecessor, the Dominion Bureau of Statistics. Statistics Canada produces, and distributes on its website, a time series of the average price of cigarettes in Canada in every month of each year from 1949 to 2012. We use those data directly. To impute an average cigarette price for every year from 1921 to 1948, we use data from time series that precede those years and data from several time series that overlap with the period 1949–2012.

Specifically, we use Statistics Canada data from the series on the average price of tobacco products, on the average price of the combined category of tobacco and alcohol, and on the average price of cigarettes in each month and year from 1949 to 2012. We also use Dominion Bureau of Statistics data on the price index for tobacco in selected months and years between 1921 and 1942, data on the average price of "food, beverages, and tobacco" in selected months and years between 1922 and 1950, and data on the price index of "consumer goods groups A & B" and "other commodities and services" from June 1922 to January 1933 and June 1936 to January 1950.[1]

To use these data, we first convert each price series to the same base year. Because data are present in intermittent months, we use linear interpolation to fill in missing values between the observed data. We then predict cigarette price in several steps. First, we regress the tobacco price index time series against the "food, beverage, and tobacco" price series and the "consumer goods groups A & B" price series together with a time trend and month dummies. We use the resulting coefficients to predict the tobacco price index for all months and years in which the tobacco price index data are missing but data on the other two series exist. We then regress the full time series on the tobacco price index against the price series for "other commodities and services" with a time trend and month dummies. We use coefficients to predict values for the remaining years for which data on the tobacco price index are missing. We fill in those missing observations with the predicted values. In the final step, we regress the cigarette price index in the years that overlap with the imputed tobacco price index (1949–1959) and use the coefficients to predict the cigarette price in each month and year before 1949.

China

We draw cigarette price data in China from the series published in *China Statistical Yearbook, 1985–2009*. That series lists the average retail price of cigarettes from 1952 to 1992 and the tobacco price index for the years 1993–2009.

Germany

We draw data on the average cigarette price from the German Statistical Office (Deutsches Statistisches Bundesamt) Fachserie 14, Reihe 9.1.1, "Absatz von Tabakwaren" Tabaksteuerstatistik (Tobacco tax statistics), Veröffentlichung Band 133 "Verbrauch und Besteuerung von verbrauchsteuerpflichtigen Waren ab 1949," *Statistical Yearbook for the German Reich* (*Statistisches Jahrbuch für das Deutsche Reich*) for 1907–1926, 1935–1940, 1941–1942, and the *Statistical Yearbook of the German Democratic Republic* (*Statistisches Jahrbuch der Deutschen Demokratischen Republik*) for 1950–1989.

Spain

We draw data on Spanish cigarette prices from multiple sources that include Castañeda (1945), Comín-Comín and Martín-Aceña (1999), Tabacalera (1992), and the Spanish Market Commission.

Turkey

The Turkish Statistical Institute maintains a time series of cigarette prices for the period 1960–2002. For the period 2002–2008, we get cigarette price data from the Regulatory Board of the Markets for Tobacco, Tobacco Products, and Alcoholic Beverages (TAPDK). For the period 1925–1959, we get data from an unpublished study by Mufit Ilter (1989) titled "Tutun and Tutun Mamullerinde Devlet Tekelince Yapilmis Olan Satis Fiat Ayarlamalari" ("Sale Price Adjustments on Tobacco and Tobacco Products Made by Government Monopoly").

United Kingdom

Our cigarette price data for the UK measure the price of 20 Capstan cigarettes (a popular brand). We got time-series data on Capstan price per pack from the Tobacco Manufacturer's Association (TMA) for the years 1922–2006. In that series, data were missing from 1980 to 1996. The TMA representative also send us a time series of the price of 20 Benson & Hedges Gold that overlapped not only with the period for which data were missing but also for many years prior to 1980. We used the two series to impute a Capstan cigarette price for the missing years. To do so, we regressed the price of Capstan cigarettes on the price of Benson & Hedges Gold plus a time trend with month dummies and predicted prices for Capstan cigarettes for the years for which the price was missing. In the years for which we observe both prices, the two prices have a correlation coefficient of more than 0.9.

United States

The US cigarette price data come from two sources. Price and tax data for the years 1954–2012 come from the *Tax Burden on Tobacco* (Orzechowski and Walker, 2012). That volume reports all state and federal taxes, the date of any changes, and the average price of cigarettes in each state in November of each year. We interpolate the price for each intervening month across all years. The data for 1926–1953 are the average retail price of cigarettes across 32 large US cities as compiled and reported in reports from the US Department of Agriculture (USDA, 1938) and US Department of Labor, Bureau of Labor Statistics (BLS, 1962, 1970). The 1938 USDA bulletin reports the average retail price of cigarettes in each year across 32 large US cities from 1920 to 1937. The BLS reports a cigarette price index for the years 1935–1968 for the same cities (with different base years). We convert the price index into nominal prices for each year. We adjust tax and price data for inflation to real December 2012 dollars using the Consumer Price Index for All Urban Consumers (CPI-U) from the BLS. To compute an average price and tax in the United States in each year, we average the tax and price in each year over all states, weighted by the share of the US population that lives in each state.

The Union of Soviet Socialist Republics, Russian Federation, and Ukraine

We draw data on USSR cigarette prices from official Soviet price lists published in 1937, 1943, 1947, 1948, 1950, 1951, 1953, 1960, 1966, 1974, 1981, and 1991. Janet Chapman (1950, 1952) reports data from some of these price lists.[2] For years for which prices were not published, we rely on price changes announced in *Pravda* as reported in Bokarev (2009). The price lists report prices for many brands of many types of cigarettes that changed over time. In early years, most prices were listed for papirosi, and almost no brands of machine-rolled cigarettes appeared. Over time, the proportion switched. By the early 1990s, papirosi had disappeared. The price lists also indicate the cost of buying loose-leaf tobacco of various types, including snuff and mahorka. The latter type is a dark tobacco leaf generally considered to be of inferior quality but with high nicotine content. It was generally very inexpensive. Many smokers used it to roll their own cigarettes. To reflect the cigarette price for the various types of tobacco, we converted all prices of snuff and roll-your-own tobacco into cost per 20 g (most manufactured cigarettes contain approximately 1 g of tobacco). We then took a simple average across all prices listed in each official price list for papirosi, manufactured cigarettes, and 20 g of snuff and mahorka tobacco.

One of the challenges we faced with regard to prices in these countries was how to adjust for inflation because no consumer price index exists for all the years in our sample, and the existing series for Russia and Ukraine are suspect. Absent a price index, we adjust prices by the average monthly wage (a method described in Kravis, 1951). We convert all prices to real terms in each year by dividing by the average monthly wage of an average worker (divided by 160 hours). This adjustment effectively converts all prices into terms of minutes of work.

Our wage data come from the sources in the References section listed under "Sources of Wage Data."[3]

Using the "real" price of cigarettes, we then linearly interpolate prices that are missing in particular years using prices in observed years that bracket the missing data. We assign these prices equally to our RLMS and ULMS samples in years before 1992.

We received cigarette price data for 1992 onward from the Russia Statistical Ministry for the Russian Federation and the Ukrainian Statistical Office for Ukraine.

NOTES

1. Paul Slater, librarian at Statistics Canada, generously sent us pdf copies of monthly price series from old reports. He can be contacted at Paul.Slater@statcan.gc.ca.
2. Wainstein (1956) and Kaplan and Wainstein (1956) also present price data, but they use the data Chapman (1950, 1952) compiled.
3. Klara Sabirianova Peter of the University of North Carolina compiled data from many of these sources and generously provided them to us. We added data for years for which they were missing from other sources. All sources are listed.

REFERENCES

Spain

Castañeda, J. 1945. *El consumo de Tabaco en España y sus Factores.* Madrid: Instituto de Estudios Políticos.

Comín- Comín, F., and P. Martín-Aceña. 1999. *Tabaculara y el Estanco del Tabaco en España 1636–1998.* Madrid: Fundación Tabacalera.

Spanish Tobacco Market Commission, Statistics. http://www.cmtabacos.es/wwwcmt/paginas/EN/webInicio.tmpl.

Tabacalera. 1992. *Series históricas de consumo de tabaco elaborado, 1957–1991.* Madrid: Tabacalera.

Turkey

Ilter, M. 1989. "Tutun and tutun mamullerinde devlet tekelince yapilmis olan satis fiat ayarlamalari" ("Sale price adjustments on tobacco and tobacco products made by government monopoly"). Unpublished manuscript.

United States

Orzechowski, W., and R. Walker. 2012. *The Tax Burden on Tobacco, Historical Compilation, Vol. 47.* Orzechowski and Walker: Arlington, VA.

US Department of Agriculture (USDA). 1938. "Annual report on tobacco statistics." Statistical Bulletin No. 67:39. Washington, DC: USDA.

US Department of Labor, Bureau of Labor Statistics (BLS). 1962. *Consumer Price Index (1957–59 = 100): Price Indexes for Selected Items and Groups, Annual Averages 1935–1961, Quarterly Indexes, March 1947–December 1961.* Washington, DC: US Government Printing Office.

USSR

Bokarev, I. U. P. 2009. "Tobacco production in Russia: The transition to communism." In *Tobacco in Russian History and Culture: From the Seventeenth Century to the Present*, edited by M. Romaniello and T. Starks, pp 132–147. New York: Routledge.

Chapman, J. G. 1950. "The regional structure of Soviet retail prices." RAND (US Air Force Project) Research Memorandum RM-425.

Chapman, J.G. 1952. "Retail prices of manufactured consumer goods in the USSR, 1937–1948." RAND (US Air Force Project) Research Memorandum RM-803-1.

Kaplan, N. M., and E. S. Wainstein. 1956. "A comparison of Soviet and American retail prices in 1950." *Journal of Political Economy* 64:470–491.

Kravis, I. B. 1951. "Techniques of comparing purchasing power among nations." *Monthly Labor Review* 72:195–197.

Wainstein, E. S. 1956. "A comparison of Soviet and United States retail prices for manufactured goods and services in 1950." RAND (US Air Force Project) Research Memorandum RM-1606.

SOURCES OF CIGARETTE PRICE DATA

Council of Ministers of the USSR. 1960."Госплан СССР №012" (Gosplan USSR No. 012); Effective 1/1/1961; Постановление Совета министров СССР от 04/05/1960 г № 470 (Council of Ministers of the USSR of 04/05/1960 No. 470); Утрачивает силу прейскурант №079-1956 (Act voided price list No. 079 passed in 1956).

Ministry of Domestic and Foreign Trade of the USSR. 1953. "Министерство внутренней и внешней торговли Союза ССР №079" (Ministry of Domestic and Foreign Trade of the USSR No. 079); effective from the date of publication; Принят приказом Минторга СССР № 300-1953 г (adopted by order of the USSR Ministry of Trade No. 300-1953).

Ministry of Trade of the USSR. 1947. "Министерство торговли Союза ССР №079" (Ministry of Trade of the USSR No.079).

Ministry of Trade of the USSR. 1948. Министерство торговли Союза ССР №113 (Ministry of Trade of the USSR No.113).

Ministry of Trade of the USSR. 1950. "Министерство торговли Союза ССР №179" (Ministry of Trade of the USSR No.179); Принят приказом Минторга СССР № 120-1950 г (adopted by order of the USSR Ministry of Trade No. 120-1950).

Ministry of Trade of the USSR. 1951. "Министерство торговли Союза ССР №079" (Ministry of Trade of the USSR No.079); effective from the date of publication; Принят приказом Минторга СССР № 125-1951 г (adopted by order of the USSR Ministry of Trade No.125-1951).

Ministry of Trade of the USSR. 1956. "Министерство торговли Союза ССР №079" (Ministry of Trade of the USSR No.079); Приложение к приказу Минторга СССР от 07/07/1956 г № 151ц (annex to the order of Ministry of Trade of the USSR of 07/07/1956 No.151ts).

National Commissariat of the USSR Trade. 1943. "Народный комиссариат торговли союза ССР" (National Commissariat of the USSR Trade); Утвержден Народным Комиссариатом Торговли Союза ССР (approved by the National Commissariat of the USSR Trade on 29/04/1942).

State Committee of the Price of the Gosplan of the USSR. 1966. "Государственный комитет цен при Госплане СССР №012" (State Committee of the Price of the

Gosplan of the USSR No. 012); Утрачивает силу прейскурант №012-1960 (Act voided price list No. 012 passed in 1960)

State Committee of the Price of the Gosplan of the USSR. 1967. "Государственный комитет цен при Госплане СССР №И-012" (State Committee of the Price of the Gosplan of the USSR No. I-012); Утрачивает силу прейскурант №012-1960 и дополнения к нему (Act voided price list No. 012 passed in 1960 and additions to it).

State Committee of the Price of the Gosplan of the USSR. 1968. "Государственный комитет цен при Госплане СССР №И-012" (State Committee of the Price of the Gosplan of the USSR No. I-012); Утрачивает силу прейскурант №012-1960 и дополнения к нему (Act voided price list No. 012 passed in 1960 and additions to it).

State Committee of the USSR Council of Ministers of the USSR. 1970."Государственный комитет цен Совета министров СССР №И-012" (State Committee of the USSR Council of Ministers prices No. I-012); Действующие на 01/07/1870 г цены помещенные в прейскурант №И-012-1968 и дополнения к нему (acting on 01/07/1970 prices price list placed on No. I- 012 passed in 1968 and its supplements).

State Committee of the USSR Council of Ministers of the USSR. 1974. "Государственный комитет цен Совета министров СССР №012" (State Committee of the USSR Council of Ministers prices No.012); Effective 1/10/1974; Постановление Госкомцен от 30/05/1974 г 878 (decision of the State Committee on 30/05/1974 No. № 878); Утрачивает силу прейскурант №012-1966 (Act voided price list No. 012 passed in 1966).

State Committee of the USSR Prices. 1980. "Государственный комитет цен СССР №И-012" (State Committee of the USSR Prices No. I-012); effective 1/10/1980; Постановление Госкомцен от 9/07/1980 г № 618 (decision of the State Committee of 29/07/1980 No. 618); Утрачивает силу прейскурант №И-012-1970 (Act voided price list No. I- 012 passed in 1970).

State Committee of the USSR Prices. 1981. "Государственный комитет цен СССР №012" (State Committee of the USSR Prices No. 012); effective 1/1/1982; Постановление Госкомцен от 04/08/1981 г № 820 (decision of the State Committee of 04/08/1981 No. 820); Утрачивает силу прейскурант №012-1974 (Act voided price list No. 012 passed in 1974).

State Committee of the USSR Prices. 1981. "Государственный комитет цен СССР №И-012" (State Committee of the USSR Prices No. I-012); effective 1/1/1982; Постановление Госкомцен от 04/08/1981 г № 820 (decision of the State Committee of 04/08/1981 No. 820); Утрачивает силу прейскурант №И-012-1980 (Act voided price list No. 012 passed in 1980).

State Committee of the USSR Prices. 1991. "Государственный комитет цен СССР №012" (State Committee of the USSR Prices No.012); Утрачивает силу прейскурант №012-1981 (Act voided price list № 012-1981).

State Committee of the USSR Prices. 1991."Государственный комитет цен СССР №И-012- 1991/С" (State Committee of the USSR prices No.I-012-1991/С); Постановление Совета министров СССР от 12/11/1990 №1134 (decision of the State Committee of 23/04/1991 No.251); Утрачивает силу прейскурант №И-012-1981 и дополнения к нему (Act voided price list number I- 012-1981 and its supplements).

SOURCES OF WAGE DATA

Bureau of Labor Statistics CSD, Trade Unions, and NLC (По данным Бюро статистики труда ЦСУ, ВЦСПС и НКТ). 1918–1920. "Labour and trade unions" (Труд и профессиональные союзы).

Bureau of Labor Statistics CSD, Trade Unions, and NLC (По данным Бюро статистики труда ЦСУ, ВЦСПС и НКТ). 1921. "Labour and trade unions" (Труд и профессиональные союзы).

Bureau of Labor Statistics CSD, Trade Unions, and NLC (По данным Бюро статистики труда ЦСУ, ВЦСПС и НКТ). 1922. "Labour and trade unions" (Труд и профессиональные союзы).

Bureau of Labor Statistics CSD, Trade Unions, and NLC (По данным Бюро статистики труда ЦСУ, ВЦСПС и НКТ). 1924. "Labour and trade unions " (Труд и профессиональные союзы).

Central Statistical Office of USSR (Центральное статистическое управление СССР). 1984. "Compilation of statistical materials" (Сборник Статистических Материалов).

Ministry of Finance of USSR Prices (Министерство Финансов СССР). 1988. "USSR state budget brief statistical compilation" (Государственный Бюджет СССР Краткий статистический сборник).

Ministry of Finance of USSR Prices (Министерство Финансов СССР). 1989. "USSR state budget brief statistical compilation" (Государственный Бюджет СССР Краткий статистический сборник).

Ministry of Finance of USSR Prices (Министерство Финансов СССР). 1981–1985. "USSR state budget statistical compilation" (Государвственный Бюджет СССР Статистический сборник).

Ministry of Finance of USSR Prices. (Министерство Финансов СССР). 1981–1985. "USSR state budget statistical compilation" (Государвственный Бюджет СССР Статистический сборник).

National Finance Commissariat (По данным Народн. Комисс. Финансов). 1922–1923. "Finance" (Финансы).

State Statistics Committee of USSR (Госкомстат СССР). 1988. "Statistical collection" (Статистический Сборник).

From website, source not identified. 1926–1930. "Chart" (Таблица).

From website, source not identified. 1926–1930. "Industrial labour" (Промышленный Труд).

From website, source not identified. 1933. "Chart" (Таблица).

From website, source not identified. 1934. "Population and labour" (Население и труд).

From website, source not identified. 1935. "Free chart" (Свободная Таблица).

From website, source not identified. 1936. "Combined section" (Сводный раздел).

From website, source not identified. 1981. "Labour" (Труд).

From website, source not identified. 1981. "The average annual number and wages of workers and employees in the national economy" (Среднегодовая Численность и Заработная плата рабочих и служащих в народном хозяйстве).

From website, source not identified. 1984. "Social development and the improvement of people's well-being" (Социальное развитие и повышение народного благосостояния).

From website, source not identified. 1985. "Improving the people's well-being" (Повышение народного благосостояния).

From website, source not identified. 1985. "Labour" (Труд).

From website, source not identified. 1987. "National income" (Национальный доход).

From website, source not identified. 1989. "Population income" (Доходы населения).

15

Derivation of Historical Smoking Prevalence

REBEKKA CHRISTOPOULOU

THE METHODS

To construct the life-course smoking trajectories we present in this book, we use retrospectively reported data on lifetime smoking status and events. As we explain briefly in the introduction, we assume that current and former smokers smoked in each year from the age they started until either the survey year (current smokers) or the age they said they quit (ex-smokers). Because we lack data on whether and when smokers might have temporarily quit, we assume that none of the smokers ever temporarily quit. Using these cross-sectional data, we then construct a longitudinal data set. In particular, for all respondents with valid responses, we construct a smoking status indicator in each year of life that equals 0 if a person does not smoke in that year and 1 if he or she does smoke. Finally, we group observations into categories by sex, and 10-year birth cohort.[1] We measure smoking prevalence rates over the life course as the mean smoking status in each year of the gender-specific cohort groups (weighted by sampling or population weights).[2]

Because our calculations rely on retrospective smoking questions, we need to account for the fact that smokers are less likely than nonsmokers to answer those questions because smokers are more likely to die from a smoking-related cause prior to the date of the survey. Due to this differential mortality, we underestimate smoking rates for old cohorts. To correct for this bias, we apply the simple formula proposed by Harris (1983) but use detailed cause-specific mortality data by age and gender, which we produce following the technique by Peto et al. (1992). In previously published work, we explain this procedure in detail and its advantages over alternative practices (Christopoulou et al., 2011; Lillard et al., 2014). In that work, we use data from the United Kingdom, United States, Russia, and Spain to show that differential mortality significantly biases smoking rates reconstructed from retrospective reports only for cohorts who, at the time of the interview, were older than 60 years. We have also made freely available online[3] fully documented STATA codes, which researchers can use to correct their own data for differential mortality bias. To save space, and given that all this material is widely accessible, we do not fully describe the methods here.

However, a note on China is necessary. China is the only country for which we have used a variant of Peto et al.'s (1992) calculation of smoking-attributable mortality in order to account for lung cancer risk associated with household energy use, specifically with the burning of coal in stoves and buildings with poor ventilation. We do not account for this for other countries because this problem is not as prevalent in other countries as it is in China and because for all other countries we lack the relevant data for the early portion of our sample period. This omission may introduce some upward bias in the adjustment in those early periods. In more recent years, domestic coal use in unvented stoves is absent or negligible in all the other countries we investigate (Smith et al., 2004).

To explain what we do differently for China, we remind the reader that Peto et al.'s (1992) method involves approximating national nonsmoker death rates from lung cancer by the death rates of a reference population of nonsmokers. Thus, we calculate mortality attributable to lung cancer in a given country as the difference between total national death rates and the respective death rates in the reference population. For other smoking-related diseases, we calculate the proportion of smoking-attributable deaths (PSAD) as follows:

$$PSAD = \frac{SIR \cdot c \cdot (RR - 1)}{SIR \cdot c \cdot (RR - 1) + 1}$$

RR denotes death rates of smokers relative to nonsmokers for the disease of interest in the reference population, and c is a constant factor that accounts for potential confounding and extrapolation bias in RR. Researchers set the value of c at less than 1 to give less weight to RR. Peto et al. (1992) set $c = 0.5$. Evidence in Thun et al. (2000), however, suggests that this value is too conservative. Following Ezzati and Lopez (2003a), we set $c = 0.7$.[4]

SIR is the smoking impact factor and is a proxy for the proportion of ever-smokers in the country of interest. For all countries apart from China, we use the standard definition for SIR: $SIR = (C - N)/(S - N)$, where C denotes lung cancer death rates in the country of study, and N and S denote nonsmoker and smoker lung cancer death rates in the reference population, respectively. For China, we use the "background adjusted SIR" as proposed by Ezzati and Lopez (2003b): $SIR = ((C - N^*)(N/N^*))/(S - N)$, where N^* now denotes nonsmoker lung cancer death rates in the country of study. Ezzati and Lopez report data on N^* in Figure 1 of their paper, which we use for our calculations.[5]

For each year, sex, and age group, the product of PSAD with the total number of deaths from the disease of interest gives the smoking-attributable number of deaths from this disease. For the years for which we have only overall mortality data, we assume that the relative mortality of smokers and nonsmokers is time invariant and equal to the mean relative mortality by cohort and gender derived from the cause-specific data. For periods with no available mortality data, we simply backcast the differential mortality adjustment factor.

THE DATA

Australia: For the period 1950–2007, we use population data and cause-specific deaths by age and gender from the World Health Organization (WHO) Mortality Database.[6] For the period 1921–1950, we use total mortality rates by birth cohort and gender from the Human Mortality Database (HMD), which is compiled by the University of California at Berkeley and the Max Planck Institute for Demographic Research in Rostock, Germany.[7]

Canada: For the period 1950–2009, we use population data and cause-specific deaths by age and gender from the WHO Mortality Database. For the period 1921–1950, we use total mortality rates by birth cohort and gender from the HMD.

China: For the period 1987–1999, we use cause-specific deaths by age and gender from the WHO Mortality Database. For the periods 1965–1986 and 2001–2009, we use total mortality rates by birth cohort and gender from the *China Statistical Yearbooks* published by the National Bureau of Statistics of the People's Republic of China. From this source, we also derive population data by age and gender for the period 1965–2009.

Germany: For the periods 1952–1990, 1969–1990, and 1991–2002, we use population data and cause-specific deaths by age and gender for West, East, and United Germany, respectively, from the WHO Mortality Database.

Russia: For the period 1965–1993, we use cause-specific deaths by age and gender from Meslé et al. (1996) and population data by age and gender from Avdeev and Monnier (1996).[8] For the period 1994–2010, we derive these data from the WHO Mortality Database. For the period 1959–1964, we use total mortality rates by birth cohort and gender from the HMD.

Spain: For the period 1950–2011, we use population data and cause-specific deaths by age and gender from the WHO Mortality Database. For the period 1908–1949, we use total mortality rates by birth cohort and gender from the HMD.

Turkey: For the years 1975–1982, 1985, and 1986, we use cause-specific deaths by age and gender from the Turkish Statistical Institute. For the years 1983, 1984, and 1987–2008, we derive these data from the WHO Mortality Database. For the period 1975–2008, we also use population data by age and gender from the Turkish Statistical Institute. For the period 1960–1974, we use total mortality rates by birth cohort and gender from the HMD.

Ukraine: For the period 1965–2000, we use population data and cause-specific deaths by age and gender from Meslé and Vallin (2003). For the period 2001–2006, we derive these data from the WHO Mortality Database. For the period 1959–1964, we use total mortality rates by birth cohort and gender from the HMD.

United Kingdom: For the period 1953–2002, we use population data and cause-specific deaths by age and gender from the WHO Mortality Database. For the period 1922–1952, we use total mortality rates by birth cohort and gender from the HMD.

United States: For the period 1933–1949, we use population data and cause-specific deaths by age and gender from the US Bureau of the Census reports. For the period 1950–2007, we draw these data from the WHO Mortality Database.

For all countries, we calculate smoking-attributable mortality using nonsmokers from the Cancer Prevention Study II (CPS-II) carried out by the American Cancer Society as the reference population. M. J. Thun, MD, MS (former Vice President Emeritus, Epidemiology, and Surveillance Research, American Cancer Society) generously provided us with the CPS-II 1982–1988 data via email (February 2010). The CPS-II sample includes more than 1 million Americans older than age 30 years starting in 1982. Like other studies, we use the CPS-II because it provides mortality rates of some of the first cohorts of men to have smoked heavily and because it conveniently disaggregates them by sex and age.

THE RESULTS

In the figures that follow, we present—for each country, cohort, and gender—the smoking prevalence rates reconstructed from our retrospective data, unadjusted (solid line) and adjusted (dotted line) for smoking-related differential mortality bias. We present results only for cohorts older than 60 years because, as mentioned previously, smoking-related mortality differences for younger cohorts are small and the adjustment has negligible effects on smoking rates. For each country, we use the Pearson test of independence for binary variables to test whether adjusted and unadjusted prevalence rates statistically differ, and we report the cohorts and periods for which we find that they do.[9]

As one would expect, for groups with very low smoking rates (e.g., most cohorts of women), the adjustment is negligible. Furthermore, in countries for which we use several waves of data, the differential mortality adjustment results in more modest differences. In fact, the earlier the year of the first available survey wave, the lower the computed adjustment. At the same time, however, the larger the number of observations that are available for each country–gender–cohort group, the more power available for the test of statistical significance of the adjustment. Thus, for a country with only one available wave of data, the size of the implied adjustment may be large but statistically insignificant, whereas for another country with several available waves of data, the size of the implied adjustment may be smaller but statistically significant (e.g., compare the size and statistical significance of the adjustment of 80- to 89-year-old males in China and Turkey).

Note that the adjustments that we present here for Russia, Spain, the United Kingdom, and the United States may differ slightly from those published in earlier work (Christopoulou et al., 2011; Lillard et al., 2014) mostly because those early results were based on different surveys or survey waves but also because of somewhat different data processing.

Australia

In Australia, we find that the difference between unadjusted and adjusted smoking prevalence is sizable for men who were 80–89 years old in 2007. As Figure 15.1 shows, at the peak prevalence rate for this group, the two rates differ by 11.5 percentage points. Unadjusted prevalence for this group is significantly underestimated in every year during the period 1941–1963 (5 percent significance level). For women and all other groups of men, the adjustment is smaller and statistically insignificant. At the

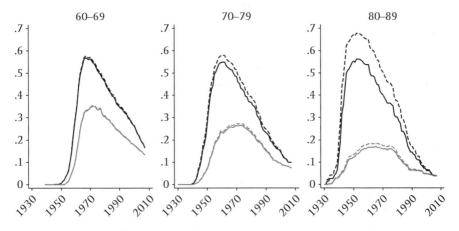

Figure 15.1 Smoking prevalence rates in Australia adjusted and unadjusted for differential mortality of males (two top lines) and females (two bottom lines) aged 60–69, 70–79, and 80–89 years in 2007.

peak prevalence rate for men who were 70–79 and 60–69 years old in 2007, adjusted and unadjusted prevalence rates differ by 3 and 0.8 percentage points, respectively. At the peak prevalence rate for women who were 80–89, 70–79, and 60–69 years old in 2007, the two rates differ by 1.6, 0.9, and 0.3 percentage points, respectively.

Canada

In Canada, we find that the difference between unadjusted and adjusted smoking prevalence is sizable for men who were 70–79 years old in 2009 and for men and women who were 80–89 years old in 2009. As Figure 15.2 shows, at the peak prevalence rate for these groups, the two rates differ by 2.8, 10.5, and 3.6 percentage

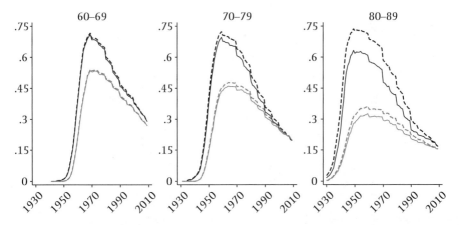

Figure 15.2 Smoking prevalence rates in Canada adjusted and unadjusted for differential mortality of males (two top lines) and females (two bottom lines) aged 60–69, 70–79, and 80–89 years in 2009.

points, respectively. Unadjusted prevalence for these groups is significantly under-estimated in every year during the periods 1948–1988, 1931–1994, and 1943–1985, respectively (5 percent significance level). For all other groups, the adjustment is smaller and statistically insignificant. At the peak prevalence rate for men who were 60–69 years old in 2009, adjusted and unadjusted prevalence rates differ by 0.8 percentage points. At the peak prevalence rate for women who were 70–79 and 60–69 years old in 2009, the two rates differ by 1.7 and 0.5 percentage points, respectively.

China

In China, we find that the difference between unadjusted and adjusted smoking prevalence is sizable for men who were 80–89 years old in 2009. As Figure 15.3 shows, at the peak prevalence rate for this group, the two rates differ by 4.2 per-centage points. Unadjusted prevalence for this group is significantly underesti-mated in every year during the period 1940–1976 (5 percent significance level). For all other groups, the adjustment is small and statistically insignificant. At the peak prevalence rate for men who were 70–79 years old in 2009, adjusted and unadjusted prevalence rates differ by 0.6 percentage points. At the peak preva-lence rate for women who were 80–89 and 70–79 years old in 2009, the two rates differ by 0.2 and 0.1 percentage points, respectively. For men and women who were 60–69 years old in 2009, the two rates are equal. As mentioned previously, this is because the earliest survey wave that we use for China was conducted in 1991. Individuals who were 42–51 years old in 1991 (and were thus interviewed when smoking-related mortality was low) are included in the cohort that reached 60–69 years of age in 2009. As a result, the share of smokers in that cohort is rep-resentative of the population.

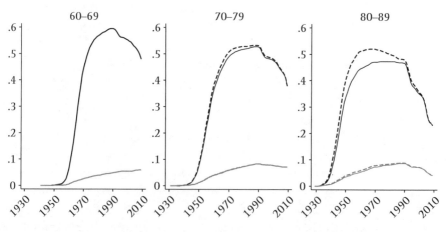

Figure 15.3 Smoking prevalence rates in China adjusted and unadjusted for differential mortality of males (two top lines) and females (two bottom lines) aged 60–69, 70–79, and 80–89 years in 2009.

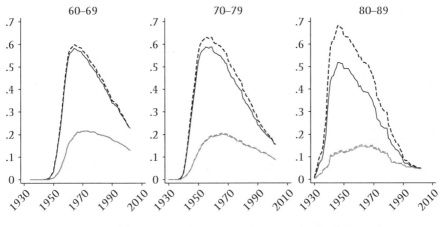

Figure 15.4 Smoking prevalence rates in Germany adjusted and unadjusted for differential mortality of males (two top lines) and females (two bottom lines) aged 60–69, 70–79, and 80–89 years in 2002.

Germany

In Germany, we find that the difference between unadjusted and adjusted smoking prevalence is sizable for men who were 80–89 years old in 2002. As Figure 15.4 shows, at the peak prevalence rate for this group, the adjustment equals 16.4 percentage points. Unadjusted prevalence for this group is significantly underestimated in every year during the period 1939–1972 (5 percent significance level). For all other groups, the adjustment is small and statistically insignificant. At the peak prevalence rate for men who were 70–79 and 60–69 years old in 2002, adjusted and unadjusted prevalence rates differ by 4.3 and 1.6 percentage points, respectively. At the peak prevalence rate for women who were 80–89, 70–79, and 60–69 years old in 2007, the two rates differ by 0.6, 0.5, and 0.2 percentage points, respectively.

Russia

In Russia, we find that the difference between unadjusted and adjusted smoking prevalence is sizable for men who were 80–89, 70–79, and 60–69 years old in 2010. As Figure 15.5 shows, at the peak prevalence rate for these groups, the two rates differ by 10.6, 6.6, and 2.6 percentage points, respectively. Unadjusted prevalence for these groups is significantly underestimated in every year during the periods 1941–1999, 1952–2002, and 1973–2000, respectively (5 percent significance level). For all cohorts of women, the adjustment is small and statistically insignificant. At the peak prevalence rate for women who were 80–89, 70–79, and 60–69 years old in 2010, adjusted and unadjusted prevalence rates differ by 0.2, 0.2, and 0.1 percentage points, respectively.

Note that, as for China, the results for Russia are based on a pooled cross section of multiple survey waves. However, unlike the results for China, we find that the differential mortality adjustment is non-negligible for the 60- to 69-year-old Russians. This difference could be explained by the difference in the scale of unadjusted smoking prevalence in the two countries (the unadjusted smoking prevalence rate of the

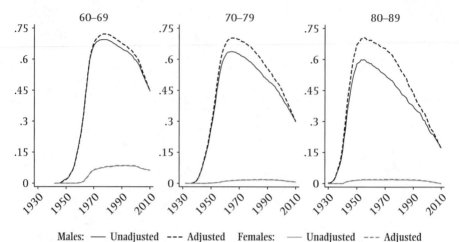

Males: —— Unadjusted --- Adjusted   Females: —— Unadjusted --- Adjusted

Figure 15.5 Smoking prevalence rates in Russia adjusted and unadjusted for differential mortality of males (two top lines) and females (two bottom lines) aged 60–69, 70–79, and 80–89 years in 2010.

60- to 69-year-old cohort in Russia is approximately 10 percentage points higher than that in China) and by the fact that, for Russia, we do not adjust smoking-attributable mortality for lung cancer risk associated with the burning of coal in unventilated residences.

Spain

In Spain, we find that the difference between unadjusted and adjusted smoking prevalence is sizable for men who were 80–89 years old in 2011. As Figure 15.6 shows, at the peak prevalence rate for this group, the two rates differ by 6.6 percentage points.

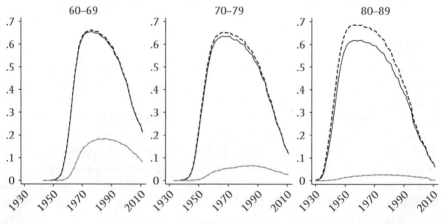

Males: —— Unadjusted --- Adjusted   Females: —— Unadjusted --- Adjusted

Figure 15.6 Smoking prevalence rates in Spain adjusted and unadjusted for differential mortality of males (two top lines) and females (two bottom lines) aged 60–69, 70–79, and 80–89 years in 2011.

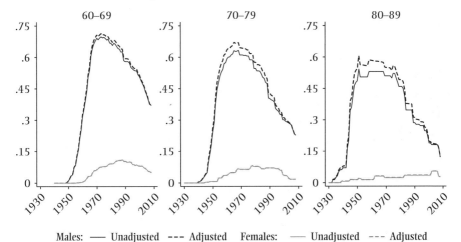

Figure 15.7 Smoking prevalence rates in Turkey adjusted and unadjusted for differential mortality of males (two top lines) and females (two bottom lines) aged 60–69, 70–79, and 80–89 years in 2008.

Unadjusted prevalence for this group is significantly underestimated in every year during the period 1936–1994 (5 percent significance level). For all other groups, the adjustment is small and statistically insignificant. At the peak prevalence rate for men who were 70–79 and 60–69 years old in 2011, adjusted and unadjusted prevalence rates differ by 1.6 and 0.5 percentage points, respectively. At the peak prevalence rate for all cohorts of women, the two rates are equal.

Note that, as for China and Russia, the results for Spain are based on a pooled cross section of multiple survey waves. However, the results for Spain more closely resemble the results for China than those for Russia. As opposed to Russia, the differential mortality adjustment in Spain and China is negligible for the 60- to 69-year-old cohorts. Again, this difference could be explained by the difference in the scale of unadjusted smoking prevalence across countries and by the fact that, for Russia, we do not adjust smoking-attributable mortality for lung cancer risk associated with the burning of coal in unventilated residences.

Turkey

In Turkey, we find that the difference between unadjusted and adjusted smoking prevalence is zero for women but non-negligible for men. As Figure 15.7 shows, at the peak prevalence rate for men who were 80–89, 70–79, and 60–69 years old in 2008, adjusted and unadjusted prevalence rates differ by 6.4, 3.9, and 1.4 percentage points, respectively. However, because of small sample sizes (especially for the oldest cohorts), the adjustment is never statistically significant.

Ukraine

For Ukraine, we lack data for the 80- to 89-year-old cohort because the ULMS only interviews individuals younger than 76 years. We find that unadjusted and adjusted

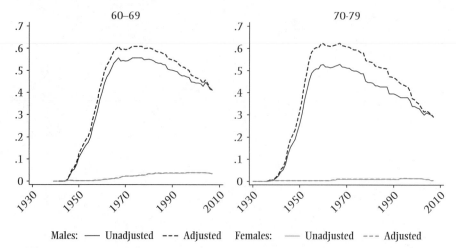

Figure 15.8 Smoking prevalence rates in Ukraine adjusted and unadjusted for differential mortality of males (two top lines) and females (two bottom lines) aged 60–69 and 70–79 years in 2007.

smoking prevalence differ for men who were 70–79 years old in 2007. As Figure 15.8 shows, at the peak prevalence rate for this group, the two rates differ by 9.5 percentage points. Unadjusted prevalence for this group is significantly underestimated in every year during the period 1954–1984 (5 percent significance level). For all other groups, the adjustment is smaller and statistically insignificant. At the peak prevalence rate for men who were 60–69 years old in 2007, adjusted and unadjusted prevalence rates differ by 5.2 percentage points. At the peak prevalence rate for women who were 70–79 and 60–69 years old in 2007, the two rates differ by 0.1 percentage points.

United Kingdom

In the United Kingdom, we find that the difference between unadjusted and adjusted smoking prevalence is sizable for men who were 80–89 years old in 2002. As Figure 15.9 shows, at the peak prevalence rate for this group, the two rates differ by 16.6 percentage points. Unadjusted prevalence for this group is significantly underestimated in every year during the period 1923–1984 (5 percent significance level). For all other groups, the adjustment is smaller and statistically insignificant. At the peak prevalence rate for men who were 70–79 and 60–69 years old in 2007, adjusted and unadjusted prevalence rates differ by 5.1 and 1.6 percentage points, respectively. At the peak prevalence rate for women who were 80–89, 70–79, and 60–69 years old in 2007, the two rates differ by 5.4, 2.7, and 0.7 percentage points, respectively.

United States

The United States is the country for which the sample size is very large because we pool together a large number of cross sections. As such, the difference between unadjusted and adjusted smoking prevalence is statistically significant for all cohorts of men and women, even though it is often less sizable than in countries in which it

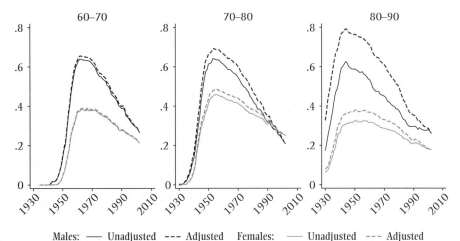

Males: —— Unadjusted --- Adjusted   Females: —— Unadjusted --- Adjusted

Figure 15.9 Smoking prevalence rates in the United Kingdom adjusted and unadjusted for differential mortality of males (two top lines) and females (two bottom lines) aged 60–69, 70–79, and 80–89 years in 2002.

is larger but statistically insignificant. As Figure 15.10 shows, at the peak prevalence rate for men who were 80–89, 70–79, and 60–69 years old in 2007, adjusted and unadjusted prevalence rates differ by 8, 4.2, and 1.1 percentage points, respectively. Unadjusted prevalence for these groups is significantly underestimated in every year during the periods 1926–1998, 1932–1999, and 1957–2000, respectively (5 percent significance level). At the peak prevalence rate for women who were 80–89, 70–79, and 60–69 years old in 2007, adjusted and unadjusted prevalence rates differ by 3.8, 2.3, and 0.9 percentage points, respectively. Unadjusted prevalence for these groups is significantly underestimated in every year during the periods 1932–2000, 1941–1998, and 1941–1997, respectively.

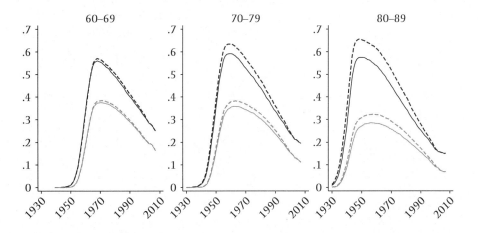

Males: —— Unadjusted --- Adjusted   Females: —— Unadjusted --- Adjusted

Figure 15.10 Smoking prevalence rates in the United States adjusted and unadjusted for differential mortality of males (two top lines) and females (two bottom lines) aged 60–69, 70–79, 80–89 in 2007.

NOTES

1. In all country-specific chapters, we define birth cohorts by age at the most recent available national survey. In the three comparative chapters, we define birth cohorts by age in 2002.

2. In some cases, when we pool together several cross sections of data to derive the smoking trajectories, due to sampling differences across survey waves, the trajectories show "bumps" at the years of survey. For clarity of exposition, we apply a standard least-squares smoothing during these years, ensuring that it does not cause level changes in the smoking trajectories.

3. See http://smoking-research.ehe.osu.edu/data-and-codes.

4. Although we do not report them here, we have also tested the sensitivity of the results to a range of correction factors (from a very conservative correction value of 0.4 to the maximum correction value of 1.0) and find that results change little. For example, when we set $c = 1$, the bias for the oldest cohort of UK women and the second-oldest cohort of UK men changes from being statistically insignificant to being marginally significant at the 10% level.

5. More details, as well as the STATA codes, are available by request.

6. Available at http://www.who.int/healthinfo/statistics/mortality_rawdata/en/index.html.

7. Available at http://www.mortality.org.

8. Available at http://www-census.ined.fr/demogrus/Demographie/Population/Structure/index.htm.

9. To be conservative, and because it better approximates the binomial distribution, for small samples we apply the Yates (1934) correction.

REFERENCES

Avdeev, A., and A. Monnier. 1996. *Mouvement de la population de la Russie: 1959–1994 Données statistiques*. Paris: Institut National d'Études Démographiques.

Christopoulou, R., J. Han, A. Jaber, and D. R. Lillard. 2011. "Dying for a smoke: How much does differential mortality of smokers affect estimated life-course smoking prevalence?" *Preventive Medicine* 52:66–70.

Ezzati, M., and A. D. Lopez. 2003a. "Measuring the accumulated hazards of smoking: Global and regional estimates for 2000." *Tobacco Control* 12:79–85.

Ezzati, M., and A. D. Lopez. 2003b. "Estimates of global mortality attributable to smoking in 2000." *Lancet* 362:847–852.

Harris, J. E. 1983. "Cigarette smoking among successive birth cohorts of men and women in the United States during 1900–80." *Journal of the National Cancer Institute* 71:473–479.

Lillard, D. R., R. Christopoulou, and A. I. Gil Lacruz. 2014. "Re: Validation of a Method for Reconstructing Historical Rates of Smoking Prevalence." *American Journal of Epidemiology* 180(6):656–658.

Meslé, F., V. Kolnikov, V. Hertrich, and J. Vallin. 1996. *Tendances récentes de la mortalité par cause en Russie, 1965–1994 Données statistiques*. Paris: Institut National d'Études Démographiques.

Meslé, F., and J. Vallin. 2003. *Mortalité et causes des décè's en Ukraine au XXe siè'cle*. Paris: Institut National d'Études Démographiques.

Peto, R., A. D. Lopez, J. Boreham, M. Thun, and C. Heath. 1992. "Mortality from tobacco in developed countries: Indirect estimation from national vital statistics." *Lancet* 339:1268–1278.

Smith, K. R., S. Mehta, and M. Maeusezahl-feuz. 2004. "Indoor air pollution from household use of solid fuels." In *Comparative Quantification of Health Risks: Global and Regional Burden of Diseases Attributable to Selected Major Risks*, edited by M. Ezzati, A. D. Lopez, C. J. L. Murray, and A. Rodgers, pp 1435–1492. Geneva: World Health Organization.

Thun, M. J., L. F. Apicella, and S. J. Henley. 2000. "Smoking vs. other risk factors as the cause of smoking-attributable mortality: Confounding in the courtroom." *Journal of the American Medical Association* 284:706–712.

Yates, F. 1934. "Contingency table involving small numbers and the X2 test." *Journal of the Royal Statistical Society* 1(Suppl):217–235.

16

Timeline of Tobacco-Related Events by Country[*]

TIMELINE OF AUSTRALIAN TOBACCO CONTROL EFFORTS

For Australia's timeline, we draw information from three main sources: Robin Walker's *Under Fire: A History of Tobacco Smoking in Australia* (Walker, 1984), Cancer Council Victoria's authoritative monograph *Tobacco in Australia* (Scollo and Winstanley, 2008), and the University of Sydney's Tobacco Control Supersite.[1] The latter also draws heavily on Cancer Council Victoria's monograph. All three sources provide a wealth of information that we only selectively repeat here. We supplement these sources with information from the Action on Smoking and Health Australia website on state and Commonwealth legislation.[2]

Health Concerns With Smoking

1840: "Professor"[3] Rennie lectures about dangers of tobacco consumption.

1936: Anti-Cancer Council of Victoria established by statute.

1950 (February): The Australian edition of *Reader's Digest* publishes article on smoking and health.

1953 (January): The Australian edition of *Reader's Digest* publishes an article titled "Cancer by the Carton," which reviewed Wynder and Graham's 1953 research showing a link between exposure to tar and cancer in mice.

1954: The *Medical Journal of Australia* warns hypertensive people not to smoke.

1955: The Central Tobacco Advisory Committee is founded to advise the government on policies related to the tobacco industry.

1955: Sir Macfarlane Burnet addresses the Australian and New Zealand Association for the Advancement of Science to warn about the dangers of smoking. Dr. John Mayo, radiologist and chairman of the Adelaide University Anti-Cancer Campaign Committee, advises all smokers to quit.

1956: The *Medical Journal of Australia* warns about the dangers of smoking, and it notes that smoking is linked to cancer and that most doctors disapprove of it.

1957: Western Australia initiates an anti-smoking campaign.

1957 (May): The Australian National Health and Medical Research Council calls on state governments to carry out anti-smoking campaigns and on the Commonwealth to establish a body to advise citizens on how to reduce risks from smoking.

---

[*] All authors contributed for each of their countries.

1961: The first tar table is published in *Choice* magazine.

1961 (October): The Australian Cancer Society is established.

1962: The Australian National Health and Medical Research Council renews its recommendations from 1957. It also recommends that the Commonwealth government ban all tobacco advertising and calls on the government to issue an official statement that smoking cigarettes contributes to lung cancer.

1962 (October): Representatives of the Australian Medical Association (AMA), Royal Australasian College of Physicians (RACP), Royal Australasian College of Surgeons (RACS), and the Anti-Cancer Council of Victoria endorse the 1962 report by the Royal College of Physicians.

1962: The *Sydney Morning Herald* calls on the government to launch a youth anti-smoking campaign.

1965 (October): The Australian Cancer Society sends deputation to the Commonwealth Minister of Health. Included in the deputation are representatives from the AMA, RACP, RACS, Australian College of Pathologists, National Heart Foundation, National Tuberculosis and Chest Association, and Australian Cancer Society. They urge the Minister of Health to declare smoking to be a health hazard, restrict television advertising of cigarettes, research cancer potential of Australian cigarettes, survey smoking habits of Australian youth, and run anti-smoking campaigns.

1965 (December): The *Commonwealth Journal of Health* publishes an article acknowledging a link between smoking and lung cancer.

1968: The *Sydney Morning Herald* ridicules conclusion of the "Education and Research Foundation of the American Medical Association" that smoking–cancer link is not proved.

1968: The Bankstown Council puts up posters warning of the dangers of smoking.

1972: The McMahon Government allocates $500,000 for each of 3 years to inform Australians about health hazards of smoking.

Health Warnings on Packs

1969: The Conference of Health Ministers approves cigarette pack warning.

1972 (September): New South Wales (NSW) introduces Cigarettes (Labeling) Bill.

1973: First health warning on cigarette packages introduced on January 1 in South Australia, Tasmania, Victoria, the Territories, and Western Australia. On June 1, NSW and Queensland follow suit . The label reads: "Warning—Smoking is a health hazard."

1985: Australia requires four rotating warning labels on cigarette packages.

1992: New labeling required on cigarette packages—detailing how health is damaged by ingestion of tar, nicotine, and carbon monoxide and explaining health risks of smoking.

2006 (March 1): The federal government requires cigarette manufacturers to print graphic images on cigarette packs. The government also requires that the mandated health warning cover 30 percent of the front and 90 percent of the back of the cigarette box. The remaining 10 percent of the space on the back of the pack must display the message "Sale to underage persons prohibited."

2012 (January 1): The federal government bans firms from printing cigarette packs with any logos, colors, or promotional text. Firms may now sell cigarettes in packs that show only the brand name and health warning messages. Cigarette pack warning labels now include the following text:

–Smoking causes peripheral vascular disease
–Smoking causes emphysema
–Smoking causes mouth and throat cancer
–Smoking clogs your arteries
–Don't let children breathe your smoke
–Smoking: A leading cause of death
–Quitting will improve your health
–Smoking harms unborn babies
–Smoking causes blindness
–Smoking causes lung cancer
–Smoking causes heart disease
–Smoking doubles your risk of stroke
–Smoking is addictive
–Tobacco smoke is toxic

Australian cigarette packaging laws also prohibit the use of terms such as "light," "mild," and "extra mild." The three major Australian tobacco manufacturers agreed to stop using these terms after a 2005 investigation by the Australian Competition and Consumer Commission of complaints of misleading and deceptive terms. This has assisted in counteracting the belief that some cigarette varieties are less harmful than others. To the same effect, although the display of carbon monoxide, nicotine, and tar content of particular brands of cigarettes used to be mandated, it is now prohibited under the government's "All Cigarettes Are Toxic" campaign.

Tobacco Product Bans

1935: The Commonwealth government bans smoking in cinemas and theaters (to reduce the risk of fire).

1977: NSW bans smoking on all metropolitan transport.

1982 (May 25): Victoria hosts the first "Smoke Out Day" to encourage smokers to quit.

1986: Limited bans on smoking in federal workplaces are introduced.

1993 (April): Fast-food chains (Hungry Jack, Kentucky Fried Chicken, and McDonald's) ban smoking.

1995 (March): The federal government bans smoking on nonstop flights to the United States and Canada.

1996 (July): The federal government bans smoking on all international flights.

1999 (January): South Australia bans smoking in all indoor dining areas.

2005 (January): Western Australia incrementally restricts smoking in public places. The process is completed July 2006.

2006: Australian states begin to implement workplace smoking bans.

2006 (January): Tasmania bans indoor smoking.

2006 (July): Western Australia bans smoking in all indoor areas of pubs, bars, and clubs. The law permits smoking in outdoor eating areas and in the international room of the Burswood Casino. The Health Ministry allows smoking at "footpath drinking establishments that do not serve food."

2006 (October 1): Tobacco sponsorship is banned at all sporting events. The 2006 Australian Motorcycle Grand Prix and the 2006 Australian Formula One Grand Prix are the last two sporting events to be sponsored.

2006 (December): Smoking is banned in all enclosed public places in Australian Capital Territory (ACT). Exempt are public places that are "open" to the outdoors. The law stipulates a place to be open if more than 25 percent of the area (measured by the surface area of the ceiling, walls, and windows) is open to the outdoors.

2007 (July 1): NSW bans smoking in enclosed public spaces. A space that has more than 25 percent of its total ceiling and wall area open to the outdoors and is 10 percent open to the elements at all times is exempt from the ban. A business owner may count windows and doors as open space only if he or she locks them open during trading hours.

2007 (July 1): Queensland bans smoking in all pubs, clubs, restaurants, workplaces, outdoor public places (e.g., patrolled beaches, children's playground equipment, major sport stadiums, and within 4 m of nonresidential building entrances), and commercial outdoor eating and drinking areas. However, there is an exemption for locations where an owner holds a hotel, club, or casino liquor license. In these cases, the owner may designate up to 50 percent of the outdoor liquor licensed area as a smoking and drinking area, but the owner may not serve or allow food, provide entertainment, or place gaming machines in the area. For any such area, the owner must establish either a 2-m-wide area or a 2.1-m-high screen—impervious to smoke—between the smoking area and any adjacent outdoor areas of the establishment that patrons usually frequent. Owners who establish an outdoor smoking area must also prepare a "smoking management plan" that complies with legislative requirements.

2007 (July 1): Victoria bans smoking in any enclosed public place. Places with 25 percent or more of the combined wall and roof space open to the outdoors are exempt. The law allows smoking on balconies, verandas, in courtyards, marquees, and on footpaths. The government will fine merchants who sell tobacco products to people younger than age 18 years. Anyone may legally possess the products.

2007 (November 1): South Australia bans smoking in enclosed public places. The law exempts places if 30 percent or more of the total wall and ceiling surfaces are open to the outdoors.

2008 (January): Tasmania bans smoking in cars with passengers younger than age 18 and fines violators $110 (paid on-the-spot).

2009 (May): Queensland bans smoking in a car in which any passenger is younger than age 16 . The government also gives local governments the power to regulate smoking at pedestrian malls and public transport waiting points such as bus stops, taxi ranks, and ferry wharves.

2009 (July 1): The Public Health (Tobacco) Act 2008 of NSW makes it illegal for a person to smoke in a car if a child younger than 16 years of age is present. The law is enforced by the NSW police and allows the police to fine the driver and every other smoker $250 (paid on-the-spot).

2010 (January 2): The Northern Territory bans smoking in all enclosed areas of restaurants, licensed clubs, and pubs.

2010 (January): Victoria makes it illegal for a person to smoke in a car if a child younger than 16 years of age is present.

2010 (December): ACT bans smoking in all outdoor eating and drinking areas. The law allows smoking in a "Designated Outdoor Smoking Area" (DOSA) if the area encompasses less than 50 percent of the total outdoor area and is separated from smoke-free areas by no less than 4 m or a nontransparent fixed wall barrier at least 3 m high. Staff may clean a DOSA only 30 minutes after the last person leaves. If authorities catch a person smoking outside a DOSA, they may fine both the individual ($200–$2,000 paid on-the-spot) and the business owner ($2,000–$10,000). No business owners apply to establish a DOSA.

Advertising and Marketing

1960: The Australian National Health and Medical Research Council recommends that the Commonwealth government restrict tobacco advertising.

1966: The Menzies government introduces a voluntary tobacco advertising code for television.

1966: The tobacco industry adopts the voluntary code for cigarette advertising.

1972: Australia begins to limit firms' advertising of cigarettes on radio and television (ban to be phased in from 1972 to 1976).

1976 (September 1): Television and radio advertising of cigarettes is banned throughout Australia.

1978: The NSW Local Government Association endorses a ban imposed by the North Sydney Council on an outdoor neon sign advertising Marlboro cigarettes.

1980: The Sydney City Council bans tobacco advertising on Council property.

1981: The Western Australian Committee on the Monitoring of the Advertising of Tobacco Products recommends that advertising should contain no photographs or illustrations and be limited to factual descriptions.

1987: Tobacco advertising is removed from taxis, delivery vehicles, and billboards.

1990: The federal government bans all tobacco advertising in print media.

1992: All tobacco advertising is banned, including the sponsorship of sporting or other cultural events (Tobacco Advertising Prohibition Act 1992). The Federal Minister for Health and Ageing is given the right to grant exemptions to events "of international significance" that "would be likely to result in the event not being held in Australia" should tobacco advertising be forbidden.

Youth Access

1882: South Australia considers the first anti-smoking bill. The bill prohibits persons younger than 16 years of age from smoking in public places, and it carries a penalty of £5 or a month in jail. The bill fails.

1896: Dr. Ross (medicine) introduces a bill in NSW to ban youth smoking. The bill fails but is resubmitted.

1897: The Women's Christian Temperance Union of NSW campaigns against tobacco and, in particular, warns shopkeepers not to sell tobacco to children.

1903: The NSW Act prohibits the sale of tobacco to juveniles.

1904: South Australia passes the Children's Protection Act, No. 875. Among other things, the Act prohibits the sale of tobacco to juveniles.

1905: The ineffectiveness of the Children's Protection Act prompts the introduction of a bill to prohibit the manufacture and sale of cigarettes. Amended to prohibit smoking by anyone younger than 21 years of age, the bill dies in committee.

1905: Queensland passes the Juvenile Smoking Suppression Act of 1905. The law bans juveniles from smoking in public; punishment is a fine or 24 hours in jail.

1917: Western Australia prohibits the sale of tobacco to children. It is the last state to do so.

1993: The legal permitted age for cigarette purchases is increased from 16 to 18 years.

Taxes, Duties, and Economic Incentives

1818: NSW Governor Macquarie levies sixpenny duty on imported tobacco.

1830: Tobacco duties constitute 8.4 percent of NSW government revenue.

1842: Tobacco duties constitute 12 percent of NSW government revenue.

1862: Import duty on unmanufactured leaf is reduced to 1 shilling per pound (2 schilling duty per pound of manufactured tobacco is kept).

1880: Victoria levies tobacco excise tax.

1884: NSW levies excise tax of 1 schilling per pound on local tobacco.

1894: Queensland levies tobacco excise tax.

1903: NSW by-law levies fine of £2 on people who spit (tobacco juice) in NSW railways.

1932: The Lyons government lowers import duties on tobacco.

1935: The excise tax is lowered for locally grown "boong twist" tobacco (1937–1938 excise tax was paid on 26,510 kg).

1935: The government reduces the excise tax on cigarettes made from Australian tobacco (small reductions) and lowers the price of cigarettes made mostly from Australian leaf.

1935: The excise on factory-made cigarettes is three times higher than the excise on cut tobacco. Roll-your-own cigarette shares are 42 percent in 1925, 54 percent in 1930, and 66 percent in 1935. (In Britain, less than 2 percent of cigarettes are hand-rolled.)

1936: The government introduces a "statutory percentage" rule for tariffs. If 2.5 percent of the tobacco used to make cigarettes is of Australian origin, manufacturers pay a lower import duty on the foreign tobacco used to produce the cigarettes. By 1982, Australian growers supply more than half of tobacco leaf used in manufacturing.

1942 (February): Tobacco rationing is introduced. Consumption is limited to the amount consumed from October 1, 1939, to September 30, 1940 (base year). Supply in subsequent months is expressed as a proportion of the base year. The supply from February 1943 to February 1944 is 65 percent. At the end of World War II, the supply is 75 percent. The Commonwealth fixed prices until September 1948, but some states continue to do so until 1954 (Victoria) and 1956 (NSW).

1942–1943: Australian servicemen in the Darwin war zone are exempted from excise duty. Elsewhere, servicemen pay normal price for cigarettes/tobacco. Servicemen are rationed to 0.5 oz. or 20 cigarettes per day in 1942 and 3 oz. per week (105 cigarettes) in 1943. In 1942, the price per pack is 15d (12.5 cents) in Australian canteens. American soldiers pay 7d (5.8 cents) because there is no excise tax.

1946 (November): The statutory percentage is reduced from 15 to 5 percent for "cut" tobacco and remains at 3 percent for cigarettes.

1953: The statutory percentage is raised by intervals, and by 1966 it is set at 50 percent.

1973: Coombs Task Force on Finance condemns boong twist tobacco and its lower excise tax.

1973: The Shield Life Assurance (insurance) company offers nonsmokers a 5 percent discount on premiums.

1974: Victoria passes Business Franchise (Tobacco) Act 1974, which levies "tobacco franchise fees" consisting of a fixed fee and a component that varies with the value of tobacco sold. This effectively levies a state tax on tobacco, and other states quickly follow suit.

1975: Western Australia passes the Business Franchise (Tobacco) Act of 1975.

1978: Northern Territory adopts the Business Franchise Act of 1978.

1980: Tasmania passes the Tobacco Business Franchise Licences Act of 1980.

1980: Legal and General Life Insurance offers discounts to nonsmokers of up to 25 percent.

1984: ACT enacts the Business Franchise (Tobacco and Petroleum Products) Act of 1984.

1986: South Australia passes the Tobacco Products (Licensing) Act of 1986.

1987: NSW enacts the Business Franchise Licenses (Tobacco) Act of 1987.

1988: Queensland passes the Tobacco Products (Licensing) Act of 1988.

1993–1995: The government raises the real excise level on tobacco products several times.

1995 (September 30): The government ends the "Tobacco Industry Stabilization Plan" (including the statutory percentage or "Local Leaf Content Scheme").

1997: The Tobacco Products Regulation Act 1997 of South Australia is passed.

1997 (August 5): The High Court of Australia rules that the states and territories do not have the power to levy tobacco franchise fees because they effectively constitute an excise tax that contravenes Section 90 of the Constitution.

1999 (November 1): The government introduces a "per stick" tobacco excise system to replace the existing weight-based system. It applies to all cigarettes with a tobacco content of up to and including 0.8 g per cigarette. An excise per kilogram of tobacco applies to all other tobacco products, including cigarettes heavier than 0.8 g of tobacco per cigarette, loose tobacco, and cigars.

2000 (July 1): The government implements the Goods and Services Tax (GST).

2008 (February): A (small) cigarette excise tax of 24.757 cents per stick is levied. Excise on tobacco products containing more than 0.8 g of tobacco is $309.47 per kilogram. Rates increase with the Consumer Price Index and are adjusted in August and February each year.

Women and Smoking

1920s: Women start to smoke in public.

1930s: Advertising begins targeting women.

General Events

1800s: Aborigines quickly take up tobacco (men and women).

1829: Western Australia is established as the Swan River Colony—renamed in 1932.

1830: Missionaries distribute tobacco to Aborigines as pay and inducement.

1830: NSW's main tobacco-growing colony is established.

1836: South Australia is established.

1846: North Australia is established.

1851: Victoria is established.

1851: A gold rush in NSW and Victoria causes the population to increase from 400,000 in 1845 to 1 million in 1896.

1860: The tobacco manufacturing industry is established and grows.

1880s: 75 percent of manufactured tobacco in NSW comes from locally grown leaf.

1882: The Bonsack machine is invented. It is capable of making 12,000 cigarettes per hour.

1890: The share of tobacco sold as cigarettes (by weight) in the Australian market is 3.1 percent.

1895: 66 percent of manufactured tobacco in NSW comes from locally grown leaf.

1900: More than 50 percent of manufactured tobacco in NSW comes from locally grown leaf.

1902: The hermetically sealed tin is developed, shifting the demand from plug to cut tobacco.

1903: The share of tobacco sold as cigarettes (by weight) in the Australian market is 10.9 percent.

1906: 18 percent of manufactured tobacco in NSW comes from locally grown leaf.

1907: Handmade cigarettes comprise 25 percent of the Australian market (3d for a pack of nine). Machine-made cigarettes costs 3d for pack of 10.

1909: W.D. & H.O. Wills captures 71 percent of the Australian cigarette market. The most popular brand is Capstan Medium Plain (56 percent of cigarettes sold).

1913: 11 percent of manufactured tobacco in Australia comes from locally grown leaf, and the share of tobacco sold as cigarettes in the Australian market is 20.5 percent.

1914: The share of Capstan Medium Plain brand rises to 75 percent of cigarettes sold.

1916–1918: Tobacco (mostly cigarettes) is shipped as 'aid' to World War I ANZAC troops.

1920: Sales of cut tobacco exceed sales of plug tobacco.

1920: W.D. & H.O. Wills' share of Australian cigarette market increases to 94 percent. The share of tobacco sold as cigarettes in the Australian market is 28.3 percent. Capstans cost 6d for a pack of 12 cigarettes.

1930: The share of tobacco sold as cigarettes in the Australian market stabilizes at 29.6 percent. Capstan Medium Plain brand constitutes 57 percent of cigarettes sold. In December, the price of Capstans is 6d for 10 cigarettes.

1930: Carreras buys a controlling interest in Victorian manufacturer, C. G. Goode Ltd (to circumvent tariffs on imported cigarettes).

1934: Cavalier captures 2 percent of the cigarette market and sells for 6d for 12 cigarettes. Coo-ee (6d for 14 cigarettes) was made from 100 percent Australian tobacco, but it was not popular. It was issued as rations to prisoners of war from 1939 to 1945 and then disappeared from the market.

1936: British Tobacco introduces the "Garrick filter tip" cigarette but fails to capture much of the market (only 2 percent by 1955).

1938: Tobacco firms launch an advertising war. Tobacco advertisements comprise 6.3 percent of total advertising space in 10 metropolitan newspapers (surpassing the 3.7 percent taken by liquor ads). It becomes second only to patent medicines.

1952: Capstan cigarettes cost 1s 1.5d for 10 cigarettes.

1954–1955: Philip Morris of America establishes Australian company (1954) and Rothmans of the United Kingdom establishes Rothmans of Pall Mall (Australia) Ltd. (1955). Demand for filter tip cigarettes takes off, and their share of the market increases from approximately 1 or 2 percent in 1955 to 75 percent by 1970.

1958: Supermarkets and chain stores discount cigarettes.

1962: The price of 20 Rothmans at "Tom the Cheap" in Melbourne is 2s 8d (26.7 cents); wholesale cost is 2s 13d (27.1 cents).

1964: "Tom the Cheap" opens Sydney store in August. It offers Rothmans cigarettes at a price so far below the wholesale price that other shopkeepers buy to resell.

1978: 30 percent of all cigarettes are sold in supermarkets and chain stores.

1999: The Commonwealth begins to tax per cigarette rather than by weight of tobacco.

TIMELINE OF CANADIAN TOBACCO CONTROL EFFORTS

In Canada, much of what went on legislatively seems to have occurred behind closed doors and involved voluntary agreements prior to the mid- to late 1980s, which saw the introduction of Bill C-204 and Bill C-51. These bills and other smoking-related events are described in Chapter 3 and in the following summary.

Health Concerns With Smoking

1962: The UK Royal College of Physicians report on smoking is published.

1963: It is declared, by the Canadian Health Minister, that smoking can contribute to lung cancer.

1964: The US Surgeon General's report on smoking is released.

1966: The Canadian Veterans' Study report is issued. A prospective study on Korean War soldiers had started in 1955.

1966: The Smoking and Health Program, an informational/anti-smoking campaign with a 5-year budget of $600,000, is founded. This is the first program of its kind in Canada.

1968–1969: The Isabelle Committee is established. This parliamentary committee studied the impact of smoking on health and made many recommendations. Included among these were a complete ban on advertising and promotion, increased efforts to educate the public on the harm of smoking, health warnings on cigarette packages, and maximum tar and nicotine levels. Their final report was issued in December 1969, and although none of the measures were implemented, the committee received much attention by the press.

1998: British Columbia files a Medicare cost recovery lawsuit against the tobacco industry. All other provinces follow this action.

2000: The Tobacco Damages and Health Care Costs Recovery Act is passed. The Act is designed with the intention of making the tobacco industry pay for health treatment needed as a result of smoking. In 2004, British Columbia's Court of Appeals upheld the legality of this act. The Supreme Court later backed up this decision.

2005: The International Tobacco Control Treaty, created by the World Health Organization (WHO) and approved in 2003, goes into effect.

Health Warnings on Packs

1972: Tobacco companies voluntarily place a (weak) warning on cigarette packages.

1988: The Non-Smokers Health Act (Bill C-204) and Tobacco Products Control Act (Bill C-51) are both enacted on May 31 (World No-Tobacco Day), although Jake Epp proposed the former earlier. The laws banned all tobacco advertising and required warnings on cigarette packaging and became quite strong legislation.

1989: As part of the Tobacco Products Control Act, it is required that 20 percent of a cigarette package's front and back include one of four health warnings. In addition, manufacturers are required to list additives and the amount in each cigarette.

1994: The Tobacco Products Control Act is amended to require one of eight new health warnings be included on cigarette packages that will take up 35 percent of the front and back of the packages.

1995: A Supreme Court decision overturns much of the 1988 legislation, such as Bill C-204 and Bill C-51, because much of their contents were ruled a violation of the Charter of Rights and Freedoms. *Tobacco Control: A Blueprint to Protect the Health of Canadians* is released by the Minister of Health in response to the Supreme Court decision. In it, the government details how it is going to approach regulating the tobacco industry from that point onward.

1997: The Tobacco Act replaced the 1988 bans, but the bill is somewhat watered down relative to the original. The Act provides standards for products, sets rules for labeling and promoting tobacco, and puts in place rules for enforcement. It also replaces the Tobacco Sales to Young Persons Act of 1994.

2001: Graphic package warnings, authorized by the Tobacco Act of 1997, begin to appear that cover 50 percent of the front and back of cigarette packages. These warnings add graphic pictures such as diseased mouths and other physical deformities to standard warnings about the dangers of smoking.

2011: Tobacco Products Labeling Regulations strengthened requirements for cigarette packages. The regulations mandate that three-fourths of the front and back of the container show graphic health warnings, that health information is included in color, and that an easy-to-read toxic emissions statement is included.

Tobacco Product Bans

1994: Ontario bans the sale of tobacco in pharmacies.

2002: Saskatchewan bans the visual display of tobacco products in all retail settings, mandating that all products be kept behind a curtain or door. The Supreme Court upholds its legality in 2005, despite the fact that the law was struck down in 2003. All other provinces and territories later follow this action.

2010: The Tobacco Act is amended to ban flavored cigarettes and all print advertising.

Advertising and Marketing

1972: A voluntary ban by the tobacco industry in broadcast media begins.

1988: See Health Warnings on Packs.

1997: See Health Warnings on Packs.

2003: An amendment to the Tobacco Act prohibits all tobacco sponsorships.

2010: See Tobacco Product Bans.

Public Smoking

1996: Vancouver becomes the first municipality to ban smoking in restaurants.

2004: Manitoba, the Northwest Territories, and Nunavut ban smoking in public places and the workplace. New Brunswick passes a similar ban for all workplaces.

2005: Newfoundland and Labrador ban smoking in all hospitality establishments. Saskatchewan passes a ban for all public places and, in 2009, bans smoking in the workplace.

2006: Nova Scotia and Ontario ban smoking in all public spaces and workplaces.

2008: Bans on all indoor public place and workplace smoking go into effect for Alberta, British Columbia, Quebec, and the Yukon.

Youth Access

1908: The Tobacco Restraint Act is passed, setting the legal age to buy cigarettes at 16 years.

1994: The Tobacco Sales to Young Persons Act raises the age to legally buy tobacco from 16 to 18 years. The Act also imposes a fine for selling tobacco to minors.

2008: A city in Nova Scotia bans smoking in cars with children. All provinces, with the exception of Quebec, later adopt this law.

Taxes, Duties, and Economic Incentives

1991: The largest increase in the federal tobacco tax occurs, raising the price of a carton of cigarettes by $6.

TIMELINE OF UK TOBACCO CONTROL EFFORTS

Health Concerns With Smoking

1950: Doll and Hill carry out the first large-scale epidemiological study of the relationship between smoking and lung cancer in the United Kingdom. Using data from interviews of 5000 patients in British hospitals, they find that of the 1357 men with lung cancer, 99.5 percent are smokers. They publish the study in the *British Medical Journal* (*BMJ*).

1962: The first Royal College of Physicians (RCP) report, "Smoking and Health," is published. It receives massive publicity. The main recommendations are to restrict tobacco advertising, increase taxes on cigarettes, further restrict the sale of cigarettes to children, restrict smoking in public places, and require companies to provide more information about the tar/nicotine content of cigarettes. For the first time in a decade, cigarette sales decline.

1964: Doll and Hill publish the results of a nationwide prospective survey on mortality in relation to smoking: 10 years of observations of British physicians. Between 1951 and 1964, approximately half the UK's doctors who smoke quit, and there was a dramatic decline in lung cancer incidence among those who quit as opposed to those who continued to smoke.

1971: Publication of the second RCP report, "Smoking and Health Now," endorses the 1970 WHO report.

1971: Action on Smoking and Health (ASH) is set up under the auspices of the RCP to make nonsmoking the norm in society and to inform and educate the public about the death and disease caused by smoking.

1975: The first report by the Independent Scientific Committee on Smoking and Health (ISCSH) on tobacco substitutes and tobacco additives is published.

1976: Professor Sir Richard Doll and Mr. Richard Peto publish the results of their 20-year prospective study of nearly 35,000 doctors' smoking habits. They conclude that one in three smokers dies from their habit.

1977: The third report of the RCP, "Smoking or Health," is published. It provides an authoritative summary of research on smoking and disease, and it makes the strongest call yet for government action to control smoking.

1978: A major article in the *BMJ* discusses the evidence that passive smoking is harmful to health; studies in the main medical journals, such as *The Lancet* and the *BMJ*, continue to show that smoking and taking the contraceptive pill raises the risk of thrombosis.

1979: The publication of a major WHO report, "Controlling the Smoking Epidemic," receives widespread press coverage.

1982: The third report of the ISCSH is published. It recommends the progressive reduction of tar levels in cigarettes over the next 4 years.

1983: The fourth RCP report, "Health or Smoking?" is published. For the first time, the report examines the health risks of passive smoking, but as before, it provides a wealth of data to support its assertion that more than 100,000 people die every year from smoking-related illness in the United Kingdom, and it calls for an end to tobacco advertising and promotion.

1988: The Independent Scientific Committee on Smoking and Health's fourth report, known as the "Froggatt Report," is published. It concludes that there is a 10–30 percent increased risk of developing lung cancer for nonsmokers exposed to other people's smoke. It recommends making nonsmoking the norm at work and in all public places where separate adequate provision for nonsmokers is not possible.

1992: The RCP's fifth report on tobacco, "Smoking and the Young," is published.

Health Warnings on Packs

1971: The first voluntary agreement between the tobacco industry and the government is drawn up. Its provisions include the following: All cigarette packs for sale in the United Kingdom should carry the words "Warning by HM Government: Smoking can damage your health"; all press and poster advertisements are to carry the reference, "Every pack carries a Government health warning"; and the formation of a scientific liaison committee consisting of scientists nominated by the industry and the Department of Health and Social Security to explore less dangerous forms of smoking and to devise a way of measuring tar/nicotine levels.

1972: 132 Members of Parliament vote in favor of a ban on cigarette advertising, and 73 vote against it. In an extension of the existing voluntary agreement, the industry agrees to include "health hints" on cigarette packs (e.g., "If you do smoke, leave a long stub"), cover up specific brand advertisements at televised sporting events, ensure that all brand ads at sports events carry a health warning, and ensure that cinema cigarette advertisements and those sent through the post carry a reference to the health warning.

1977: A new voluntary agreement with the tobacco industry stipulates a slightly strengthened health warning to appear on packs and ads; advertising of high tar brands to be stopped immediately, and advertising of middle-to-high tar brands to be stopped by 1978; no new brands in these categories to be introduced; a new, stronger code of advertising practice to be introduced; and a code of practice for sponsorship to be discussed with the Minister for Sport.

1991: The government announces a series of new, larger health warnings for tobacco packaging, in line with European Commission (EC) requirements.

This is the first time that health warnings are legally required, as opposed to covered in the voluntary agreements. There will be two health warnings on the packs from now on instead of one, and they will include "Smoking kills" and "Protect children: don't make them breathe your smoke." They will cover 6 percent of the relevant face of the pack. The minimum requirement under the terms of the European Union (EU) directive is 4 percent.

2001: EU directive requiring larger, bolder health warnings on tobacco packaging becomes law. Measures to be phased in beginning September 30, 2002, include increasing the amount of the main pack that health warnings must cover from 30 to 40 percent; a reduction in maximum tar yields from 12 to 10 percent, with maximum yields imposed also for nicotine and carbon monoxide; removal of misleading descriptors such as "light" and "mild"; and a requirement by tobacco companies to disclose ingredients and additives by brand.

2003: New, large health warnings start to appear on cigarette packs as required by the EU tobacco product directive. The stark messages include "Smoking clogs the arteries and causes heart attacks and strokes" and the first warning about addiction: "Smoking is highly addictive, don't start."

Advertising and Marketing

1962: The Tobacco Advisory Committee (subsequently Council, and now known as the Tobacco Manufacturers' Association), which represents the interests of the tobacco industry, agrees to implement a code of advertising practice for cigarettes, which is intended to take some of the glamor out of cigarette advertisements. The code is based on the former International Television Association (ITA) code governing cigarette advertisements on television.

1965: After considerable debate, and after consultation with the ITA, the government uses the powers vested in it under the terms of the 1964 Television Act to ban cigarette advertisements on television.

1969: The Health Education Council's first anti-smoking campaign is launched: Posters asking, "Why learn about lung cancer the hard way?" appear.

1972: See entry under "Health Warnings on Packs."

1975: Code of Advertising Practice of cigarettes is taken out of the hands of the industry and is monitored by the Advertising Standards Authority (ASA). Imperial Tobacco, which controls two-thirds of the UK market, agrees unilaterally to remove brand names and logos from racing cars participating in UK races.

1975: In response to the government's 1974 proposals, the industry agrees to withdraw advertising from cinema programs and end the advertising of free samples. Following discussions with the industry and the Department of Health, the ASA agrees to devise a new, stricter code governing cigarette advertising.

1977: See entry under "Health Warnings on Packs."

1978: The Independent Broadcasting Authority publishes a Code of Advertising Standards that regulates all commercial TV and radio broadcasting. Cigarettes and cigarette tobacco are "unacceptable products" not to be advertised on commercial radio.

1980: The government announces a new voluntary agreement with the tobacco industry, which is only in force for a very short time. Four new health warnings are introduced, and more space is allocated to them on posters. The industry agrees to cut its expenditure on poster advertising by 30 percent. It also agrees to take steps not to put posters within view of schools, although the clause is vaguely worded.

1982: The government announces two new voluntary agreements on advertising and sponsorship. The sponsorship agreement permits the industry to increase the prize money offered in sporting events to £6 million. All advertisements for these events will have to carry a health warning. The advertising restrictions are yet to be decided, but the industry announces its intention to spend £3 million a year on health-promotion activities.

1982: The government announces a new voluntary agreement with the tobacco industry to regulate advertising and promotion. Advertising materials at point-of-sale and over a certain size will have to carry a health warning, and video cassettes will not be allowed to carry cigarette advertising. Health warnings are modified, and the rotation system that formerly applied is discontinued. The industry offers to reduce expenditure on cinema and poster ads by 50 and 40 percent, respectively. The feature of the agreement that draws widespread and bitter criticism from the media and public alike is the industry's offer to pay £11 million over the 3½ years the agreement is to run to fund the Health Promotion Research Trust, which will offer grants to research a wide variety of health-related topics, except anything connected with tobacco use.

1985: The new voluntary agreement on tobacco advertising and promotion is announced. A ban on tobacco advertising in cinemas and six new health warnings are introduced. The new warnings are as follows: "Smoking can cause fatal diseases"; "Smoking can cause heart disease"; "Smoking when pregnant can injure your baby and cause premature birth"; "Stopping smoking reduces the risk of serious diseases"; "Smoking can cause lung cancer, bronchitis and other chest diseases"; and "More than 30,000 people die each year in the UK from lung cancer." Tobacco advertising is banned in certain women's magazines with 200,000 readers, of whom at least one-third are aged 16–24 years, and so is advertising for brands with a tar level of 18 mg or higher. The industry agrees to spend £1 million per year on publicity to make it clear that children younger than age 16 years must not be sold cigarettes.

1985: The government signs a new voluntary agreement with the tobacco industry on sports sponsorship.

1989: It is announced that beginning in October 1991, it will be against the law to advertise tobacco on television anywhere in the EC. This will have the effect of banning cigar and pipe tobacco commercials from British television.

1990: Members of the European Parliament vote in favor of banning tobacco advertising.

1991: A new voluntary agreement is published that has a provision for new legally required health warnings on advertisements. Other provisions include a reduction over 5 years to half the number of shopfront advertisements that were counted in July 1991; minor tightening of the rules surrounding direct mailing; an extension of the controls on advertising in women's magazines, with no advertising allowed in new publications until total readership and readership by young women have been ascertained; and no tobacco advertising allowed in publications for which one-third of the readership is young women aged between 16 and 24 years.

1994: The details of the new Voluntary Agreement on tobacco advertising and promotion, announced in May 1994, are published. Measures include increasing the size of health warnings on posters and banning tobacco advertising on billboards within 200 m of school entrances.

2002: The EU directive on tobacco advertising is adopted. It is limited in scope, covering only transborder advertising and sponsorship. However, it allows for member states to adopt stronger measures.

2003: The first phase of the Tobacco Advertising and Promotion Act is implemented. This brings an end to tobacco advertising on billboards and in the print media, and it bans direct mail, Internet advertising, and new promotions.

2005: The final part of the Tobacco Advertising and Promotion Act 2002, banning tobacco sponsorship of global sports such as Formula One motor racing, comes into effect. An EU directive banning cross-border tobacco advertising and sponsorship takes effect at the same time.

Tobacco Product Bans

1988: The government announces that it is to ban Skoal Bandits and other forms of sucking tobacco from sale in the United Kingdom, with effect from March 1990.

1990: The government ban on oral snuff products comes into force.

Smoke Constituents Labeling

1973: The first tar/nicotine tables, in which information on the tar and nicotine levels in all generally available cigarettes is given, are published. The lowest is 4 mg, and the highest is 38 mg. The average tar yield of cigarettes then on sale is 20.6 mg.

1974: The second edition of the tar tables is published, dividing cigarettes into high, middle-to-high, middle, low-to-middle, and low tar categories.

Public Smoking

1969: The *Radio Times* implements its own ban on cigarette advertising.

1974: British Rail and British Airways increase the proportion of accommodation for nonsmokers.

1979: Main post offices are made smoke-free.

1984: Following a fire possibly caused by a cigarette at Oxford Circus tube station, London Regional Transport bans smoking on all Underground trains.

1985: London Regional Transport bans smoking at all stations wholly or partly underground.

1987: Following the King's Cross underground fire, in which 31 people died, London Underground immediately bans smoking throughout the network and bans tobacco advertising. British Rail also bans smoking on a section of commuter line that runs through a deep tunnel in central London.

1988: IBM announces that it will make its 60 UK buildings entirely smoke-free beginning in September. British Airways bans smoking on domestic flights.

1991: The Department of the Environment publishes a voluntary code of practice on smoking in public places. If the public is present by necessity (health premises, banks, post offices, local government premises, etc.), no smoking should be the norm. If the public is present by choice (e.g., cafes, restaurants, pubs, and community centers), separate provision should be made for smokers and nonsmokers, unless this is impractical, in which case no smoking should be the norm.

2004: A complete public smoking ban goes into effect in Ireland.

2006: Scotland becomes the first country in the United Kingdom to implement smoke-free legislation. Smoking is now banned in virtually all workplaces and enclosed public places, including pubs and clubs.

2007: The smoke-free legislation is implemented in Wales (April 2) and in Northern Ireland (April 30); England goes smoke-free on July 1.

Youth Access

1908: The UK Children Act prohibits the sale of tobacco to children younger than age 16 years based on the belief that smoking stunts children's growth.

1933: The Children's Act is repealed and replaced by the Children and Young Persons Act. Under Section 7 of the Act, it is made illegal to sell cigarettes to children younger than age 16 years.

1986: The Protection of Children (Tobacco) Act makes it illegal to sell any tobacco product to children younger than age 16 years (previously the law applied only to smoking tobacco).

1992: The Children and Young Persons (Protection From Tobacco) Act 1991 comes into force. This tightens up existing legislation on the sale of cigarettes to children younger than age 16 years. The new law makes it illegal to sell single cigarettes and also requires warning notices, stating that it is illegal to sell tobacco to anyone younger than the age of 16 years, to be displayed at all points of sale including vending machines.

2007: The government announces that the legal age for the purchase of tobacco will be raised to 18 years beginning October 1, 2007.

TIMELINE OF US TOBACCO CONTROL EFFORTS

The events listed here constitute only a small subset of tobacco-related events in US history. Interested readers should consult the sources we used to compile this list. Our sources were as follows: http://ash.org; http://no-smoking.org; http://www.cdc.gov/tobacco/data_statistics; http://www.cdc.gov/tobacco/; and http://www.epi.umn.edu/research/tobctime.shtm.

Health Concerns With Smoking

1906: The Food and Drugs Act of 1906 becomes the first federal food and drug law, although there is no express reference to tobacco products. Definition of a drug includes medicines and preparations listed in *US Pharmacopeia* or *National Formulary*. A 1914 interpretation advised that tobacco be included only when used to cure, mitigate, or prevent disease.

1914 (amended 1938): The Federal Trade Commission (FTC) Act of 1914 empowers the FTC to "prevent persons, partnerships, or corporations . . . from using unfair or deceptive acts or practices in commerce." Between 1945 and 1960, the FTC completed seven formal cease-and-desist order proceedings for medical or health claims (e.g., a 1942 complaint countering claims that Kool cigarettes provide extra protection against colds or that they cure colds).

1938: The Federal Food, Drug, and Cosmetic Act (FFDCA) of 1938 supersedes the 1906 Act. Definition of a "drug" now includes "articles intended for use in the diagnosis, cure, mitigation, treatment, or prevention of disease in man or other animals" and "articles (other than food) intended to affect the structure or any function of the body of man or other animals." The Food and Drug Administration (FDA) has asserted jurisdiction in cases in which the manufacturer or vendor has made medical claims.

1950: Articles published in US medical journals by Wynder and Graham, Schrek et al., and Levin et al. link smoking to cancer. (Doll and Hill do the same in Britain.)

1960: The Federal Hazardous Substances Labeling Act (FHSA) of 1960 authorizes the FDA to regulate substances that are hazardous (toxic, corrosive, irritant, strong sensitizers, flammable, or pressure-generating) because such substances may cause substantial personal injury or illness during, or as a result of, customary use.

1963: The FDA expresses its interpretation that tobacco does not fit the "hazardous" criteria stated previously and withholds recommendations pending the release of the report of the Surgeon General's Advisory Committee on Smoking and Health.

1964: "Smoking and Health: Report of the Advisory Committee to the Surgeon General," the first major US report on smoking and health, is published and concludes that cigarette smoking is a cause of lung cancer.

1967: Executive Director John F. Banzhaf III and a distinguished body of physicians, attorneys and other prominent citizens who see the need for an effective organization to represent nonsmokers' rights form Action on Smoking and Health (ASH) to defend and enforce the "fairness doctrine" ruling and also to add legal action as a new weapon in the war on smoking. Although its income is tiny compared to that of the big national health organizations also active in the field, ASH is a major factor in the war against smoking. For this reason, and because of its location in the nation's media center, ASH also emerges as a major spokesperson for nonsmokers on radio and television and in the print media. Unlike the many smaller state, local, and specialty anti-smoking organizations with which it cooperates closely, ASH is active with regard to all aspects of the problems of smoking and nonsmokers' rights, and it has a truly national focus. The group plays a major role in establishing the legal concept of the right of nonsmokers to be free from exposure to tobacco smoke. John F. Banzhaf III is the lawyer who successfully lobbied for a law that required TV networks and stations to air anti-smoking messages at no charge.

1967: Delegates from 34 countries attend the first World Conference on Smoking and Health in New York.

1967: "The Health Consequences of Smoking: A Public Health Service Review" is published by the US Surgeon General.

1968: "The Health Consequences of Smoking: 1968 Supplement to the 1967 Public Health Service Review" is published by the US Surgeon General.

1970: The Controlled Substances Act of 1970 is ratified to prevent the abuse of drugs, narcotics, and other addictive substances. It specifically excludes tobacco from the definition of a "controlled substance."

1971: "The Health Consequences of Smoking: A Report of the Surgeon General: 1971" is published.

1972: "The Health Consequences of Smoking: A Report of the Surgeon General: 1972" is published.

1976: The Toxic Substances Control Act of 1976 is passed to "regulate chemical substances and mixtures which present an unreasonable risk of injury to health or the environment." The term "chemical substance" does not include tobacco or any tobacco products.

1976: An amendment to the Federal Hazardous Substances Labeling Act of 1960 states that the term "hazardous substance" shall not apply to tobacco and tobacco products (passed when the American Public Health Association petitioned the Consumer Product Safety Commission (CPSC) to set a maximum level of 21 mg of tar in cigarettes).

1977: The "Great American Smokeout" is launched and soon becomes a national event.

1980: The Surgeon General reports that cigarette smoking is a major threat to women's health.

1981: Insurance companies begin to offer discounts on life insurance premiums to nonsmokers.

1983: "The Health Consequences of Smoking—Cardiovascular Disease: A Report of the Surgeon General: 1983" is published.

1984: "The Health Consequences of Smoking—Chronic Obstructive Lung Disease: A Report of the Surgeon General: 1984" is published.

1984: The FDA approves Nicorette, a nicotine-based chewing gum, as a smoking cessation aid.

1986: In separate reports, the National Research Council of the National Academy of Sciences (NAS) and the U.S Public Health Service in conjunction with the Surgeon General both conclude that secondhand tobacco smoke causes lung cancer and lung cancer deaths among nonsmokers.

1987: The federal government permits a federally qualified health maintenance organization (HMO) to require smokers to pay a higher premium than nonsmokers.

1988: The Surgeon General reports that nicotine is a drug that can be as addictive as heroin.

1987: A new medical study reports that involuntary or passive smoking kills approximately 46,000 American adults per year.

1990: "The Health Benefits of Smoking Cessation: A Report of the Surgeon General: 1990" is published.

1991: Nicotine patches are approved for prescription sale.

1992: The Supreme Court holds that cigarette manufacturers could be held liable to smokers for making false statements or conspiring to misrepresent or conceal the hazards of smoking.

1993: The Environmental Protection Agency officially determines that secondhand tobacco smoke is a "Group A carcinogen" that kills an estimated 3000 Americans each year from lung cancer alone and creates widespread and very serious risks for children.

1993: The US Supreme Court holds that it is "cruel and unusual punishment" to expose prisoners to levels of tobacco smoke that place their health at risk.

1994: The FDA proposes to regulate nicotine as a drug.

1996: The Liggett Group, the smallest of the nation's five major tobacco companies, offers to settle the Castano class action, the largest and most visible tobacco liability case, taking responsibility for tobacco-related diseases and death for the first time.

1996: The FDA approves nicotine gum and two nicotine patches for over-the-counter sale.

1998: The Master Settlement Agreement is reached after the US Department of Justice (DOJ) sues the tobacco industry to recover billions of government dollars spent on smoking-related health care, accusing cigarette makers of a "coordinated campaign of fraud and deceit."

2000: "Reducing Tobacco Use: A Report of the Surgeon General: 2000" cites tobacco use as the "number one cause of preventable disease and death" in the United States. According to Dr. David Satcher, the Surgeon General, "Tobacco use will remain the leading cause of preventable illness and death in this nation and a growing number of other countries until tobacco prevention and control efforts are commensurate with the harm caused by tobacco use."

2000: Lorillard and Liggett tobacco companies reach a tentative $8 billion settlement for individual tobacco suits.

2001: "Women and Smoking: A Report of the Surgeon General: 2001" is published.

2002: The Centers for Disease Control and Prevention estimates that smoking health and productivity costs reach $150 billion per year.

2003: The Framework Convention on Tobacco Control is unanimously adopted at the World Health Assembly in Geneva, Switzerland. ASH is identified as playing a crucial role during the development of this first legally binding tobacco treaty.

2004–2014: Over a 10-year period, the US Surgeon General publishes five reports on smoking (2004, 2006, 2010, 2012, and 2014).

2009: Congress passes the Family Smoking Prevention and Tobacco Control Act of 2009, which gives the FDA the authority to regulate "modified risk tobacco products" (MRTPs). If a firm wants to sell a product as an MRTP, it must apply to the FDA for permission. The FDA plans to require that firms produce evidence that a particular product will impose fewer health costs than existing products.

Health Warnings on Packs

1964: The FTC proposes to require health warnings indicating that cigarette smoking is "dangerous to health and may cause death from cancer and other diseases."

1965: The Federal Cigarette Labeling and Advertising Act of 1965 requires the following package warning label: "Caution: Cigarette Smoking May Be Hazardous to Your Health" (other health warnings prohibited). The law implements a 3-year prohibition of any labels on cigarette advertisements and requires the FTC to report to Congress annually on the effectiveness of cigarette labeling, current cigarette advertising and promotion practices, and to make recommendations for legislation. In addition, the Act requires that the Department of Health, Education, and Welfare provides an annual report to Congress on the health consequences of smoking.

1969: The Public Health Cigarette Smoking Act of 1969 requires a package label stating, "Warning: The Surgeon General Has Determined that Cigarette Smoking Is Dangerous to Your Health" (other health warnings prohibited), and temporarily preempts an FTC requirement of health labels on advertisements. The DOJ prohibits cigarette advertising on television and radio, and states and localities are prevented from regulating or prohibiting cigarette advertising or promotion for health-related reasons.

1970: See entry under "Advertising and Marketing."

1972: The Consumer Product Safety Act of 1972 transfers authority from the FDA to regulate hazardous substances as designated by the Federal Hazardous Substances Labeling Act to the CPSC. The term "consumer product" does not include tobacco and tobacco products.

1983: See entry under "Advertising and Marketing."

1984: The Comprehensive Smoking Education Act of 1984 preempts other package warnings and institutes four rotating health warning labels (all listed as Surgeon General's Warnings) on cigarette packages and advertisements: "Smoking causes lung cancer, heart disease and may complicate pregnancy"; "Quitting smoking now greatly reduces serious risks to your health"; "Smoking by pregnant women may result in fetal injury, premature birth, and low birth weight"; and "Cigarette smoke contains carbon monoxide." The Department of Health and Human Services (DHHS) is required to publish a biennial status report to Congress on smoking and health. The law also creates the Federal Interagency Committee on Smoking and Health and requires the cigarette industry to provide a confidential list of cigarette additives (brand-specific quantities not required).

1986: The Comprehensive Smokeless Tobacco Health Education Act of 1986 preempts other health warnings on packages or advertisements (except billboards), institutes three rotating health warning labels on smokeless tobacco packages and advertisements ("This product may cause mouth cancer"; "This product may cause gum disease and tooth loss"; and "This product is not a safe alternative to cigarettes"), and prohibits smokeless tobacco advertising on television and radio. The DHHS is required to publish a biennial status report to Congress on smokeless tobacco and has to conduct a public information campaign on the health hazards of smokeless tobacco. The FTC is to provide reports to Congress on smokeless tobacco sales, advertising, and marketing. Smokeless tobacco companies have to provide a confidential list of additives and a specification of nicotine content in smokeless tobacco products.

Advertising and Marketing

1964: The FTC proposes a rule to strictly regulate the imagery and copy of cigarette ads to prohibit explicit or implicit health claims.

1965: See entry under "Health Warnings on Packs."

1966: John F. Banzhaf III files a complaint with the FCC, arguing that stations broadcasting cigarette commercials should be required to provide free time for the opposing view.

1967: In response to Banzhaf's petition, the FCC rules that the fairness doctrine applies to cigarette commercials, and that radio and television stations must devote hundreds of millions of dollars worth of broadcast time to anti-smoking messages.

1968: The US Court of Appeals upholds, in the case *Banzhaf v. FCC*, the fairness doctrine ruling requiring broadcasters to carry anti-smoking messages.

1968: ASH files a complaint with the FTC charging the Tobacco Institute with ghost writing and deceptively promoting pro-smoking articles in *True* and *National Enquirer*. The FTC upholds the complaint, and it urges a ban on cigarette commercials.

1969: ASH files a complaint with the FTC charging several tobacco companies with widely promoting filter cigarettes in so-called "gas derby" based on an article they knew was misleading. Gas derby ceases.

1969: The FCC rules that stations cannot present all anti-smoking messages during non-prime hours and must present a significant number during prime time when cigarette commercials are presented.

1969: The US Supreme Court agrees with a brief filed by ASH and lets stand the *Banzhaf v. FCC* decision, upholding the application of the fairness doctrine to require reply time to cigarette commercials.

1969: See entry under "Health Warnings on Packs."

1970: Congress bans cigarette advertising on television and radio and requires a stronger health warning on cigarette packages: "Warning: The Surgeon General Has Determined that Cigarette Smoking is Dangerous to Your Health."

1971: Fairness doctrine anti-smoking messages end as cigarette advertising on radio and television ends.

1973: The Little Cigar Act of 1973 bans little cigar advertisements from television and radio (authority to DOJ).

1975: The FTC, in response to ASH's petition, sues the six major cigarette manufacturers concerning their billboard ads.

1983: The FTC determines that its testing procedures may have "significantly underestimated the level of tar, nicotine, and carbon monoxide that smokers received from smoking" certain low-tar cigarettes. The Brown and Williamson Tobacco Company is prohibited from using the tar rating for Barclay cigarettes in advertising, packaging, or promotions because of problems with the testing methodology and consumers' possible reliance on that information. The FTC authorizes revised labeling in 1986.

1984: See entry under "Health Warnings on Packs."

1985: The FTC acts to remove the R. J. Reynolds advertisements "Of Cigarettes and Science," in which the Multiple Risk Factor Intervention Trail (MRFIT) results were misinterpreted.

1986: See entry under "Health Warnings on Packs."

1999: Philip Morris begins $100 million ad campaign touting its charitable contributions.

2003: The first stage of the Tobacco Advertising and Promotion Act 2002 is put into effect, banning new tobacco sponsorship agreements and advertising on billboards, in the press, and free distributions. The ban includes direct mail, Internet advertising, and promotions.

Tobacco Product Bans

1893: Washington becomes the first of what will eventually be 15 states to ban the sale of cigarettes in some manner. The US Circuit Court declares the law unconstitutional and repeals it in 1895.

1897: Iowa bans the manufacture, sale, exchange, and disposition of cigarettes and cigarette papers.

1900: Tennessee and North Dakota outlaw the sale of cigarettes.

1907: Washington again bans the sale of cigarettes and cigarette papers. The law is extended to ban possession in 1909; it is repealed in 1911.

1921: Fifteen states ban the sale of cigarettes.

1959: Trim Reducing-Aid Cigarettes (contained the additive tartaric acid, which was claimed to aid in weight reduction) are seized for libel. The FDA asserts jurisdiction over alternative nicotine-delivery products.

1975: Cigarettes are discontinued in K-rations and C-rations given to soldiers and sailors.

1983: The federal cigarette tax increases. Revenues are used to finance cancer research in New Jersey.

Public Smoking

1936: Milwaukee, Wisconsin becomes the first US city to make all forms of public transportation (street cars, buses, etc.) completely smoke-free.

1948: Berkeley, California becomes the second US city with 100 percent smoke-free public transit.

1967: John F. Banzhaf III asks the Federal Aviation Administration to order airlines to segregate smokers from nonsmokers.

1969: ASH collects evidence that ambient tobacco smoke is a health hazard, and it files a petition with the Civil Aeronautics Board seeking separate smoking and nonsmoking sections aboard aircraft.

1971: United Airlines becomes the first carrier to offer separate smoking and nonsmoking sections.

1973: The Civil Aeronautics Board—the agency charged with the power to regulate the economic aspect of air transportation and to supervise air carriers as well as their property, property rights, equipment, facilities, and franchises—begins requiring separate smoking and nonsmoking sections on airplanes.

1981: The Merit Systems Promotions Board of the Civil Service and the Department of Labor rule that employers must make reasonable accommodations to persons sensitive to tobacco smoke.

1986: The National Academy of Sciences (NAS) publishes "The Airliner Cabin Environment: Air Quality and Safety." In the publication, NAS reports that the nation's flight attendants are exposed to smoke levels similar to those of a person living with someone smoking a pack a day, and it recommends a "ban on smoking on all domestic commercial flights."

1987: Public Law 100-202 bans smoking on domestic airline flights scheduled for 2 hours or less.

1992: The International Civil Aviation Organization passes a resolution urging its 152 member countries to go completely smoke-free by July 1, 1996.

1994: The Occupational Safety and Health Administration (OSHA) proposes regulation to prohibit smoking in the workplace, except in separately ventilated smoking rooms.

2002: Smoking bans pass in Nassau County and Dutchess County, New York, as well as in Oregon and Hawaii.

2003: Florida, Maine, Connecticut, Alabama, Oklahoma, and the state of New York pass statewide smoking bans for indoor public places, including worksites, offices, hospitals, bars, and restaurants. Some businesses remain exempt.

2004: On the first anniversary of New York City's smoking ban, studies find no adverse financial impact on bars and restaurants. Report highlights from the finance, health, small business, and economic development agencies for New York City include the following: Employment in NYC's restaurant/bar industry is the highest in more than a decade; tax receipts in restaurants and bars are up 8.7 percent; bar permits/licenses are up by 234 percent; bar/restaurant air quality is significantly better (cotinine pollution levels are down 85 percent); the popularity of the law is higher than that of the New York Yankees; compliance is almost 100 percent; and smoking bans passed in Hennepin, Ramsey, and Beltrami Counties.

Youth Access

1992: Courts begin making widespread use of a legal principle to protect children from smoking in the home.

1994: The Pro-Children Act of 1994 requires that all federally funded children's services become smoke-free. The Act expands upon a 1993 law that banned smoking in Women, Infants, and Children (WIC) clinics.

1994: "Youth and Tobacco: Preventing Tobacco Use Among Young People: A Report of the US Surgeon General: 1994" is published.

1996: On August 23, 1996, President Clinton announces the nation's first comprehensive program to prevent children and adolescents from smoking cigarettes or using smokeless tobacco and beginning a lifetime of nicotine addiction. The FDA will regulate the sale and distribution of cigarettes and smokeless tobacco to children and adolescents. The provisions of the FDA rule are aimed at reducing youth access to tobacco products and the appeal of tobacco advertising to young people. In addition, the FDA proposes to require the major tobacco companies to educate young people about the real health dangers associated with tobacco use through a multimedia campaign.

1997: The FTC charges R. J. Reynolds Tobacco Company with unfair advertising practices for the use of the "Joe Camel" campaign to pitch cigarettes to children and youth. R. J. Reynolds files a suit against the FTC alleging harassment.

TIMELINE OF TOBACCO-RELATED EVENTS IN GERMANY

The events listed here constitute a subset of tobacco-related events in Germany. Interested readers should consult the sources we used to compile this list. In addition to sources listed in the text, we acquired information from the following: The 2009 Tobacco Atlas accessed through the Deutsches Krebsforschungszentrum (German Cancer Research Center) website[3]; "Tobacco or Health in the European Union" accessed through the European Commission, Public Health website[4]; and the European Public Health Alliance website on the implementation of EU directives.[5]

History

1573: Tobacco was introduced into German lands.

1600s: Mercenary soldiers in the Thirty Years War (1618–1648) spread tobacco consumption habits.

1680s: Hugenots flee religious persecution in France and are recruited to Brandenburg to cultivate tobacco (Weiss and Herbert, 1854).

1910s: The American Tobacco Company and Imperial Tobacco begin to buy controlling shares of German tobacco manufacturers. After the US Supreme Court dismantles the American Tobacco Company, the British American Tobacco Company (BAT) continues the strategy.

World War I: The United States and United Kingdom are declared hostile nations. This declaration derails BAT's attempt to gain control of the German industry. Reemtsma develops into the dominant German tobacco firm.

1933: The National Socialist German Workers Party (NSDAP) gains majority (1932), forms government, and starts policy of protecting and building German industries.

1939 (September): The German army invades Poland, starting World War II.

1945 (May 8): The Nazi-led German government surrenders, ending World War II. Four Allied powers each occupy and oversee reconstruction of a part of Germany.

1949 (October 6): The Soviet occupying force formally establishes the German Democratic Republic (East Germany) as a separate nation. It will remain divided for 40 years.

1953 (June 17): Soviet occupation forces fire on unarmed East German workers at the Brandenburg Gate in Berlin. The workers aimed to rally with West German workers.

1950s: Residents of East Germany flee to West Germany, numbering approximately 8000–10,000 people per day.

1957 (January 1): The state of Saarland joins West Germany.

1961 (August 13): The Berlin Wall is erected. During the next 39 years, 70 people die trying to escape.

1989 (November 10–12): The East German government stops preventing East Germans from crossing into West Berlin. The Wall is opened at Potsdamer Platz.

1989 (December 22): The Brandenburg Gate opens.

1990 (March 18): The first free elections are held in the German Democratic Republic.

1990 (July 1): Former East and West Germany form a monetary and economic union.

1990 (October 3): East and West Germany are unified.

2003: The Framework Convention on Tobacco Control (FCTC) is unanimously adopted at the World Health Assembly in Geneva, Switzerland. On October 24, Germany signs the FCTC.

2004 (December 16): The German Parliament ratifies the FCTC. The agreement becomes legally binding 90 days later (March 16, 2005).

Advertising Bans

1941 (December): The Nazi government restricts tobacco advertising (but does not completely ban it).

1975: The German Food and Commodities Act prohibits advertising tobacco products on television and radio, advertising the physical act of smoking as harmless or healthy, and advertising smoking as a means of stimulating well-being.

1989: The EC adopts a proposal designed to harmonize the laws of the member states on tobacco advertising.

1991 (October): EU Directive 89/552/CEE bans tobacco television advertising in all EU member states.

1998: EU Directive 98/43/EC bans all tobacco advertising. The German government sues to invalidate the directive, arguing a failure of the EC to consider the cross-border implications of the ban.

1999 (August 31): The State Broadcasting Treaty prohibits sponsorship of radio and television programs by tobacco companies.

2000 (October 5): A court rules in favor of Germany and annuls EU Directive 98/43/EC.

2002 (July 23): The Youth Protection Act prohibits tobacco advertising in cinemas before 6 pm.

2003 (May 26): The EU adopts Tobacco Advertising Directive 2003/33/EC that again bans all tobacco advertising.

2003 (September): Germany challenges the validity of the directive. It argues that EU lawmakers exceeded their powers under the internal market provisions of the EU Treaty (Article 95). Owners of a Nürburgring motor racing circuit lodge a parallel challenge. They argue that the ban on tobacco sponsorship unlawfully imposes economic damage.

2004 (July 23): The Act to Enhance the Protection of Young People Against the Dangers of Alcohol and Tobacco Consumption prohibits distribution of free cigarettes and specifies that cigarette packs must contain at least 17 pieces.

2006 (February 1): The EC sends Germany a "reasoned opinion" for failing to adopt national laws to implement the provisions of the Tobacco Advertising Directive. It gives them 2 months to comply.

2006 (December): The European Court of Justice dismisses Germany's challenge of the Tobacco Advertising Directive 2003/33/EC.

2007 (January 1): The Tobacco Advertising Directive of the European Union (2003/33/EC) is superseded by § 21a of the Draft Tobacco Act. This prohibits advertising tobacco products in newspapers and magazines that are not exclusively intended for professionals in the tobacco trade, advertising tobacco products in "information society services" such as the Internet, and sponsorship of radio programs and cross-border events by undertakings whose principal activity is the manufacture or sale of tobacco products.

Taxes

1628: The city of Köln levies the first documented tobacco tax—an import duty on pipe tobacco (Schäfke, 1984).

1906: The first modern tobacco tax is introduced.

1948 (August): Occupation administrators lower cigarette and tobacco taxes.

1951 (July): The newly elected West German government again lowers cigarette tax.

1953 (June): The West German government lowers the cigarette tax and establishes a lower tax on manufactured tobacco products containing a minimum quantity of domestically grown tobacco.

1957 (April): The West German government again lowers the cigarette tax. Except for one other time in 1968, this is the last time the tax will be lowered.

1972 (September): The West German government reintroduces a specific tax levied on each cigarette. It simultaneously lowers the ad valorem tax rate levied on the final retail price.

1977 (January): The West German government raises the ad valorem tax rate.

1980 (January): The West German government requires that when calculated together, the specific and ad valorem cigarette taxes be an amount greater than a minimum per cigarette. This structure of taxes is maintained.

2004 (March and December): The ad valorem tax rate increases.

Information

1920s: German scientists begin to accumulate evidence about exposure to smoke
(environmental and through smoking), cancer, and disease (see Seyfarth,
1924; Lickint, 1929).

1939: Franz Müller (1939) publishes a medical dissertation showing the link
between smoking and lung cancer. It was one of the first studies to use a
healthy "control" group and to acknowledge the role of sample selection
bias. Fritz Lickint publishes *Tabak und Organismus: Handbuch der gesamten
Tabakkunde*" (*Tobacco and the Organism*; 1939). He surveys 8000 articles
published worldwide that investigated correlations between tobacco
consumption and health.

1943: Eberhard Schairer and Erich Schöniger (1943) publish a sophisticated
statistical analysis of smoking and lung cancer. They conclude that smoking
causes lung cancer.

Cigarette Content

2001 (January 1): EU Directive 2001/37/EC (Tobacco Products Directive)
requires that, by January 1, 2004, the yield of cigarettes released for free
circulation, marketed, or manufactured in the member states shall not be
greater than 10 mg of tar per cigarette, 1 mg of nicotine per cigarette, and 10
mg of carbon monoxide per cigarette.

2001: BAT and Germany (each separately) sue the EU Parliament and the
Council of the European Union to challenge two different provisions of the
content requirement.

2002 (December 10): The Court dismisses both cases on the grounds that
Germany failed to lodge the case within the deadline for lawsuits and that,
contrary to BAT's claim, the measures in the directive sought to improve the
functioning of the internal market.

Anti-smoking Campaigns/Organizations

1904: The "Association for the Protection of Non-smokers" is formed.

Pre-World War I: The "Bundes Deutscher Tabakgegner" (Association of German
Tobacco Opponents) is formed. It is renamed during the Weimar Republic
as the "Deutscher Bund zur Bekämpfung der Tabakgefahren" (German
Association to Combat the Dangers of Tobacco).

1930s: Under the National Socialists, part of the "Deutscher Bund zur
Bekämpfung der Tabakgefahren" was adopted by the Ministry of the Interior
and named "Reichsarbeitsgemeinschaft für Rauschgiftbekämpfung" (Reich
Association for the Control of Drug Abuse). Another arm was absorbed
into the "Deutschen Gesellschaft für Lebensreform" (German Society for
Life Reform). Also, industrial policies of the Nazi party favor Reemtsma,
solidifying its position as the dominant German tobacco firm.

1941 (May): State Secretary and Reich Health Leader Dr. Leonardo Conti meets
with representatives of the Health Ministry, the Reich Office Against the

Dangers of Alcohol and Tobacco, and the Reich Press and the Propaganda Ministry. They agree to press for national anti-smoking campaigns to combat smoking health risks.

1941 (July): The Propaganda Department of the Third Reich issues guidelines on anti-smoking campaigns and authorizes limited campaigns aimed at women and youth.

1971: The "Ärztlichen Arbeitskreises Rauchen und Gesundheit" (Medical Action Group on Smoking and Health) is founded.

1988: "Nichtraucher-Initiative Deutschland" (Non-smoking Initiative, Germany) is founded. With 4000 members, it is currently the largest nationwide association dedicated to the protection of nonsmokers' rights.

1992: The "Koalition gegen das Rauchen" (Coalition Against Smoking) is founded. In 2003, it is renamed the "Aktionsbündnis Nichtrauchen" (Action Alliance for Non-smoking). It represents 10 nongovernmental health organizations during legislative debate in each parliamentary session.

Smoking Bans

1936: The state of Mecklenburg–West Pomerania bans smoking in public for boys and girls; transgressions are punishable by 2 weeks in jail or a fine of 150 Reichsmark.

1940 (March): The government prohibits smoking in public by youth younger than 18 years.

2007 (July 20): The Federal Non-smoking Protection Act prohibits smoking in public federal institutions, public transport, and passenger stations of public transport. The law allows for the establishment of smoking areas.

2007 (August 1): The smoking ban is adopted by the states of Baden–Wuerttemberg, Mecklenburg–West Pomerania, and Lower Saxony.

2007 (October 1): The smoking ban is adopted by the state of Hesse.

2008 (January 1): The smoking bans are adopted by the states of Bavaria, Berlin, Brandenburg, Bremen, Hamburg, Mecklenburg–West Pomerania, North Rhine–Westphalia, Saxony–Anhalt, and Schleswig–Holstein.

2008 (February): The smoking ban is adopted by Saxony (February 1), Rhineland–Palatinate, and Saarland (February 15).

2008 (July 1): The smoking ban is adopted by the states of North Rhine–Westphalia and Thuringia.

2008 (July 30): The Federal Constitutional Court rules that smoking in restaurants is constitutional, but only if certain accommodations are met. One-room dining establishments with a guest area of less than 75 square meters may allow smoking, provided that no persons younger than 18 years of age are permitted, no "prepared food" will be served, and the operation is clearly marked as a smoking restaurant. Nightclubs, to which only persons older than the age of 18 years may have access, can set up smoking rooms. However, these may not be located on the dance floor.

2009: Smoking bans are modified in the states of Bremen (January 1), Baden–Wuerttemberg (March 3), Rhineland–Palatinate (May 26), Bavaria (August 1), and Mecklenburg–West Pomerania (December 17).

2010: Smoking bans are modified in Hamburg and Saxony (both January 1).

2011: The smoking ban is modified in Saxony–Anhalt (February 26).

2013: Smoking bans are modified in the states of Bremen (January 1), Thuringia (April 9), and North Rhine–Westphalia (May 1).

TIMELINE OF SPANISH TOBACCO CONTROL EFFORTS

The Spanish legislative system is structured under three different domains for different levels of geographical aggregation: autonomous communities (also called regions), the whole nation, and the European Union. When Spain adopted its constitution in 1978, it granted the Spanish autonomous communities the legal authority to regulate health markets and commerce that affects health (including the sale and consumption of tobacco). Under the constitution, a regional law may not weaken a state law. For example, if the federal law bans the sale of tobacco products to people younger than 18 years, the regional law might impose a minimum legal purchase age of 20 years but may not allow local firms to sell to people younger than 18 years. Since Spain joined the EU in 1986, its regulation of tobacco markets and consumption has been guided by EU regulations. The EU sometimes encourages and sometimes requires that its members harmonize their legal and economic systems to conform to a common standard. Whether the regulations must be similar to or exactly match each other varies with the type of activity that is being regulated. For example, the EU cannot dictate how member states set or run fiscal policies. Instead, the EU recommends a set of model policies (e.g., value added tax (VAT) and special indirect taxes) that member states may or may not adopt. Each EU member passes its own legislation to determine the sanctions for violators (although state legislators usually adapt their own laws to the EU communitarian directives). The EU strives to harmonize regulations across its members, including the sanctions that violators face (Communication of the European Commission: COM/2006/823). We next summarize anti-tobacco laws implemented in Spain and organize them by topic. Unless otherwise noted, all regulations are issued by Spain's central government.

Health Concerns With Smoking

1978: Spain endorses the recommendations of WHO that urges nations to reduce tobacco consumption by limiting advertising and increasing taxes.

1996: The EU passes a resolution to recommend that its members adopt a set of tobacco control policies. The policies include health education in schools, an increase in the minimum age at which people may legally buy tobacco products, and limits on places where people may smoke in public.

1999: The EU Council reviews tobacco consumption levels and the effectiveness of tobacco control policies.

2002: The EU focuses on youth smoking and recommends that members restrict where, when, how, and to whom firms may market and sell tobacco products, with an emphasis on the marketing and sale of tobacco to adolescents and youth.

2003: Spain adopts the Spanish National Plan for Tobacco Prevention and Control (2003–2007).

2003: WHO member states ratify the WHO Framework Agreement to control tobacco.

2006: The Spanish Ministry of Health, Social Affairs, and Equity establishes the Spanish Observatory for Smoking Prevention to monitor the efficiency of Spanish tobacco control policies.

Constituents of Cigarette Smoke

1979: The government stipulates that firms may label cigarettes as low-nicotine cigarettes only if each cigarette contains less than 1 mg of nicotine, and they may label cigarettes as low-tar cigarettes only if each cigarette contains less than 16 mg of tar. In addition, firms must list tar and nicotine content on cigarette packs.

1992: The government lowers the maximum permissible tar content to 15 mg per cigarette. The same law stipulates that, by 1997, firms may not market any cigarette that has more than 12 mg of tar per cigarette. To market a cigarette as a "low tar/low nicotine" cigarette, a firm must manufacture each cigarette so it contains no more than 10 mg of tar and no more than 0.8 mg of nicotine.

2004: Maximum permissible levels of nicotine and tar are lowered to 1 mg of nicotine and 10 mg of tar per cigarette. The new regulation further stipulates that each cigarette produces no more than 10 mg of carbon monoxide when it is smoked. Manufacturers and importers must provide public authorities with the evidence showing that their products comply with these requirements.

Health Warnings on Packs

1992: The government requires that firms print a warning label on each cigarette pack that reads, "Health authorities warn that smoking seriously damages health" and that it is easy for smokers to see and read the label.

2004: The government modifies the warning label requirement forcing firms to print the following on each pack of cigarettes: (1) "Tobacco products may be harmful to health and create addiction"; (2) one of the following: "Smoking kills," "Smoking might kill," or "Smoking seriously harms your health and the health of those around you"; and (3) one more sentence, selected from a list, that similarly warns about the general health risk associated with smoking. The government also increases the amount of the pack surface that firms must devote to health warnings from 5 percent to 70 percent.

2010: The government removes the sentence "Smoking might kill" from the list of sentences from which firms may choose to meet the labeling requirement and adds the requirement that firms print visual images that show the physical consequences of smoking. Firms must also print on cigarette packs that it is illegal to sell tobacco products to minors.

Advertising and Marketing

1979: The Spanish government regulates when and how firms may advertise tobacco products on television and radio. For example, firms may not advertise before 9:00 pm. The government also bans advertising on educational programs or programs financed through public funding.

1989: An EU directive called "Television Without Frontiers" bans all tobacco advertising on television and sponsorship of programs by tobacco firms (Directive 89/552/EEC). To comply, the Spanish government makes it illegal for firms to advertise tobacco (at any time) on television and makes it illegal for firms to advertise (in print or on billboards) in any place where tobacco consumption is not allowed (e.g., education centers). The Spanish national law is legislated in 1988, but it enters into force in 1989 (Spanish National Law 34/1988, November 11).

1994: The government makes it illegal for firms to indirectly promote tobacco (e.g., through product placement or through celebrity endorsements) (Spanish National Law 25/1994, July 12). The government also makes it illegal for firms to develop and market orally ingested tobacco products other than those products that already exist that are smoked and chewed. Edible products include powdered tobacco or other types of tobacco (Royal Decree 1185/1994, June 3).

1998: A directive extends the 1989 directive to all direct and indirect advertising of tobacco products and also sponsorship of events on behalf of tobacco products. Member states have to implement the new directive no later than July 30, 2001. Member states have the possibility to delay the application for press advertising until July 30, 2002, and until July 30, 2003, for sponsorship. In addition, for world-level events, the member states may authorize the continued sponsorship of existing activities for a further period of 3 years, ending at the latest on October 1, 2006. All court judgments related to tobacco advertisements today are based on this directive.

2005: Following an EU directive, Spain bans print, radio, and Internet tobacco advertising. The law also makes it illegal for firms to sponsor cultural and sport events in EU member countries. In an important exemption, tobacco firms may sponsor a Formula One race (and broadcast the race from local television stations) if the race takes place outside the EU. Spain makes it illegal to advertise tobacco on tobacco vending machines.

2006: The government makes it illegal for firms to sell cigarettes in packs of fewer than 20 pieces. The law specifically bans firms from selling individual cigarettes. In addition, firms may locate tobacco vending machines only inside buildings or in newsstands that workers directly control. The law also bans firms from selling any other products in tobacco vending machines and requires that firms post visible health warnings on the machines.

Organization of the Industry

1636: The government establishes the royal monopoly to sell tobacco.

1886: The government transfers operating authority over the tobacco monopoly to the joint authority of the Bank of Spain and a leasing company called Compañía Arrendataria de Tabacos.

1945: The government grants the tobacco monopoly to Tabacalera, a private company.

1998: Spain ends the tobacco monopoly and allows firms to freely enter and exit the industry, but the government still restricts tobacco imports. Tobacco dealers and sellers must also pay additional fees on imported cigarettes. At the same time, the government establishes the Spanish Tobacco Market Commission. Its charge is to safeguard the success of the domestic tobacco industry.

2007: Restrictions on tobacco imports are dropped.

Taxes, Duties, and Economic Incentives

1979: The government relabels the Tobacco Monopoly Rent as an indirect tax.

1986: With its entry into the EU, Spain's citizens must pay the VAT. The initial VAT rate on tobacco products is 12 percent. The tobacco retail trade has the structure of a monopoly because the retailers are dealers of the state. Retailers will dispense tobacco products under the conditions determined by the Spanish Ministry of Economy and Finance. The retailer commission is 8.5 percent of the selling price for all tobacco products except for cigars, in which case the retailer commission might be as high as 9 percent. Spouses and family members, up to 3 grades, might inherit retailer concession.

1992: The VAT increases to 16 percent. The government replaces the specific luxury tax on tobacco products with two new taxes: an ad valorem tax equal to 48.5 percent of the product's value and a specific tax of 150 pesetas (0.90 euros) on every 1000 cigarettes. The new taxes help align Spain's fiscal structure with that of the EU.

1996: The specific tax increases twice to 2.50 euros and to 3 euros on every 1000 cigarettes.

1998: There are some changes in retailer conditions. For example, concessions are now granted for only 25 years.

2002: The specific tax increases to 3.91 euros on every 1000 cigarettes.

2005: The specific tax increases to 3.99 euros on every 1000 cigarettes, and the ad valorem tax increases to 54.95 percent.

2006: The specific tax increases twice—to 6.20 and 8.20 euros on every 1000 cigarettes—as does the ad valorem tax—to 55.95 and 57 percent. To compensate loses, retailers might get an additional transitory margin of 0.25 percent of the selling price from February 2006 to June 2006. A minimum tax of of 116.7 euros per 1000 cigarettes is established for packages less than 3.66 euros. This tax was created after a price war for controlling market shares with cheap products.

2009: The specific tax increases to 10.20 euros on every 1000 cigarettes.

2010: The VAT increases to 18 percent.

2011: The specific tax increases to 12.70 euros on every 1000 cigarettes.

2012: The specific tax increases to 19 euros on every 1000 cigarettes, and the ad valorem duty decreases to 55 percent. Duty on pipe tobacco is standardized with that on fine-cut tobacco, and the minimum tax increases to 119.1 euros per 1000 cigarettes.

Public Smoking

1989: The EU Council and Health Ministries of EU member countries agree to ban smoking in places open to the public, such as school centers, hospitals, and public transportation. They also consider the option of spaces specifically designed for smoking, and they argue that in cases of ambiguity, the rights of the nonsmoker should prevail.

2006: The government bans smoking in almost all public places. The law exempts restaurants and bars but makes it illegal for anyone younger than 16 years to frequent smoking areas of a restaurant.

2011: The government bans smoking in all public places and in public and private workplaces.

Youth Access

1989: Spain bans smoking in schools and makes it illegal for anyone to sell or distribute tobacco products in public schools.

1991: Catalonia becomes the first Spanish autonomous community to increase the minimum age at which people may legally buy tobacco products from 16 to 18 years. After this, other Spanish autonomous communities do the same. With the target of preventing youth tobacco use, regional governments regulate not only the minimum legal age but also the places where it is illegal to consume or to sell tobacco products.

2006: The central government makes it illegal for youth of 17 years or younger to buy tobacco products. The law only affects the two autonomous communities (Asturias and Castilla la Mancha) that still allow young people aged 16 and 17 years (respectively) to buy tobacco products. Firms have to warn on cigarette packs that it is illegal to sell cigarettes to anyone younger than 18 years.

TIMELINE OF CHINESE TOBACCO CONTROL EFFORTS

Advertising and Marketing

1987: Article 20 of the Regulation on Advertising Management bans radio, television, and newspaper tobacco advertising.

1992: Articles 18 and 19 of the Law of China on Monopoly of Tobacco Sales extends advertising ban to magazines. In addition, the law requires firms to print the tar content and the phrase "Smoking is hazardous to health" on cigarette packs.

1995: The Law of China on Advertising is passed. Article 18 extends the advertising ban to films and also determines that advertisements for tobacco should carry the indication of "Smoking is harmful to your health." The law also bans poster tobacco advertising in any kind of waiting rooms, cinemas, theaters, conference halls, stadiums and gymnasiums, or other similar public places.

1996: Articles 6 and 10 of the Provisional Guideline on Tobacco Advertising prohibit firms from using images of smoking activities and juveniles in advertisements. Warning labels are required to cover at least 10 percent of an advertisement's surface.

2005: Approval of the FCTC comprehensively bans all advertising and promotion of tobacco, including sponsorship of events by tobacco companies.

Youth Access

1981: Article 6 of the Code of Conduct for Middle School Students prohibits middle school students from smoking.

1991: The Behavior Guideline for Elementary School Students is established. Article 20 prohibits elementary school students from smoking.

1999: The Law of China to Prevent Crimes by Minors is passed. Article 15 makes it illegal for firms to sell cigarettes to minors.

Public Smoking

1991: Article 28 of the Implementation Guideline for the Public Place Hygiene Management Regulation bans smoking in cinemas, theaters, music halls, stadiums, libraries, museums, art galleries, shopping stores, bookstores, hospital waiting rooms, and public transport waiting rooms.

1992: The Law of China on Protection of Minors is put into effect. Article 27 bans smoking in classrooms, bedrooms, living rooms, and others places of child care centers. The ban also applies to nurseries and primary and middle schools.

1992: The Law of China on Monopoly of Tobacco Sales is passed, further limiting where people can smoke. Specifically, Article 5 bans or limits smoking on public traffic vehicles and in public places.

1997: Article 3 of the Regulation of China on Prohibiting Smoking on Public Transport and in Waiting Rooms extends the 1991 ban to all waiting rooms, meeting rooms, reading rooms, and other public places of train stations, ferry terminals, and airports.

2008: Several provisions on the Scope of No-Smoking Public Places in Beijing (in Article 3) suggest setting up designated smoking areas in public places and prohibiting smoking outside of these smoking areas.

2011: Rules for the Implementation of the Public Place Hygiene Management Regulation ban smoking in all enclosed public places.

TIMELINE OF USSR TOBACCO CONTROL EFFORTS

Historical/Political Events

1917: The Russian Revolution of 1917 and rebirth of the Ukrainian state occur.

1939: World War II begins; the Carpatho-Ukrainian state is created, and the Hungarian occupation of the Transcarpathia region begins (–1944).

1941–1944: German–Romania occupies Ukraine; Ukrainian Insurgent Army (1942); "Galicia" division (1943).

1943–1944: The Red Army fights to regain Ukraine.

1945: World War II ends.

1963: "Corn fever" food shortages force the USSR to violate its long-standing policy of peacetime self-sufficiency. It begins to import grain from abroad, especially from Canada.

1970s: Urbanization starts gaining steam in the 1960s and especially the 1970s: A majority of the ethnic Ukrainians live in urban areas (53 percent in 1979). Only 37 percent are employed in agriculture in 1970 (vs. 53 percent in 1959).

1985: Mikhail Gorbachev is elected the General Secretary of the Communist Party of the Soviet Union. He implements perestroika and glasnost (i.e., restructuring and openness, respectively).

1991 (December 7–8): The Commonwealth of Independent States Treaty is signed by Ukraine, Russia, and Belarus, dissolving the USSR.

Consumption Bans

Early 1980s: Smoking is banned in most public buildings. It is sometimes allowed in designated nonsmoking areas. In addition, the age at which smoking is permitted is raised from 14 to 16 years.

1985–1987: Mikhail Gorbachev's well-known health campaign, focused largely on reducing alcohol consumption but also on reducing cigarette consumption by reducing the supply of leaf tobacco and manufactured cigarettes, begins.

Health Information

1928: The Ministry of Health Protection establishes the Institute for Health Education in Moscow to promote "sanitary enlightenment."

1930: The Institute for Health Education issues a series of posters to discourage smoking.

1935–1966: Few anti-smoking posters are published during these years.

1967–1980: A second wave of anti-smoking posters occurs.

Market Structure

Late 1940s: American firms flood the European market with cheap cigarettes, many of which make their way into aid packages to the USSR.

1947: Limited advertising starts in the Soviet Union. It grows in volume over time.

1960: The Sino-Soviet split results in increased Soviet demand for tobacco from the West.

1963–1969: Lyndon B. Johnson's administration in the United States pursues trade relations with the Eastern Bloc. Western tobacco companies begin to pursue the Soviet market in earnest, stepping up their efforts to penetrate Bloc markets in whatever way possible. Although they are unable to penetrate the market and sell cigarettes directly to consumers, they manage to instill the notion that Western blends (e.g., Marlboro, Winston, and Kent [BAT]), filters, and styles of packing are attractive. They press this marketing campaign through the 1960s and especially the 1970s.

1964: Justus Heymans, representative of Philip Morris International, goes on a fact-finding mission to Moscow.

1965: Filtered cigarettes appear and quickly become popular. By 1982, one-third of all cigarette sales are filtered brands.

Mid-1960s: Eastern Bloc countries begin to import American (and also German) cigarettes in limited quantities, primarily for sale in major hotels and hard-currency stores.

Mid-1960s: Local manufacturers slowly begin to adopt American technologies, including filters and the practice of "blending" tobacco.

1967–1968: The USSR gets a windfall of hard currency because the price of oil rises. It buys large amounts of modern rotary equipment for tobacco production.

1972: The Nixon administration in the United States initiates and pursues a policy of trade with the Eastern Bloc.

1973: An R. J. Reynolds trade delegation meets and establishes trade relations with Bulgartabak. Their agreement opens the Iron Curtain to trade. R. J. Reynolds licenses Winston cigarette brands for domestic production and sale at a price almost double the price of domestic brand counterparts. They go on sale in early 1974.

1975 (August): Philip Morris licenses Marlboro cigarette brands for domestic production and sale at a price double that of their domestic brand counterparts. Their licensing agreement includes the joint development of other brands.

1970s: As part of the licensing agreements, the USSR acquires equipment and training from the Western firms to modernize its tobacco leaf processing, cigarette making, and packaging.

1975–1977: Together with Philip Morris, the Russian firm Iava produces the cigarette "Soiuz-Apollo" to commemorate the joint space mission of Soviet and American cosmonauts.

1977–1986: Philip Morris signs a new licensing agreement that ensures that Marlboro cigarettes will be domestically produced and sold for 9 more years in the USSR. Annual production averages 1 billion cigarettes.

Late 1970s–early 80s: Light cigarettes are introduced.

1980: The USSR buys 10 billion internationally branded cigarettes. Intended for Olympic Games guests, they are quickly sold throughout the USSR.

1981: Inflation leads Brezhnev's government to dramatically increase cigarette prices. The price of a pack of 25 Belomorkanal cigarettes rises from 22 kopeks in 1961 to 35 kopeks in 1981; the price of a pack of 20 Prima cigarettes rises from 14 kopeks in 1961 to 20 kopeks in 1981.

1981: Imports of foreign-produced cigarettes are allowed, including the R. J. Reynolds' brand Winston.

1986 (April 26): The meltdown of Chernobyl Nuclear Reactor No. 4 causes smokers to be concerned that cigarette tobacco is radioactive.

Late 1980s: Shortages in tobacco products lead to a decrease in consumption.

1989–1991: Socialist governments resign in Eastern European countries. The USSR tobacco crisis continues.

1990–1991: Philip Morris and R. J. Reynolds ship 34 billion cigarettes to the former Soviet Union (FSU). This constitutes their single largest export order.

Early to mid-1990s: Transnational tobacco companies enter the markets in the former Soviet Union. They spend heavily on marketing campaigns, production and distribution, and reduce prices of their brands. They quickly capture 60–90 percent of market sales.

Health Warning Labels

1971: Iava prints the first USSR health warning labels on its cigarette packs.

1978: The USSR institutes an anti-smoking (and anti-alcohol) campaign. It tests a warning label on a small batch of cigarette packs that reads, "The Ministry of Health warns that smoking is hazardous to your health." Eventually, this appears on all cigarette packs.

TIMELINE OF RUSSIAN FEDERATION TOBACCO CONTROL EFFORTS

Regulatory Events/Market Structure

1992: The tobacco state monopoly is dissolved.

1997: 21 tobacco companies merge to form "Tabakprom."

2008: The government signs the FCTC.

2010: The government signs "The Concept of the Government Policy on Combatting Tobacco Use for 2010–2015." This introduces measures to encourage people to consume less tobacco with the aim of minimizing the health impact of smoking and tobacco use.

Advertising and Marketing Restrictions

1995: Federal Law No. 108-FZ of the Russian Federation prohibits advertising from using images of people smoking or the opinions or participation of persons who are popular among youth younger than 21 years. It prohibits advertising on radio or television between 7 am and 10 pm; in printed radio and television guides, cinema or video services, or publications targeted for minors; on the first or last page of newspapers or magazines; and within 100 m of children's, scholastic, medical, sporting, or cultural organizations.

1996: Federal Law No. 108-FZ of the Russian Federation prohibits all television and radio tobacco advertising.

2001: Federal Law No. 87-FZ of the Russian Federation bans selling tobacco to minors and regulates the packaging and labeling of tobacco products. It provides no specific language about tobacco advertising, promotion, and sponsorship; instead, it states that "tobacco and tobacco articles shall

be advertised in compliance with advertisement legislation of the Russian
Federation." Also, firms may not sell cigarettes in packs of less than 20
cigarettes, and vending machine cigarette sales are banned.

2008: Technical Regulations for Tobacco Products No. 268-FZ establish
requirements for tobacco products, definitions of tobacco products, and rules
and forms used to assess whether tobacco products comply with the law. In
addition to this, the government requires that the maximum retail price be
printed on every cigarette pack.

Content Restrictions

2001: Tar and nicotine contents are limited to 14 mg of tar and 1.2 mg of nicotine
per filtered cigarette and 16 mg of tar and 1.3 mg of nicotine per unfiltered
cigarette.

Smoking Bans

2001: Federal Law No. 87-FZ of the Russian Federation bans smoking on buses,
in taxis, and on air flights of 3 hours or less. It also requires special smoking
areas in trains, water transport, health care facilities, education facilities,
government facilities, indoor workplaces and offices, theaters, and cinemas.
Smoking by youth younger than 18 years is prohibited.

Taxes

1995: An excise tax is levied on tobacco products.

2003: Tax reform increases the fixed (or specific) tax and introduces a new ad
valorem tax. This leads to the only significant increase in real cigarette prices
in the 2000s.

2007: A new excise tax system is introduced. It is based on the maximum retail
price (vs. the wholesale price) and the minimum excise tax rate.

2007: Taxes are levied on previously untaxed loose tobacco, snus, and chewing
tobacco.

Warning Labels

1995: Federal Law No. 108-FZ of the Russian Federation requires that
advertising include a warning about the dangers of smoking. Radio and
television advertising must include a health warning of not less than 3 seconds
of air time, and print advertisements must include health warnings that cover
at least 5 percent of the area of the advertisement.

2001: Warning labels are required on not less than 4 percent of the surface
area on each large side of the pack and must list tar and nicotine
content.

TIMELINE OF UKRAINIAN TOBACCO CONTROL EFFORTS

Advertising/Marketing Restrictions

1992: "The basics of legislation on health protection" Article 32 prohibits tobacco advertising in all forms, but the law lacks an enforcement mechanism. It is largely ignored.

1994: Presidential Decree 723/94 prohibits advertising of tobacco products that are "unhealthy for human beings."

1996: Tobacco advertising is prohibited on national and cable television and radio, in publications targeted at youth of 17 years or younger, in public transportation, on billboards located within 300 m of educational facilities, and at social/cultural events with large attendance. Print advertising must contain health warnings that cover at least 5 percent of the surface area.

1998: Ukrainian youth younger than 18 years may not buy or sell tobacco (enforcement in doubt).

2002: Tobacco sales to youth younger than 18 years are prohibited.

2003: Law on Advertisement (amended in 2003) Article 21 prohibits tobacco companies from sponsoring events with tobacco brand names; it requires that print advertising include a health warning that covers at least 15 percent of the surface area.

Content Restrictions

1997: Legislation sets maximum tar levels at 15 mg per filtered cigarette and 22 mg per unfiltered cigarette; maximum nicotine level is set at 1.3 and 1.5 mg per filtered and unfiltered cigarette, respectively.

Smoking Bans

1997 (April): Smoking is banned in health care facilities.

2002: Smoking is prohibited in buildings and on the territory of preschool, educational institutions, health protection institutions, and at sport competition venues.

2005 (October): Law of Ukraine No. 2899-IV bans smoking in work and public places, with an exemption granted if the owners and tenants of buildings and premises designate separate smoking areas.

2006 (July): At least 50 percent of the area of public places must be smoke-free.

Taxes

1993 (January): A tax on cigarettes is set at 70 percent of the retail price, and an excise duty on imported cigarettes is set at 150 percent of the retail price.

1993 (December): The tax is lowered to 60 percent of the retail price for filtered cigarettes and to 45 percent of the retail price for unfiltered cigarettes.

1994 (February): The excise tax rate on domestically produced cigarettes is lowered to 50 and 35 percent of the retail price of filtered and unfiltered cigarettes, respectively.

1995: The excise tax rate on domestically produced cigarettes is lowered to 40 and 10 percent of the retail price of filtered and unfiltered cigarettes, respectively.

1995 (November/December): The excise duty on imported cigarettes is eliminated. A new tax is levied at a rate of 6 ECU per 1000 cigarettes.

1996 (February): The tax is set at 2 ECU per 1000 filtered cigarettes and 0.5 ECU per 1000 unfiltered cigarettes. This translated into a rate on domestic filtered and unfiltered cigarettes of 4.8 and 1 UAH per 1000 cigarettes, respectively.

1997 (February): The tax on unfiltered cigarettes is raised to 1 ECU per 1000.

1998 (February): The tax on unfiltered cigarettes is raised to 2 ECU per 1000.

1998 (August): The tax is raised to 3 and 2.3 ECU per 1000 filtered and unfiltered cigarettes, respectively.

1998 (December): The tax is set at 2.5 ECU per 1000 cigarettes for both filtered and unfiltered cigarettes.

1999 (July): A new cigarette tax is levied to fund supplemental pension insurance. The tax is set at 2.5 and 1.5 UAH per 1000 filtered and unfiltered cigarettes, respectively.

1999 (November): The tax is set at 10 UAH per 1000 filtered cigarettes and 7 UAH per 1000 unfiltered cigarettes (until July 1, 2000).

2001 (January): The tax for unfiltered cigarettes is lowered to 5 UAH per 1000 cigarettes.

2013 (March): The cabinet passes resolution No. 188 to require excise tax labels for tobacco from UAH 0.055 to 0.142 (effective April 1).

TIMELINE OF TURKISH TOBACCO CONTROL EFFORTS

Health Warnings on Packs

1981: The government requires the cigarette warning label "Attention: Affects your health" to appear on all cigarette packages.

1986: TEKEL changes warning label to read, "Cigarette smoking is harmful to health."

1991: Warning label wording is changed to read, "Cigarette smoking is dangerous to health."

1996: Warning label wording is changed to read, "Legal Warning: Harmful to Health." This must appear on all cigarette packages (domestic and imported).

2005: The Regulatory Committee for Tobacco, Tobacco Products and Alcoholic Beverages Market (TAPDK) allows firms more flexibility in the warning label that they print. Firms may choose from 14 different labels. They must also print a graphic image that shows the health consequences of excessive smoking.

Advertising and Marketing

1977: The Turkish Court of Accounts (Sayistay) decides TEKEL cannot distribute free cigarettes to its civil servants but can discount the price at which it sells cigarettes to its employees. The price to employees is 0.75 of the regular price. TEKEL is allowed to distribute free cigarettes to its production facility employees.

1984: To reduce smuggling, the government lets TEKEL import cigarettes. TEKEL maintains the monopoly right to import, price, and distribute foreign and domestic tobacco products.

1985: To compete with foreign brands, TEKEL launches an advertising campaign.

1986: The government lets domestic companies (other than TEKEL) import cigarettes from abroad.

1991: The government lets multinational tobacco companies open production facilities in Turkey. When annual production exceeds 2000 tons, they may also distribute and sell their products.

1996: The government passes Law No. 4207, the Prevention and Control of Harm from Tobacco Products, making it illegal for firms to advertise tobacco and to run marketing campaigns to promote tobacco use or tobacco products.

2006: The government makes it illegal to sell cigarettes on the Internet.

2007: The State Council (Danistay) invalidates the Internet sales ban on legal grounds.

2008: The government passes Law No. 5727, which bans tobacco gifts, promotions, and samples to distributors and/or customers; the publication of advertisements or any other material using their names, brands, and logos in the press; the production of any chewing gum, confectionary, toys, clothing, accessories, or anything that looks like cigarettes; the sale of cigarettes individually or in small packs; the sale on the Internet; throwing away of packs, filters, paper, or other by-products where others can see them; any form of display of company names, brands, or logos; sponsoring events with company names or brand logos; the organization of campaigns that could promote smoking; the use of company names, brands, or logos on any type of clothing or accessories; and the display of company names, brands, or logos on their commercial vehicles.

Public Smoking

1991: The government bans smoking in public transportation vehicles.

1996: The government passes the Prevention and Control of Harm from Tobacco Products Act (Law No. 4207), which makes it illegal for people to consume tobacco at educational institutions, in enclosed areas, and in public transportation.

2008: The government passes Law No. 5727 to make it illegal to consume tobacco in the following places: indoor areas of public workplaces; indoor areas of buildings that are privately owned by legal entities and used for educational, health, commercial, social, cultural, sports, or entertainment purposes, including hallways with room for more than one person (except private houses); in intercity, railway, sea, and air mass transportation vehicles, including private taxis; and the indoor and outdoor areas accepted as part of the premises of preschool educational institutions, primary and secondary schools, including private establishments preparing students for various

examinations, and cultural and social service buildings. The law allows
tobacco to be consumed in designated areas of care facilities for the elderly,
psychiatric hospitals and prisons, and decks of ships or railway carriages
carrying passengers between cities or on international routes.

2009: A separate provision of Law No. 5727 prohibits the use of tobacco products
in restaurants and entertainment establishments such as cafes, cafeterias,
and bars.

Youth Access

1996: Law No. 4207 makes it illegal to sell tobacco products to anyone younger
than 18 years.

2008: Law No. 5727 makes it illegal to offer tobacco products to anyone
younger than 18 years and makes it illegal for them to occupy designated
smoking areas.

NOTES

1. Available at http://www.tobacco.health.usyd.edu.au/australian-tobacco-timeline
(accessed in 2010).
2. Available at http://www.ashaust.org.au/lv3resources_tobacco_legislation-htm/.
3. Available at http://www.dkfz.de/de/tabakkontrolle/download/Publikationen/sonst-Veroeffentlichungen/Tabakatlas_2009.pdf.
4. Available at http://ec.europa.eu/health/archive/ph_determinants/life_style/tobacco/documents/tobacco_fr_en.pdf.
5. Available at http://www.epha.org/a/1889.

REFERENCES

Lickint, F. 1929. "Tabak und Tabakrauch als Ätiologischer Factor des Carcinoms." *Zeitschrift für Krebsforschung* 30:349–365.

Lickint, F. 1939. *Tabak und Organismus: Handbuch der gesamten Tabakkunde.* Stuttgart: Hippokrates.

Müller, F. H. 1939. "Tabakmissbrauch und Lungencarcinom." *Zeitschrift für Krebsforschung* 49:57–85.

Schäfke, W. 1984. *Blauer Dunst: Vier Jahrhunderte Tabak in Köln.* Köln, Germany: Druck und Verlagshaus Wienand.

Schairer, E., and E. Schöniger. 1943. "Lungenkrebs und Tabakverbrauch." *Zeitschrift für Krebsforschung* 54:261–269.

Scollo, M. M., and M. H. Winstanley. 2008. *Tobacco in Australia.* Melbourne: Cancer Council Victoria.

Seyfarth, C. 1924. "Lungenkarzinome in Leipzig." *Deutshe Medizinische Wochenschrift* 50:1497–1499.

Walker, R. 1984. *Under Fire: A History of Tobacco Smoking in Australia.* Melbourne: Melbourne University Press.

Weiss, C. M., and H. W. Herbert. 1854. *History of the French Protestant Refugees, Volume 1 from the Revocation of the Edict of Nantes to Our Own Days.* New York: Stringer & Townswend.

AUTHOR INDEX

SUBJECT INDEX